Thrombosis and Cancer

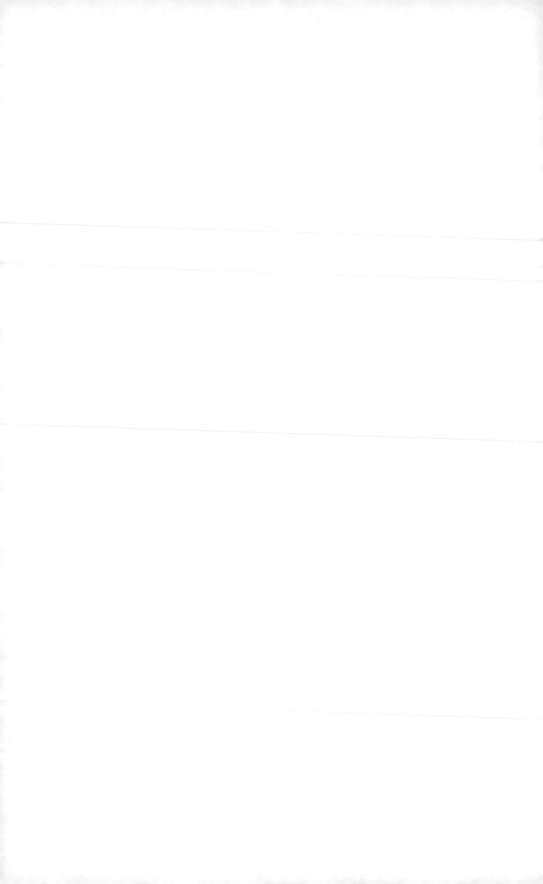

Thrombosis and Cancer

Edited by

Gilles Lugassy MD
Department of Hematology
Barzilai Medical Center
Ashkelon
Israel

Anna Falanga MD
Hematology–Oncology Department
Ospedali Riuniti di Bergamo
Bergamo
Italy

Ajay K Kakkar BSc PhD FRCS
Imperial College
Hammersmith Hospital
Du Cane Road
London
W12 0NN
UK

Frederick R Rickles MD
The Departments of Medicine, Pediatrics and Pharmacology
The George Washington University
Washington DC
Federation of American Societies for Experimental Biology
Bethesda
USA

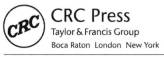

CRC Press
Taylor & Francis Group
Boca Raton London New York

CRC Press is an imprint of the
Taylor & Francis Group, an **informa** business

CRC Press
Taylor & Francis Group
6000 Broken Sound Parkway NW, Suite 300
Boca Raton, FL 33487-2742

© 2004 by Taylor & Francis Group, LLC
CRC Press is an imprint of Taylor & Francis Group, an Informa business

No claim to original U.S. Government works

Visit the Taylor & Francis Web site at
http://www.taylorandfrancis.com

and the CRC Press Web site at
http://www.crcpress.com

Contents

Contributors

Rupert Bauersachs
Department of Internal Medicine
Division of Angiology
JW Goethe University
Frankfurt am Main
Germany

Hans Klaus Breddin
International Institute of
  Thrombosis and Vascular
Diseases e.V.
Ferdinand-Schrey-Weg 6
D-60598 Frankfurt am Main
Germany

Benjamin Brenner
Thrombosis and Hemostasis Unit
Department of Hematology and
  Bone Marrow Transplantation
Rambam Medical Center
Bruce Rappaport Faculty of
  Medicine
Haifa 31096
Israel

Harry R Büller
Department of Vascular Medicine
Academic Medical Center
Meibergdreef 9
Amsterdam 1105 AZ
The Netherlands

Maria Benedetta Donati
Center for High Technology
  Research and Education in
  Biomedical Sciences
Catholic University
Loc. Tappino
86100 Campobasso
Italy

Anna Falanga
Hematology–Oncology
  Department
Ospedali Riuniti di Bergamo
Largo Barozzi, 1
24128 Bergamo
Italy

Patricia M Fernandez
Assistant Professor
Department of Pharmacology
The George Washington University
  Medical Center
Ross Hall 712E
2300 Eye Street NW
Washington, DC, 20037
USA

Ron Hoffman
Thrombosis and Hemostasis Unit
Department of Hematology and
  Bone Marrow Transplantation
Rambam Medical Center
Bruce Rappaport Faculty of
  Medicine
Haifa 31096
Israel

Russell D Hull
601 South Tower – Foothills
   Hospital
1403 – 29 Street NW
Calgary, Alberta
   Canada T2N 2T9

Ajay K Kakkar
Department of Surgical Oncology
   and Technology
Imperial College
Hammersmith Hospital
Du Cane Road
London
W12 0NN
UK

Simon Karpatkin
Department of Medicine
New York University Medical
   Center
550 First Avenue; Room 439
New York, NY 10016-6481
USA

Abraham Klepfish
Blood Bank
Wolfson Medical Center
Holon
Israel

Clara PW Klerk
Department of Vascular Medicine
   Room F4-277
Academic Medical Center
Meibergdreef 9
1105 AZ Amsterdam
The Netherlands

Marcel Levi
Department of Medicine (F-4)
Academic Medical Center
Meibergdreef 9
1105 AZ Amsterdam
The Netherlands

Mark Levine
McMaster University
Faculty of Health Sciences
1200 Main Street
Hamilton, Ontario
Canada L8V 1C3

Roberto Lorenzet
'Antonio Taticchi' Unit for
   Atherosclerosis and Thrombosis
Istituto Ricerche Farmacologiche
   Mario Negri
Consorzio Mario Negri Sud
66030 S Maria Imbaro
Italy

Gilles Lugassy
Department of Hematology
Barzilai Medical Center
Ashkelon
Israel

Marina Marchetti
Hematology–Oncology
   Department
Ospedali Riuniti di Bergamo
Largo Barozzi, 1
24128 Bergamo
Italy

Manuel Monreal
Professor of Medicine
Servicio de Medicina Interna
Hospital Universitari Germans Trias
   i Pujol
Carretera del Camyet s.n.
08916 Badalona, Barcelona
Spain

Hans-Martin MB Otten
Department of Clinical
   Epidemiology and Medical
   Technology Assessment
Academic Hospital Maastricht
Maastricht
The Netherlands

Steven R Patierno
Departments of Pharmacology
    and Urology
The George Washington University
    Medical Center
Ross Hall 712E
2300 Eye Street NW
Washington, DC, 20037
USA

Gloria A Petralia
Department of Surgical Oncology
    & Technology
Imperial College
Hammersmith Hospital
Du Cane Road
London
W12 0NN
UK

Andrea Piccioli
Department of Medical and
    Surgical Sciences
University of Padua
Via Ospedale Civile 105
35128 Padua
Italy

Graham F Pineo
601 South Tower – Foothills
    Hospital
1403 – 29 Street NW
Calgary, Alberta
Canada T2N 2T9

Paolo Prandoni
Department of Medical and
    Surgical Sciences
University of Padua
Via Ospedale Civile 105
35128 Padua
Italy

Martin H Prins
Department of Internal Medicine
Slotervaart Hospital
Amsterdam
The Netherlands

Frederick R Rickles
The Department of Medicine,
    Pediatrics and Pharmacology
The George Washington University
Federation of American Societies
    for Experimental Biology
9650 Rockville Pike
Bethesda, MD 20814-3998
USA

Ami Schattner
Department of Medicine
Kaplan Hospital
Rehovot
Israel

Susanne M Smorenburg
Department of Cell Biology and
    Histology
Academic Medical Center
University of Amsterdam
Meibergdreef 9
Amsterdam 1105 AZ
The Netherlands

Alfonso Vignoli
Hematology–Oncology
    Department
Ospedali Riuniti di Bergamo
Largo Barozzi, 1
24128 Bergamo
Italy

Boris Yoffe
Department of Hematology
Barzilai Medical Center
Ashkelon
Israel

Preface

One hundred and forty years ago, Armand Trousseau described the occurrence of unexplained episodes of migratory thrombophlebitis in patients with visceral cancer, and concluded that spontaneous coagulation is common in cancer patients because of a 'special crisis' in their blood. It is now common knowledge that thromboembolic disease is often the earliest manifestation, and almost the most frequent complication of cancer.

Thromboembolism is the second cause of death among patients with overt malignancy. Evidence of thromboembolism is seen in up to half of all cancer patients at autopsy, particularly in tumours of the pancreas, lung and gastrointestinal tract. Recent studies have investigated the mechanisms by which cancer causes thrombosis, and emphasized the importance of the coagulation system in angiogenesis and tumour metastasis.

It is the purpose of this book to provide comprehensive and timely coverage of our current knowledge of cancer-associated thrombosis, its pathogenesis, clinical features, prevention and therapy. All the contributors of this book are acknowledged specialists in their field, and conducted large clinical trials in oncology and thrombosis.

We hope this book will be of interest to general practitioners, internists, oncologists, haematologists and to all physicians involved in the management of cancer patients.

Gilles Lugassy
Anna Falanga
Ajay K Kakkar
Frederick R Rickles

1

Thrombosis and cancer: A short history of Trousseau's syndrome

Martin H Prins and Hans-Martin MB Otten

Historical background

After the concept of continuous circulation of blood within a contained system had been established by William Harvey (1578–1657), others, such as Boerhaave (1668–1738), Morgagni (1682–1771) and especially Virchow (1821–1902), made important contributions to the field of thrombosis within the system, both arterial and venous.[1,2] The association between cancer and venous thromboembolism (VTE) was recognized in the nineteenth century, and Armand Trousseau (1801–1867) is often considered to be the first scientist who described this association. However, a careful literature analysis revealed that, already in 1823, Bouillaud had described three patients with deep venous thrombosis and cancer.[3] He discussed several causes of peripheral edema of the legs and suggested that in the three cancer patients the edema was secondary to obliteration of the veins by a 'caillot fibrineux' caused by an obstructing 'tumeur cancéreuse'. He did not mention a general association between cancer and phlegmasia alba dolens. White had given this name to thrombosis in the supposition that it was a painful inflammation of the lymphatic veins. In a review about phlegmasia alba dolens, Bouchut proposed, on the basis of necropsy studies, to change the name to 'spontaneous obliteration of the veins', but it took several decades before this point of view was accepted.[4] In 1856, Rudolf Virchow wrote a monograph about the obstruction of pulmonary arteries.[2] Among animal experiments and various case reports, he presented five patients with different kinds of cancer succumbing to pulmonary embolism. All patients had signs or symptoms of cancer before the final embolic event and had clinical and, at autopsy, confirmed deep venous thrombosis. In most cases, the diagnosis of cancer could be confirmed only postmortem because they lacked the diagnostic tools of the present time. On the basis of these observations, he concluded 'dass gerade der marasmus und die kachexie, welche gewönlich mit blutarmuth vergesellschaft sind, zu spontanen gerinnungen des blutes in den peripherischen venen führen, und da gerade ... wiederum ablösungen von gerinnselstücken und verstopfungen der lungenarterie geschehen' ('already the weightloss and cachexia, that usually accompany anemia, can lead to clotting of the blood in the peripheral veins, and that already ... dislodging of pieces of these clots and occlusions of the pulmonary arteries happen'). This means he already appreciated the relation between chronic illness, including cancer, and VTE.

In 1860, a pupil of Trousseau, Joseph Werner, published a thesis entitled 'Phlegmasia Alba Dolens'. In this thesis, he mentioned the association between 'les affections cancéreuses' and VTE.[5] In the introduction to his dissertation, he stated that Trousseau had been informing his pupils about this association since 1843. In lessons, published in the much cited book *Clinique médicale de l'Hôtel-Dieu de Paris*, Trousseau explicitly reported on the relation between cancer and VTE.[6] Ever since, many case reports and necropsy studies have been published. Interestingly, studies to investigate the frequency of VTE, its consequences and the possible interactions with other risk factors for VTE in these patients are scarce.

In the past, the idea was generated that Trousseau linked deep venous thrombosis to occult cancer. For instance, Sproul wrote 'He [Trousseau] was specially interested in the frequency with which thrombosis of one or more peripheral veins was the first indication of the presence of a malignant tumour'.[7] This quotation cannot be confirmed by reading Trousseau's lessons—in particular, not the pages Sproul referred to.[8,9] The patients Trousseau presented all had overt signs of cancer at the time the venous thrombosis became symptomatic. The first to report the observation of VTE as a sign of truly occult malignancy were Illtyd James and Matheson, in 1935.[10] Note this salient detail: they mentioned that Trousseau himself succumbed to carcinoma of the stomach, thrombophlebitis being the initial symptom.

Up to 1951, an association between occult cancer and VTE was based only on case reports and necropsies, not quite the evidence physicians would currently require for guiding their clinical practice.[11-13] In 1951, the first cohort study was published, a retrospective investigation on the prognosis and morbidity of thrombophlebitis.[14] Unfortunately, the authors did not have objective tests at their disposal to confirm the diagnosis of deep venous thrombosis. In addition, 27% of the patients were lost to follow-up. Nevertheless, of the 67 patients with VTE, 6 (9%) appeared to have an underlying, occult malignancy. Hereafter, some studies were published on the relation of occult malignancy and venous thrombosis.[15–17] However, it took another 30 years for the first proper cohort study to appear.[18]

Definitions

A difficulty in reading the earlier reports is related to varying terms for (deep) venous thrombosis and the lack of objective tests for this condition as well as for pulmonary embolism. Fortunately, in the period that coincides with most cohort studies, objective diagnostic tests were available; consequently, we limited our analysis to those studies that used phlebography or ultrasonography to confirm deep venous thrombosis, and perfusion–ventilation lung scanning and/or pulmonary angiography for pulmonary embolism.[19–22]

The term 'occult' malignancy poses another difficulty. As described before, it was not always possible in earlier days to diagnose cancer prior to death because of insufficient diagnostic tools, even if there were definite signs or symptoms that could be related to cancer, and that currently would undoubtedly lead to the performance of tests to detect a concealed malignancy. Even in apparently healthy patients who present with thrombosis, usually a screen of 'simple' tests is performed, such as hematological parameters, liver and kidney function, or chest radiograph. It is questionable whether patients with cancer detected by these simple tests are still to be considered as harboring truly occult cancer.

Patients with known cancer at time of VTE

In total, 13 cohort studies have been published that adequately report the prevalence of known cancer in consecutive patients with a new diagnosis of VTE. In most studies, the prevalence range was 10–20% (Table 1.1). In another, population-based study, this prevalence was comparable: 17.5%.[23] The low prevalence in the study of Sanella and O'Connor can be explained by the setting in which they worked and by 'spectrum' bias.[24] The study was performed in a surgical and radiological department and contained many surgical patients (85 of 237). In addition, many patients (54) had thrombosis secondary to paraplegia or hemiparesis. A similar mechanism might be present in the cohort of O'Connor et al.[25]

The high prevalence (24.1%) in the study of Rajan et al might be caused by the failure to distinguish between patients with truly occult cancer and those with symptomatic but at that time yet-undiagnosed cancer.[26] A selective referral, 'popularity bias', might explain the extremely high prevalence observed in the study of Monreal et al.[27]

Table 1.1 Patients with known cancer at time of VTE.

Reference	Patients with VTE	Known cancer[a]
Bastounis 1996[37]	368	57 (15.5)
Carson 1992[38]	399	73 (18.3)
Griffin 1987[39]	128	15 (11.7)
Goldberg 1987[35]	420	50 (11.9)
Gore 1982[18]	128	15 (12.0)
Monreal 1988[40]	104	10 (9.6)
Monreal 1991[27]	163	50 (30.7)
Monreal 1997[32]	832	147 (17.7)
O'Connor 1984[25]	127	6 (4.7)
Prandoni 1992[41]	342	49 (14.3)
Rajan 1998[26]	348	84 (24.1)[b]
Rance 1997[42]	928	119 (12.8)
Sanella 1991[24]	237	9 (3.8)

[a]Percentages in parentheses.
[b]Including concomitant cancer.

Concomitant diagnosis of VTE and cancer

Because of the association between cancer and VTE, investigators became interested in the prevalence of concomitant cancer in (idiopathic) VTE. In patients presenting with VTE, the prevalence of concomitant cancer, defined as cancer not known before VTE and discovered by routine investigation (history taking; physical examination; and simple laboratory tests such as ESR, whole-blood count, liver and kidney function tests, urinalysis, and chest radiograph), varied considerably among the studies (Table 1.2). This variation might relate to the depth of the routine examinations and to the characteristics of the included patients. Another part of the explanation is the variability of definition used for secondary thrombosis and differences in threshold of suspicion. It seems that some of the differences can also be explained by the age of the patients. The studies of Ahmed and Mohyuddin[28] and Subira et al[29] that both found a zero prevalence contained almost exclusively patients younger than 40 years. They did not find any concomitant cancer in this age category.

Seven other studies have investigated the prevalence of concomitant cancer and differentiated between secondary and idiopathic VTE. In these studies, risk of concomitant cancer was increased among patients with idiopathic VTE by a factor of 3–19. The larger series report a significantly increased risk by a factor of 3–4. The prevalence of concomitant cancer in patients with secondary VTE was low and in general comparable with the 2–3% prevalence expected in the general population after middle age.[30]

Table 1.2 Patients with concomitant diagnosis of VTE and cancer.

Reference	Type of study	Screening for cancer	Prevalence of concomitant cancer in patients with VTE[a]		
			All VTE	Secondary VTE	Idiopathic VTE
Ahmed 1996[28b]	Retrosp.	NM	0/196 (0.0)	0/83 (0.0)	0/113 (0.0)
Subira 1999[29c]	Retrosp.	Routine	0/40 (0.0)	0/30 (0.0)	0/10 (0.0)
Ackar 1997[43]	Prosp.	Extensive[d]	18/232 (8.0)	5/154 (3.0)	13/78 (17.0)
Bastounis 1996[37]	Prosp.	Routine	13/293 (4.4)	4/207 (1.9)	7/86 (8.1)
Monreal 1988[40]	Retrosp.	Routine	6/104 (5.8)	1/83 (1.2)	5/21 (23.8)
Monreal 1991[27]	Prosp.	Routine	8/113 (7.1)	4/82 (4.9)	4/31 (12.9)
Monreal 1997[32]	Prosp.	Routine	11/685 (1.6)	4/573 (0.7)	7/112 (6.3)
Prandoni 1992[41]	Prosp.	Routine	5/260 (1.9)	0/107 (0.0)	5/153 (3.3)
Rance 1997[42]	Retrosp.	Routine	26/809 (3.2)	8/530 (1.5)	18/279 (6.5)
Cornuz 1996[33]	Retrosp.	Routine	— —	16/142 (11.3)	
Girolami 1999[44]	Prosp.	Routine	— —	15/343 (4.4)	
Sanella 1991[24]	Retrosp.	Routine	— —	3/21 (14.3)	

Retrosp. = retrospective; Prosp. = prospective; NM = not mentioned.
[a]Percentages in parentheses.
[b]Most patients younger than 40 years.
[c]Only patients younger than 40 years.
[d]Routine plus tumor markers, abdominal and pelvic CT scan, mammography >40 years, prostate ultrasonography >60 years, and in some thoracic CT scan.

Diagnosis of cancer after VTE

When cells dedifferentiate into cancer cells, it takes at least 2 (up to 8) years for the cancer to become detectable, considering the doubling time of cancer cells and the volume needed to be detected.[31] It has been estimated that it takes an additional 2 years for these cancers to become symptomatic. Thus, it is plausible that a cancer detected within 3 years after VTE was already present at the time of VTE. Therefore, we considered malignancies detected up to 3 years after VTE, not known before VTE and not detected by routine investigations (see last paragraph) at the time of VTE to be occult at the time of VTE. Table 1.3 summarizes the results of 14 cohort studies investigating the prevalence of occult cancer. The prevalence of occult cancer in patients with idiopathic VTE, aged 40 years or more, was roughly 4–10%. In all studies that allow comparison, this figure is higher than in patients with secondary thrombosis. It is interesting to note that three studies with extensive screening procedures for cancer at the time of thrombosis tend towards a lower incidence of a diagnosis of cancer later.[24,27,32] In the study performed by Cornuz et al, a low index of suspicion led to additional testing in 80 of 136 patients. Cancer was diagnosed in 16 of them.[33] Thus, extensive screening was performed in the majority of the patients who

Table 1.3 Patients with diagnosis of cancer within 3 years after VTE, occult at the time of VTE.

Reference	Type of study	Screening for cancer at admission	Prevalence of occult cancer in VTE patients[a]		
			All VTE	Secondary VTE	Idiopathic VTE
Aderka 1986[34]	Prosp.	Routine	11/83 (13.3)	2/48 (4.2)	9/35 (25.7)
Prandoni 1992[41]	Prosp.	Routine	13/250 (5.2)	2/105 (1.9)	11/145 (7.6)
Hettiarach 1997[45]	Prosp.	NM	13/326 (4.0)	3/171 (1.8)	10/155 (6.5)
Monreal 1991[27]	Prosp.	Extensive[b]	1/113 (0.9)	0/82 (0.0)	1/31 (3.2)
Monreal 1997[32]	Prosp.	Extensive[c]	8/659 (1.2)	4/563 (0.7)	4/96 (4.2)
Monreal 1988[40]	Retrosp.	Routine	3/94 (3.2)	0/73 (0.0)	3/21 (14.3)
Rajan 1998[26]	Retrosp.	Routine	21/264 (8.0)	8/112 (7.1)	13/152 (8.6)
Subira 1999[29d]	Retrosp.	Routine	0/40 (0.0)	0/30 (0.0)	0/10 (0.0)
Ahmed 1996[28e]	Retrosp.	NM	3/196 (1.5)	0/83 (0.0)	3/113 (2.7)
Gore 1982[18]	Retrosp.	NM	15/113 (13.3)	—	—
Girolami 1999[44]	Prosp.	Routine	—	—	28/328 (8.5)
Cornuz 1996[33]	Retrosp.	Routine	—	—	3/122 (2.6)
O'Connor 1984[25]	Retrosp.	Routine	—	—	0/17 (0.0)
Sanella 1991[24]	Retrosp.	Extensive[f]			1/21 (4.7)

Including routine screening by history taking, physical examination, measurement of ESR, complete blood count, liver- and renal function tests, urinalysis, and chest radiograph.
[a] Percentages in parentheses.
[b] Included extensive serum protein electrophoresis (SPE), CEA, abdominal (abd.) ultrasonography in all, and abd. CT scan and upper gastrointestinal endoscopy in most.
[c] Included extensive SPE, CEA, PSA, abd. ultrasonography or abd. CT scan.
[d] Only patients younger than 40 years.
[e] Most patients younger than 40 years.
[f] Included extensive abd. CT scan.

were followed for 1 year. Although these results are suggestive, it would be premature to conclude that such extensive screening did indeed identify occult malignancies.

The study of Rajan et al showed a remarkably high prevalence of cancer in the group with secondary VTE, compared with other studies, a finding which cannot be explained.[26]

If VTE does indeed flag for occult malignancy, it could be expected that the incidence of cancer would be increased in the first years after VTE, and would subside thereafter. Indeed, in the study of Aderka et al, the incidence in the first 3 years was 13.3% as compared with 4.2% thereafter.[34] A similar trend was seen in the study of Goldberg et al[35] (5.7% versus 0.3%).

Moreover, the population-based studies of Baron et al[23] and Sørensen et al[36] point in the same direction, with standardized incidence ratios of newly diagnosed cancer, as compared with the normal population, of 4.4 and 2.1, respectively, during the first year after the diagnosis of thrombosis and only 1.3 and 1.1, respectively, in the period thereafter. This indicates that 6–12 months after VTE the incidence of cancer becomes comparable to that of the normal population.

Detection of occult cancer by extensive screening

Four studies have systematically evaluated the added value of extensive screening on cancer detection (Table 1.4). The frequency of additional malignancies detected by extensive screening was impressively high (13% and 33%) in the studies that included only patients with idiopathic VTE. Although the figures differ, the conclusions are the same: more malignancies are detected by extensive screening. Sanella and O'Connor were the only ones not to exclude recurrent VTE patients.[24] Routine screening discovered a high number of cancer patients in these studies, probably because of a low threshold of suspicion. Nevertheless, extensive screening had a substantial additional yield. It is of interest that most cancer was detected by non-(or minimally) invasive tests, such as blood testing for prostate-specific antigen (PSA) or carcinoembryonic antigen (CEA) and CT scans. Although Sannella and O'Connor report a potential advantage in life expectancy for only one of seven patients with cancer detected by extensive screening, Monreal et al published more positive results.[24,27,32] In the study published in 1991, two out of three, and in the study published in 1997, 9 out of 15 patients could be treated as intentionally curative, because of extensive screening, while two others profited from palliative surgery. It should be noted, however, that an effect on survival cannot be assessed by these nonrandomized studies.

Table 1.4 Difference in detection of cancer in patients with VTE in relation to screening method.

Reference	Prevalence of cancer detected by[a]	
	Routine screening	Routine and extensive screening
Bastounis 1996[37]	13/293 (4.4)	22/293 (7.5)[b]
Monreal 1991[27]	8/113 (7.1)	12/113 (10.6)
Monreal 1997[32c]	7/112 (6.3)	22/112 (19.6)
Sanella 1991[24c]	4/21 (19.0)	11/21 (52.4)

[a]Percentages in parentheses.
[b]6/207 (2.9%) in secondary VTE and 16/86 (18.6%) in idiopathic VTE.
[c]Only idiopathic VTE.

Conclusion

Although the exact mechanism has not been entirely elucidated, cancer is a risk factor for VTE. About 10–20% of patients with VTE suffer from a known cancer. The prevalence of cancer diagnosis concomitant with VTE is low in patients with secondary VTE and comparable to the prevalence in the general population. Patients with idiopathic VTE seem to have a 3–19-fold increased risk of concomitant cancer.

The prevalence of occult cancer, defined as cancer occurring after VTE that could not be detected by routine examinations at the time of VTE, is 4–10% in patients with idiopathic VTE aged over 40 years, within the first 3 years after VTE. This is three- to fivefold higher than in patients with secondary VTE and than expected in patients with the same baseline characteristics. These figures are influenced by the composition of the investigated cohorts, the age of the patients and the definition of secondary VTE. The recent discovery of risk factors for VTE, such as factor V Leiden and prothrombin G20210A mutant, might have consequences for the formation of the groups of idiopathic and secondary VTE. This could have an effect on the magnitude of the figures mentioned before. The subsiding incidence of cancer with time since VTE is in concordance with the theory that idiopathic VTE flags for cancer.

By extensive, mainly noninvasive, screening methods, it is possible to detect significantly more patients with cancer than by routine examination and laboratory investigations alone. Although some reports suggest that cancers detected by extensive screening are suitable for curative treatment, it is unclear whether such extensive screening results in longer survival.

References

1. Lyons AS, Keiner M. The seventeenth century, circulation of the blood. In: Rawls W, ed. Medicine. An Illustrated History (Abrams: New York, 1987)432–7.

2. Virchow R. Weitere Unter-suchungen über die Verstopfung der Lungenarterie und ihre Folgen. In: Virchow R, ed. Gesammelte Abhandlungen zur wissenschaftlichen Medizin. (Meidinger Sohn: Frankfurt am Main, 1856)227–380.

3. Bouillaud B. De l'Oblitération des veines et de son influence sur la formation des hydropisies partielles: considérations sur la hydropisies passives en général. Arch Gen Med 1823; 1:188–204.

4. Bouchut V. Pathologie Interne. Mémoire sur la phlegmatia alba dolens. Gazette Médicale de Paris 1844; 13:297–303.

5. Werner J. De la phlegmasia alba dolens. (Faculté de médecine de Paris, 1860).

6. Trousseau A. Phlegmasia alba dolens. In: Trousseau A, ed. Clinique medicale de l'Hôtel-Dieu de Paris. (Baillière: Paris, 1865)654–712.

7. Sproul E. Carcinoma and venous thrombosis: the frequency of associations of carcinoma in the body or tail of the pancreas with multiple venous thrombosis. Am J Cancer 1938; **34**:566–85.

8. Trousseau A. Ulcère chronique simple de l'estomac. In: Peter M, ed. Clinique médicale de l'Hôtel-Dieu de Paris. (Baillière: Paris, 1877) 80–107.

9. Trousseau A. Phlegmatia alba dolens. In: Peter M, ed. Clinique médicale de l'Hôtel-Dieu de Paris. (Baillière: Paris, 1877)695–739.

10. Illtyd James T, Matheson N. Thrombo-phlebitis in cancer. Practitioner 1935; **134**:683–4.

11. Haward W. Phlebitis and thrombosis. Lancet 1906; i:650–5.

12. Barker N. Thrombophlebitis complicating infectious and systemic diseases. Proc Staff Meetings Mayo Clin 1936; **11**:513–17.

13. Hoerr S, Harper J. On peripheral thrombophlebitis. JAMA 1957; **164**: 2033–4.

14. Ackerman R, Estes J. Prognosis in idiopathic thrombophlebitis. Ann Intern Med 1951; **34**:902–10.

15. Woolling K, Shick R. Thrombophlebitis: a possible clue to cryptic malignant lesions. Proc Staff Meetings Mayo Clin 1956; **31**:227–33.

16. Anlyan W, Shingleton W, Delaughter G. Significance of idiopathic venous thrombosis and hidden cancer. JAMA 1956; **161**: 964–6.

17. Lieberman J, Borrero J, Urdaneta E et al. Thrombophlebitis and cancer. JAMA 1961; **177**:542–5.

18. Gore JM, Appelbaum JS, Greene HL et al. Occult cancer in patients with acute pulmonary embolism. Ann Intern Med 1982; **96**:556–60.

19. Hull R, Hirsch J, Sackett DL et al. Clinical validity of a negative venogram in patients with clinically suspected venous thrombosis. Circulation 1981; **64**:622–5.

20. Lensing AW, Prandomi P, Brandjes D et al. Detection of deep-vein thrombosis by real-time B-mode ultrasonography. N Engl J Med 1989; **320**:342–5.

21. Biello DR, Mattar AG, McKnight RC et al. Ventilation–perfusion studies in suspected pulmonary embolism. Am J Roentgenol 1979; **133**: 1033–7.

22. Dalen JE, Brooks HL, Johnson LW et al. Pulmonary angiography in acute pulmonary embolism: indications, techniques, and results in 367 patients. Am Heart J 1971; **81**:175–85.

23. Baron JA, Gridley G, Weiderpass et al. Venous thromboembolism and cancer. Lancet 1998; **351**: 1077–80.

24. Sanella NA, O'Connor DJ, Jr. 'Idiopathic' deep venous thrombosis: the value of routine abdominal and pelvic computed tomographic scanning. Ann Vasc Surg 1991; **5**:218–22.

25. O'Connor NT, Cederholm-Williams SA, Fletcher EW et al. Significance of idiopathic deep venous thrombosis. Postgrad Med J 1984; **60**: 275–7.

26. Rajan R, Levine M, Gent M et al. The occurrence of subsequent malignancy in patients presenting with deep vein thrombosis: results from a historical cohort study. Thromb Haemost 1998; **79**:19–22.

27. Monreal M, Lafoz E, Casals A et al. Occult cancer in patients with deep venous thrombosis. A systematic approach. Cancer 1991; **67**:541–5.

28. Ahmed Z, Mohyuddin Z. Deep vein thrombosis as a predictor of cancer. Angiology 1996; **47**:261–5.

29. Subira M, Mateo J, Souto JC et al. Lack of association between venous thrombosis and subse-

quent malignancy in a retrospective cohort study in young patients. Am J Hematol 1999; **60**:181–4.

30. Coebergh JWW. Incidence and prognosis of cancer in the Netherlands: studies based on cancer registries. University of Rotterdam, 1991. Thesis, 191–5.

31. Fingert H, Campisi J, Pardee A. Cell proliferation and differentiation. In: Holland J et al, eds. Cancer Medicine. (Williams and Wilkins: Baltimore, 1997)3–18.

32. Monreal M, Fernandez-Llamazares J, Perandreu J et al. Occult cancer in patients with venous thromboembolism: which patients, which cancers. Thromb Haemost 1997; **78**:1316–18.

33. Cornuz J, Pearson SD, Creager MA et al. Importance of findings on the initial evaluation for cancer in patients with symptomatic idiopathic deep venous thrombosis. Ann Intern Med 1996; **125**:785–93.

34. Aderka D, Brown A, Zelikovski A et al. Idiopathic deep vein thrombosis in an apparently healthy patient as a premonitory sign of occult cancer. Cancer 1986; **57**:1846–9.

35. Goldberg RJ, Seneff M, Gore JM et al. Occult malignant neoplasm in patients with deep venous thrombosis. Arch Intern Med 1987; **147**:251–3.

36. Sørensen HT, Mellemkjaer L, Steffensen FH et al. The risk of a diagnosis of cancer after primary deep venous thrombosis or pulmonary embolism. N Engl J Med 1998; **338**:1169–73.

37. Bastounis EA, Karayiannakis AJ, Makri GG et al. The incidence of occult cancer in patients with deep

venous thrombosis: a prospective study. J Intern Med 1996; **239**: 153–6.

38. Carson JL, Kelley MA, Duff A et al. The clinical course of pulmonary embolism. N Engl J Med 1992; **326**:1240–5.

39. Griffin MR, Stanson AW, Brown ML et al. Deep venous thrombosis and pulmonary embolism. Risk of subsequent malignant neoplasms. Arch Intern Med 1987; **147**: 1907–11.

40. Monreal M, Salvador R, Soriano V et al. Cancer and deep venous thrombosis. Arch Intern Med 1988; **148**:485.

41. Prandoni P, Lensing AW, Buller HR et al. Deep-vein thrombosis and the incidence of subsequent symptomatic cancer. N Engl J Med 1992; **327**:1128–33.

42. Rance A, Emmerich J, Guedj C et al. Occult cancer in patients with bilateral deep-vein thrombosis. Lancet 1997; **350**:1448–9.

43. Ackar A, Laaban JP, Horellou MH et al. Prospective screening for occult cancer in patients with venous thromboembolism. Thromb Haemost 1997; **78**:3835 (abst).

44. Girolami A, Prandoni P, Zanon E et al. Venous thromboses of upper limbs are more frequently associated with occult cancer as compared with those of lower limbs. Blood Coagul Fibrinolysis 1999; **10**: 455–7.

45. Hettiarachchi RJK, Lok J, Prins MH et al. Undiagnosed malignancy in patients with deep vein thrombosis. Incidence, risk indicators, and diagnosis. Cancer 1998; **83**:180–5.

2

Pathogenesis of thrombosis in cancer

Anna Falanga, Marina Marchetti, and Alfonso Vignoli

Introduction

Tumor growth is associated with the development of a hypercoagulable state and an increased risk of thrombosis in the host. A high incidence of thromboembolic disease in patients with cancer has been early reported by postmortem studies, particularly in patients who died of mucinous carcinoma of the pancreas, lung and gastrointestinal tract.[1,2] In addition, histological analyses have shown the presence of fibrin or platelet plugs in and around many types of tumors, suggesting a local activation of coagulation.[3]

Thromboembolic disease can be the earliest clinical sign of a tumor. This observation, originally reported by the French clinician Armand Trousseau, over a century ago, was confirmed in recent years by controlled prospective clinical trials, which clearly demonstrate that patients with deep-vein thrombosis (DVT), in the absence of known risk factors (that is, 'idiopathic' thrombosis), have a substantial likelihood of having cancer.[4] These cancers may be occult or at a very early stage.[5]

On the other hand, patients with already diagnosed cancer have a significantly higher risk of developing 'secondary' thrombosis in specific conditions (that is, in the presence of additional risk factors). In this setting, the role of antitumor therapies is important. Indeed, both surgery and chemotherapy increase the cancer-associated risk of developing thrombosis.[6]

Thromboembolic disorders in cancer patients include venous and arterial thrombosis, and the clinical manifestations of disseminated intravascular clotting, that is, thrombotic microangiopathy and disseminated intravascular coagulation (DIC). Severe DIC is generally associated with acute leukemia and is characterized by life-threatening hemorrhages caused by an excessive consumption of clotting factors and platelets.[7]

However, even in the absence of manifest thrombosis, cancer patients with solid tumors and leukemia commonly present with abnor-

malities in laboratory coagulation tests, underlying a subclinical hypercoagulable condition, characterized by varying degrees of blood-clotting
activation.[6,8,9] The results of laboratory tests demonstrate that a process
of fibrin formation and removal is continuous during the development of
malignancy. Plasma markers of clotting activation, such as
thrombin–antithrombin (TAT) complex, prothrombin fragments 1 and 2,
fibrinopeptide A, and D-dimer, are all elevated in patients with cancer,[10-14] and elevated levels may be related to the stage of the disease
(Figure 2.1). It is important to remember that fibrin formation can play a
role not only in thrombogenesis but also in tumor progression.[15] Fibrin
deposits on potentially metastatic blood-borne malignant cells mediate
the attachment of these cells to the vascular endothelium, thus favoring
extravasation and the formation of distant metastases. Pharmacological
interventions to block thrombogenicity in malignancy could be important
not only for reducing thromboembolic complications, but also for
improving the treatment of cancer.

In this chapter, we will review the development of our knowledge of
the interactions between malignant disease and the hemostatic system
in order to provide useful information on the pathogenetic mechanisms
of thrombotic complications in cancer patients.

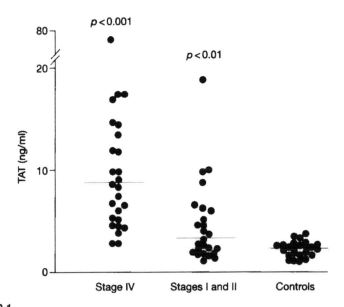

Figure 2.1

Plasma levels of TAT complex in breast-cancer patients with disseminated (stage IV) or localized (stages I and II) disease and in healthy control subjects.

Pathogenetic mechanisms

The activation of blood coagulation and the thrombotic diathesis of patients with cancer is multifactorial, and the mechanisms include non-specific factors, tumor-specific activities, and anticancer therapies (that is, chemo- and radiotherapy, and surgery). General mechanisms for clotting activation in malignancy are related to the host response to the tumor and include the acute-phase reactants and necrosis (that is, inflammation), abnormal protein metabolism (that is, paraproteinemia), and hemodynamic disorders (that is, venous stasis). However, a prominent role in the hemostatic system activation in this disease is attributed to tumor-specific, clot-promoting mechanisms, which include a series of prothrombotic properties of tumor cells. Of particular interest are also a number of procoagulant effects triggered by chemotherapy.

Tumor-cell prothrombotic mechanisms

The principal prothrombotic properties of tumor cells can be classified into two general categories. The first is represented by the capacity of tumor cells to interact with host blood cells, such as endothelial cells lining the blood vessels, leukocytes, and platelets. This interaction can occur directly, by means of adhesion mechanisms (cell–cell interaction), or indirectly, by means of inflammatory cytokines; in both cases, this interaction results in the activation of the vascular cells, with downregulation of their anticoagulant properties and upregulation of their procoagulant properties.

The second category of tumor prothrombotic mechanisms is represented by the capacity of the tumor cell to produce and release its own procoagulant and fibrinolytic activities, besides proinflammatory cytokines. Figure 2.2 is a schematic representation of all these properties.

Cancer-cell interaction with blood cells

The interaction of tumor cells with host cells represents a mechanism by which tumors can manipulate the hemostatic defense system and thereby induce thromboembolic events. Several tests are available that measure circulating markers reflecting the activation status of the hemostatic system. Studies on these parameters demonstrate the occurrence of activation/perturbation of different cellular hemostatic mechanisms, in vivo, in cancer patients. Indeed, findings of elevated levels of plasma markers of endothelial activation (for example, von Willebrand factor, thrombomodulin, soluble E-selectin, tissue-type plasminogen activator [t-PA], and its inhibitor [PAI-1])[16] indicate the involvement of endothelial

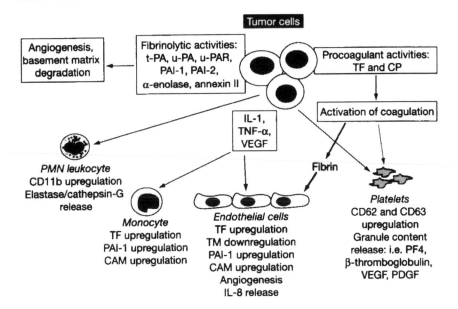

Figure 2.2

Tumor-cell interactions with the hemostatic system. Tumor cells express cellular procoagulants (TF, CP, an FV receptor, and an FXIII-like activity) that activate the clotting cascade; fibrinolysis proteins (u-PA, t-PA, and PAI) and receptor (u-PAR); and cytokines, including IL-1β, TNF-α, and VEGF, that induce endothelium thrombogenicity and angiogenesis. They also interact (directly or through soluble mediators) with other blood cells, that is, endothelial cells, PMN leukocytes, monocytes, and platelets.

hemostasis, especially during chemotherapy[17–19] and antiangiogenic therapy.[20] Furthermore, the increase in tissue factor (TF) procoagulant activity expressed by circulating mononuclear cells demonstrates that this cellular compartment is equally activated.[21] Recently, the occurrence of polymorphonuclear leukocyte (PMN) activation has also been shown in patients with myeloproliferative disorders.[22] Finally, the detection by flow cytometry of high levels of platelet membrane-specific glycoproteins (such as P-selectin and CD63), which are exposed upon activation, provides evidence for platelet activation, in vivo, in malignant conditions.[23]

Cancer and endothelial cells

The endothelium, a continuous cellular monolayer lining the blood vessels, has a broad range of important homeostatic roles. Among these, it participates in the control of primary hemostasis, blood coagulation and fibrinolysis, and platelet and leukocyte interactions with the vessel wall. The endothelial cells are also the target of many drugs and exogenous toxic substances.[24]

Tumor cells can convert the normal anticoagulant endothelium to a prothrombotic and proadhesive one by releasing proinflammatory cytokines. Tumor-cell-derived cytokines, including tumor necrosis factor α (TNF-α) and interleukin-1 β (IL-1β), can induce the expression of endothelial TF,[25] and downregulate the expression of endothelial cell thrombomodulin, the surface high-affinity receptor for thrombin; the thrombomodulin–thrombin complex activates the protein C system, which, in turn, functions as a potent anticoagulant. Taken together, TF upregulation and thrombomodulin downregulation lead to a prothrombotic condition of the vascular wall.[26–28] The same cytokines also stimulate endothelial cells to produce the fibrinolysis inhibitor PAI-1, further contributing to the prothrombotic potential of endothelial cells.[29] In addition, as discussed below, another tumor-cell-derived cytokine, vascular endothelial growth factor (VEGF), can induce the expression of TF by endothelial cells, with implications in tumor neovascularization.[30]

The changes induced by cytokines on the vascular wall not only lead to a prothrombotic state of the endothelium, but may also contribute to an enhancement of the metastatic potential through changes in the adhesion molecules of endothelial cells, which become more capable of attracting tumor cells and supporting their extravasation.[31] The malignant cells attached to the vessel wall may play a key role in promoting localized clotting activation and thrombus formation by releasing their cytokine content and favoring the adhesion and arrest of other cells, including leukocytes and platelets.

The tumor cell's capacity to adhere to both resting and cytokine-stimulated endothelium is well described, and adhesion molecule pathways specific to different tumor-cell types have been identified.[32] We found that NB4 cells, a human acute promyelocytic cell line, adhere to endothelial cells preferentially by the interaction of their surface integrin VLA-4 with its counterreceptor VCAM-1 expressed on endothelial cells, which is sensitive to inflammatory stimuli, including IL-1β. Furthermore, in vitro treatment of NB4 cells with all-*trans*-retinoic acid (ATRA) significantly increases the expression of surface integrins, and this effect translates into an actual increase of NB4 capacity to adhere to endothelium monolayers.[33] Increased adhesion of acute promyelocytic leukemia (APL) blast cells to the vascular endothelium is considered important in the pathogenesis of the ATRA syndrome, a rare side effect occurring in patients with APL receiving ATRA, and characterized by pulmonary distress symptoms and organ infiltration by leukemic cells. However, more recently, we could show that ATRA also affects adhesion molecule expression by endothelial cells, and observed that ATRA significantly reduces the levels of VCAM-1 induced by IL-1β on the endothelium. As a result of this effect, the adhesion of NB4 cells to activated endothelial cells is reduced by 40% in the presence of ATRA (Figure 2.3). Therefore, the proadhesive effect of ATRA on leukemic cells may be in some

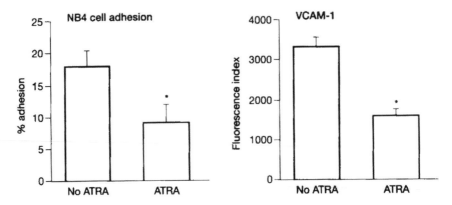

Figure 2.3

ATRA reduces the adhesion of NB4 cells to endothelial cells (left panel) and the expression of VCAM-1 by endothelial cells (right panel).[109] Endothelial cell monolayers were treated for 24 hrs with 100 U/ml IL-1β or 100 U/ml IL-1β plus 1 μmol/l ATRA. Adhesion of NB4 cells to endothelium was evaluated by a fluorimetric assay. Endothelial cell expression of VCAM-1 was assessed by a cytofluorimetic assay, with an FITC-conjugated anti-VCAM-1 antibody (Bender MedSystems, Vienna, Austria). Values are reported as fluorescence index = (% positive cells) × (mean intensity fluorescence channel).

instances counteracted by an antiadhesive effect of ATRA on endothelial cells.

Cancer and platelets

Patients with metastatic cancer may exhibit increased platelet activation, as also indicated by enhancement of platelet turnover and decrease in platelet survival time. These platelet abnormalities may be due to a greater destruction of the lysosomal membranes and to an involvement of platelets in the low-grade intravascular clotting activation detectable in the majority of cancer patients.[34] Clinical and experimental evidence suggests that platelets may play a role in tumor-cell dissemination via the bloodstream. The most convincing evidence is that experimental thrombocytopenia reduces hematogenous tumor metastasis in animal models, an effect that is reversed upon platelet infusion.[35] Tumor cells can induce platelet activation and platelet aggregation directly or by released factors, such as ADP, thrombin, and a cathepsin-like cysteine proteinase.[36,37] Once activated, platelets increase their capacity to interact through specific adhesive mechanisms with other vascular cells, that is, endothelial cells and leukocytes, but also with blood-borne tumor cells.[38,39] In addition, activated platelets aggregate and release their granule contents, as shown by both in vitro and in vivo studies.[39] Elevated levels of β-thromboglobulin and platelet factor-4 have been detected in patients with active malignant disease compared with those in complete remission.[40] As mentioned above, the presence of circulating activated platelets has also been shown in cancer patients, by detecting on their surface the platelet activation-dependent antigens P-selectin and CD63,[23] and by the finding of increased factor VIII antigen and ristocetin cofactor, enhanced ADP-induced platelet aggregation, and reduced sensitivity of platelets to prostacyclin.[41–43]

Another emerging role of platelets in tumor biology is suggested by recent observations indicating that platelets may participate in angiogenesis in many ways. The physiological importance of each of these effects, as well as of the net contribution of platelets to angiogenesis, is yet to be fully established. Upon activation, platelets were found to release VEGF and PDGF, which play an important role in the angiogenic process.[44]

Cancer and leukocytes

In normal inflammation (that is, in response to tissue injury), a multifactorial network of chemical signals activates and directs the migration of leukocytes from the venous system to the damaged site. Recent data have expanded the concept that inflammation is a critical component of tumor progression.[45] Leukocytes also constitute an integral part of the cell infiltrate of the tumor mass. This is because tumor cells produce various cytokines and chemokines that attract leukocytes. The inflammatory component of a developing neoplasm may include a diverse leukocyte population, such as PMN, dendritic cells, macrophages, and mast cells, as well as lymphocytes. Experimental and in vitro studies have shown that PMN may function to promote tumor growth and metastasis.[46–48] A recent in vitro study has demonstrated that tumor-cell-derived factors could activate PMN function by upregulating the expression of adhesion molecules (that is, the β_2 integrin CD11b/CD18) by PMN, which attach to tumor cells and facilitate tumor-cell migration through the endothelium.[49] Upon activation, PMN not only increase their expression of CD11b, but also release reactive oxygen species and intracellular proteases that possess several activities on endothelial cells and platelets and may modify the hemostatic balance towards a pro-thrombotic state.[50] We could observe the presence of activated circulating PMN in patients with myeloproliferative disorders (that is, polycythemia vera and essential thrombocythemia), as demonstrated by the finding of increased expression of cell membrane PMN-CD11b, and increased content and release of endogenous elastase and myeloperoxidase. In these patients, the increase in PMN activation markers was closely related to the increase in plasma markers of hypercoagulation and endothelial cell activation.[22]

Like endothelial cells, monocytes do not constitutively express TF, but generate and expose this procoagulant on their surface when exposed to activating molecules, including bacterial endotoxins, inflammatory cytokines, and complement proteins. In vitro studies show that tumor cells and tumor-cell products can induce the expression of TF by monocytes.[51] Mononuclear cell activation may occur in vivo as well. Indeed, tumor-associated macrophages harvested from experimental and human tumors express significantly more TF than control cells.[51,52] This mechanism might contribute to the activation of the patient hemostatic system and to localized fibrin deposition within tumor tissues. Furthermore, circulating monocytes from patients with different types of cancer have been shown to express increased TF activity.[21] The generation of procoagulant activity by monocyte/macrophages in vivo is conceivably one mechanism explaining clotting activation in malignancy.[51] Of interest also is the evidence that tumor-associated macrophages respond to tumor-derived mediators not only by expressing TF, but also by increasing their fibrinolytic enzyme production.[53]

Cancer-cell procoagulants, fibrinolysis proteins, and cytokines

Cancer-cell procoagulant activities

The production of procoagulant activities by tumor cells promotes fibrin formation at sites of extravasation and in the tumor microenvironment at the extracellular level.[54,55] The best-characterized tumor-cell procoagulants are TF and cancer procoagulant (CP). Other tumor-cell procoagulant activities include a factor V receptor associated with vesicles shed from tumor-cell plasma membranes, which binds factor V, thus facilitating the assembly of prothrombinase complex,[56] and a factor XIII-like activity that promotes the cross-linking of fibrin.[57]

TF, the primary activator of normal blood coagulation, is a 47-kDa glycoprotein that forms a complex with factor VII (FVII) and FVIIa to trigger blood coagulation by proteolytically activating FX and FIX.[58,59] The expression of TF by normal vascular cells, that is, endothelial cells and monocytes/macrophages, is tightly controlled. In normal conditions, TF is not expressed by these cells, but it can be induced by proinflammatory stimuli such as the cytokines IL-1β and TNF-α, and bacterial lipopolysaccharides.[51,59] Unlike normal cells, constitutive expression of TF is observed in malignantly transformed cells. In addition to its central role in maintaining normal hemostasis, TF is involved in the enhancement of tumor growth and metastasis.[60] The specific role of TF in experimental metastasis is shown by the fact that nonmetastatic tumor cells, transfected to hyperexpress TF, become highly metastatic.[61] Overexpression of TF by tumor cells markedly increases the production of VEGF;[62] and the two proteins appear to colocalize at sites of angiogenesis.[33] The prometastatic and angiogenic effects of TF are not entirely mediated via clotting activation, but may depend on signalling through the cytoplasmic domain, suggesting a 'noncoagulation role' for TF in cancer disease.[63]

CP is a 68-kDa cysteine proteinase (EC 3.4.22.26) with 674 amino-acid residues and no detectable carbohydrates.[64] Unlike TF, CP directly activates FX independently of FVII and cleaves the FX heavy chain at a different site than other known FX activators.[65,66] CP has been found in extracts of neoplastic cells and in amnion–chorion tissues, but not in extracts of normally differentiated cells.[64,67–70] CP antigen has been identified in cancer patients' sera and found to be elevated in 85% of the study subjects.[71] These findings have been confirmed by determining the procoagulant activity of CP in the sera of patients with cancer.[72]

TF and CP have been identified in several human and animal tumor tissues.[55,56,73] In recent years, many studies have focused on the procoagulant activity expressed by leukemic cells. Several authors have identified TF in these cells.[58,74,75] Falanga and colleagues have reported the finding of CP in blasts of various acute myelogenous leukemia phenotypes, with the greatest expression in the APL subtype.[70,76,77] Interestingly, in patients with acute myeloid leukemias, CP was detected in the bone marrow and in mononuclear cells at the onset of the disease, but not in cells from the same subjects upon complete remission.[70] These findings support the hypothesis that undifferentiated cells may express CP, while it is repressed once normal differentiation occurs. Recent data show that differentiating treatment with ATRA induces the complete remission of human APL and a rapid resolution of the associated coagulopathy.[78] In vitro and in vivo studies have shown that ATRA reduces TF and CP in APL cells.[68,77] Our group has shown that ATRA can modulate the hypercoagulable state in patients with breast cancer too.[10] We have also observed that breast-cancer cells express TF, which is inhibited by ATRA, like APL cells.[79,80]

Cancer-cell fibrinolytic proteins

The activation of the fibrinolytic system is important in the maintenance of proper hemostasis after blood coagulation.[81] Fibrinolysis is also a key component in tumor biology, as it is essential in releasing tumor cells from their primary site of origin, in neoangiogenesis, and in promoting cell mobility and motility.[82,83] Tumor cells can express all the proteins regulating the fibrinolytic system, including the urokinase-type plasminogen activator (u-PA), the tissue-type plasminogen activator (t-PA), and the fibrinolysis inhibitors PAI-1 and PAI-2.[84] Among the activators, u-PA is the most widely expressed within malignant lesions.[85] Furthermore, cancer cells can carry the specific plasminogen activator receptor (u-PAR) on their membranes.[86] The presence of these receptors favors the assembly of all the fibrinolytic components on tumor-cell surface membranes, facilitating the activation of the fibrinolytic cascade.[86] The expression of these activities by leukemic cells is believed to play a role in the pathogenesis of the bleeding symptoms of this disease.[78] The finding of impaired plasma fibrinolytic activity (by global tests, that is, the euglobulin lysis area on fibrin plates) in patients with solid tumors represents another tumor-associated prothrombotic mechanism.[87] Fibrinolytic proteins are under evaluation as potentially valuable predictors of disease-free interval and long-term survival in malignant disease.[84] Mostly, in breast cancer, u-PA and PAI-1 are tumor biological prognostic factors validated at the highest level of evidence with regard to their clinical utility; numerous studies showed that patients with low levels of u-PA and PAI-1 have a significantly better survival rate than patients with high levels of either factor, particularly in node-negative breast cancer.[88]

Cancer-cell-derived cytokines

Cytokines are low-molecular-weight polypeptides that act as pleiotropic mediators of inflammation. Experimental and clinical evidence has suggested that cytokines may play a role also in the onset of hemostatic abnormalities in various disease states, including septicemia-induced coagulopathy, veno-occlusive disease of the liver after bone-marrow transplantation, the prothrombotic state associated with atherosclerotic vessels, and the thrombotic tendency of cancer patients.[89] Tumor cells produce inflammatory cytokines, including TNF-α, IL-1β, and VEGF. The role of TNF-α and IL-1β in regulating a number of hemostatic functions (that is, the expression of TF, TM, PAI-1, and adhesion molecules) of endothelial cells and monocytes has been elucidated in a previous section. In addition to those cytokine activities, the production of VEGF by malignant cells may significantly affect the functions of microvascular vessels in proximity to the tumor and may play an important role in tumor-induced angiogenesis.[33,90] Furthermore, VEGF is chemotactic for macrophages and can induce the TF procoagulant activity of monocytes and endothelial cells.[91] Interestingly, the expression of TF by tumor cells upregulates the transcription of VEGF in these cells.[63] Finally, TF modulates the expression of VEGF by endothelial cells, a function that can have important implications in tumor neovascularization.[33] Regulation of VEGF synthesis by TF in malignant cells and vascular cells provides an important link in cancer patients between activation of coagulation, inflammation, thrombosis, and tumor progression and metastasis.[92]

Antitumor drug prothrombotic mechanisms

The role of antitumor therapies (that is, chemo-, hormone and radiotherapy) in increasing the thrombotic risk in malignancy has been demonstrated by retrospective and prospective clinical studies.[93–95] For several years, thrombotic complications have been described in association with specific chemotherapeutic agents, such as L-asparaginase, mitomycin C, cisplatin, or high-dose chemotherapy conditioning regimens for bone-marrow transplantation.[93] Importantly, prospective controlled studies have now shown that conventional chemotherapy commonly used for breast cancer can increase the risk of thromboembolism,[94] and that prophylaxis with low-dose warfarin in these patients can significantly decrease this risk.[96] In addition, hormone therapy with tamoxifen can also be a risk factor in breast cancer. The combination of chemotherapy with tamoxifen has been associated with more thrombotic complications than chemotherapy alone in premenopausal women.[95] The use of hematopoietic growth factors (that is, granulocyte and granulocyte/monocyte colony-stimulating factors, G-CSF and GM-CSF) may also be implicated in hypercoagulation and clot formation in this disease.[50,97]

The pathogenesis of thrombosis during chemotherapy is not entirely understood, but the following mechanisms have been identified: (1) the damage to tumor cells caused by the antitumor drugs, (2) their toxic effect on host cells, (3) the suppression of anticoagulants and fibrinolysis, and (4) the induction of apoptosis.

Tumor-cell damage

The first mechanism is due to the release of procoagulants and cytokines by tumor cells that have been damaged by chemotherapy. This mechanism is considered responsible for the exacerbation of DIC observed in laboratory and clinical data upon starting chemotherapy in acute leukemia.[7] In addition, the downregulation of TF and CP in the blast cells of patients with APL, paralleled by a reduction in laboratory and clinical signs of hypercoagulation in these subjects, provides strong evidence of a role for procoagulant activities in the pathogenesis of DIC.[10] The release of cytokines in response to chemotherapy may also have important implications for increasing the thrombotic risk. This was suggested by Bertomeu et al,[98] who demonstrated that plasma samples collected from women with breast cancer after chemotherapy contained higher levels of mediators (probably cytokines) able to increase the reactivity of endothelial cells to platelets.

Endothelium and monocyte toxicity

Another mechanism involves the direct damage exerted by chemoradiotherapy on vascular endothelium. Two categories of chemotherapeutic agents have been identified on the basis of an in vitro assay to detect the sublethal effects of drugs on endothelial integrity in tissue culture.[99] The differences may depend on the different mechanisms of drug cytotoxicity. Radiation therapy can also cause endothelial injury, as demonstrated by the release of von Willebrand protein from human umbilical vein endothelial cells irradiated with doses up to 40 Gy.[100] In animal studies, bleomycin has been implicated in determining morphological damage to vascular endothelium of the lung, which may result in pulmonary thrombosis and fibrosis. Furthermore, doxorubicin, in some experimental models, directly affects glomerular cells, impairing their permeability and leading to a nephrotic syndrome, accompanied by hypercoagulation and increased thrombotic tendency.[101] The clinical counterpart of this experimental condition has not yet been completely clarified. However, profound changes in plasma markers of endothelial damage are reported in patients receiving chemotherapy.[17–19] It has been observed that some chemotherapeutic agents can directly stimulate the expression of TF procoagulant activity by macrophages and monocytes.[102] Therefore, chemotherapy can induce a procoagulant response from host cells.

Suppression of anticoagulants and fibrinolysis

Falls in the levels of naturally occurring inhibitors of blood coagulation such as antithrombin, protein C, and protein S, have been repeatedly reported after chemotherapy.[103] This is a recognized mechanism of acquired thrombophilia. The defect in natural anticoagulants is likely to be a consequence of the direct hepatotoxicity of radio- and chemotherapy. However, there are few studies analyzing the levels of fibrinolytic proteins during chemotherapy, and data from these studies are contradictory. In one series of patients, a significant reduction in t-PA levels occurred, which was associated with an increase in PAI-1 activity and reduction of the fibrinolytic activity.[104] In contrast, other authors have not found evidence of fibrinolysis impairment during anticancer treatments.[105–107]

Induction of apoptosis

The last mechanism involves the potential thrombogenic role of apoptosis induced in tumor cells by chemotherapeutic agents. Apoptosis, the well-characterized form of programmed cell death, is involved in many biological processes. The relationship between cellular procoagulant activity and chemotherapeutic drug-induced apoptosis has been described by Wang et al in various human tumor cell lines.[108] They found a significant correlation between thrombin generation, TF activity, and the degree of apoptosis, hypothesizing that the exposure of phosphatidylserine on the cell surface membrane during apoptosis is essential for both thrombin generation and TF activation.

However, we may note that the proapoptotic activity of antineoplastic drugs is not always associated with an increase in the procoagulant activity of tumor cells. Indeed, apoptosis induced by differentiating agents, such as ATRA in the model of APL cells, is accompanied by a downregulation of cellular procoagulant activities.[69,78,109]

Summary and conclusions

The development of cancer is associated with activation of coagulation. The results of laboratory tests clearly demonstrate that fibrin formation and dissolution are continuous at different rates in these patients, who are at increased risk of secondary thrombosis. It is important to remember that fibrin formation is also involved in the processes of tumor spread and metastasis.

The pathogenesis of hemostatic disorders in cancer is complex and reflects the interaction of different mechanisms involving the activation of various hemostatic components, such as the coagulation and fibrinolytic systems, vascular endothelium, leukocytes, and platelets. Tumor cells possess the capacity to interact with all parts of the hemostatic system. They can directly activate the coagulation cascade by producing their own procoagulant factors, or they can stimulate the prothrombotic properties of other blood-cell components. Additional mechanisms of blood-clotting activation are started by the initiation of antitumor therapies.

In the last 10 years, research studies have greatly improved our knowledge of tumor-promoted prothrombotic functions. Understanding the molecular basis of the underlying mechanisms may help to identify better-targeted strategies to prevent thromboembolism in cancer patients. Furthermore, pharmacological modulation of malignant-cell hemostatic properties not only may affect the tumor-associated thrombotic risk, but also may offer the ability to interfere with the progression of the disease.

References

1. Rickles FR, Edwards RL. Activation of blood coagulation in cancer: Trousseau's syndrome revisited. Blood 1983; 62:14–31.

2. Donati MB. Cancer and thrombosis: from phlegmasia alba dolens to transgenic mice. Thromb Haemost 1995; 74:278–81.

3. Bini A, Mesa-Tejada R, Fenoglio JJ et al. Immunohistochemical characterization of fibrin(ogen)-related antigens in human tissues using monoclonal antibodies. Lab Invest 1989; 60:814–21.

4. Monreal M, Prandoni P. Venous thromboembolism as first manifestation of cancer. Semin Thromb Hemost 1999; 25:131–6.

5. Prandoni P, Lensing AWA, Buller HR et al. Deep-vein thrombosis and the incidence of subsequent symptomatic cancer. N Engl J Med 1992; 327:1128–33.

6. Rickles FR, Levine MN. Epidemiology of thrombosis in cancer. Acta Haematol 2001; **106**: 6–12.

7. Barbui T, Finazzi G, Falanga A. The impact of all-*trans*-retinoic acid on the coagulopathy of acute promyelocytic leukemia. Blood 1998; **91**:3093–4102.

8. Falanga A, Barbui T, Rickles FR et al. Guidelines for clotting studies in cancer patients. Thromb Haemost 1993; **70**:343–50.

9. Falanga A, Ofosu FA, Delaini F et al. The hypercoagulable state in cancer: evidence for impaired thrombin inhibition. Blood Coagul Fibrinolysis 1994; Suppl: S19–S23.

10. Falanga A, Iacoviello L, Evangelista V et al. Loss of blast cell procoagulant activity and improvement of hemostatic variables in patients with acute promyelocytic leukemia given all-*trans*-retinoic acid. Blood 1995; **86**:1072–84.

11. Lindhal AK, Sandset PM, Abilgaard U. Indices of hypercoagulation in cancer as compared with those with acute inflammation and acute infarction. Haemostasis 1990; **20**: 253–62.

12. Seitz R, Rappe N, Kraus M et al. Activation of coagulation and fibrinolysis in patients with lung cancer: relation to tumour stage and prognosis. Blood Coagul Fibrinolysis 1993; **4**:249–54.

13. Kakkar AK, DeRuvo N, Chinswangwatanakul V et al. Extrinsic-pathway activation in cancer with high factor VIIa and tissue factor. Lancet 1995; **346**:1004–5.

14. Falanga A, Levine MN, Consonni R et al. The effect of very low dose warfarin on markers of hypercoagulation in metastatic breast cancer: results from a randomized trial. Thromb Haemost 1998; **79**:23–7.

15. Donati MB, Poggi A, Semeraro N. Coagulation and malignancy. In: Poller L, ed. Recent Advances in Blood Coagulation, (Churchill Livingstone: Edinburgh, 1981) 227–59.

16. Gadducci A, Baicchi U, Marrai R et al. Pretreatment plasma levels of fibrinopeptide A (FPA), D-dimer (DD), and von Willebrand factor (vWF) in patients with ovarian carcinoma. Gynecol Oncol 1994; **53**: 352–6.

17. Licciardello JTW, Moake JL, Rudi CK et al. Elevated plasma von Willebrand factor levels and arterial occlusive complications associated with cisplatin-based chemotherapy. Oncology 1985; **42**:296–300.

18. Bazarbachi A, Scrobohachi ML, Gisselbrecht C et al. Changes in protein C, factor VII and endothelial markers after autologous bone marrow transplantation: possible implications in the pathogenesis of veno-occlusive disease. Nouv Rev Fr Hematol 1993; **35**:135–40.

19. Catani L, Gugliotta L, Vianelli N et al. Endothelium and bone marrow transplantation. Bone Marrow Transplant 1996; **17**:277–80.

20. Kuenen BC, Levi M, Meijers JC et al. Analysis of coagulation cascade and endothelial cell activation during inhibition of vascular endothelial growth factor/vascular endothelial growth factor receptor pathway in cancer patients. Arterioscler Thromb Vasc Biol 2002; **22**: 1500–5.

21. Semeraro N, Montemurro P, Conese M et al. Procoagulant activity of mononuclear phagocytes from different anatomical sites in patients with gynaecological malignancies. Int J Cancer 1990; **45**: 251–4.

22. Falanga A, Marchetti M, Evangelista V et al. Polymorphonuclear leukocyte activation and hemostasis in patients with essential thrombocythemia and polycythemia vera. Blood 2000; **96**: 4261–6.

23. Wehmeier A, Tschope D, Esser J et al. Circulating activated platelets in myeloproliferative disorders. Thromb Res 1991; **61**:271–8.

24. Cines DB, Pollak ES, Buck CA et al. Endothelial cells in physiology and in the pathophysiology of vascular disorders. Blood 1998; **91**:3527–61.

25. Bevilacqua MP, Pober JS, Majeau GR et al. Recombinant tumor necrosis factor induces procoagulant activity in cultured human vascular endothelium: characterization and comparison with the actions of interleukin-1. Proc Natl Acad Sci USA 1986; **83**:4533–7.

26. Moore KL, Esmon CT, Esmon NL. Tumor necrosis factor leads to the internalization and degradation of thrombomodulin from the surface of bovine aortic endothelial cells in culture. Blood 1989; **73**:159–65.

27. Falanga A, Marchetti M, Giovanelli S et al. All-*trans*-retinoic acid counteracts endothelial cell procoagulant activity induced by a human promyelocytic leukemia-derived cell line (NB4). Blood 1996; **87**:613–7.

28. Maiolo A, Tua A, Grignani G. Hemostasis and cancer: tumor cells induce the expression of tissue factor-like procoagulant activity on endothelial cells. Haematologica 2002; **87**:624–8.

29. Van Hinsbergh VWM, Bauer KA, Kooistra T et al. Progress of fibrinolysis during tumor necrosis factor infusion in humans. Concomitant increase of tissue-type plasminogen activator, plasminogen activator inhibitor type-1, and fibrin(ogen) degradation products. Blood 1990; **76**:2284–9.

30. Contrino J, Hair G, Kreutzer DL et al. In situ detection of tissue factor in vascular endothelial cells: correlation with the malignant phenotype of human breast disease. Nat Med 1996; **2**:209–15.

31. Honn KV, Tang DG, Chen YQ. Adhesion molecules and site-specific metastases. In: Neri Serneri GG, Abbate R, Genuini G, eds. Thrombosis: An Update. (Scientific Press: Florence, 1992)269–303.

32. Giavazzi R, Foppolo M, Dossi R et al. Rolling and adhesion of human tumor cells on vascular endothelium under physiological flow conditions. J Clin Invest 1993; **92**:3038–44.

33. Marchetti M, Falanga A, Giovanelli S et al. All-*trans*-retinoic acid increases the adhesion to endothelium of the acute promyelocytic leukemia cell line NB4. Br J Haematol 1996; **93**:360–6.

34. Donati MB, Poggi A. Malignancy and haemostasis. Br J Haematol 1980; **44**:173–82.

35. Gasic GJ, Gasic TB. Plasma membrane vesicles as mediators of interactions between tumor cells and components of the hemostatic and immune system. In: Jamieson GA, ed. Interactions of Platelets and Tumor Cells. (AR Liss: New York, 1982)429–32.

36. Grignani G, Jamieson GA. Platelets in tumor metastasis: generation of ADP by tumor cells is specific but not unrelated to metastatic potential. Blood 1988; **71**:844–9.

37. Varon D, Brill A. Platelets cross-talk with tumor cells. Haemostasis 2001; **31**(Suppl 1):64–6.

38. Felding-Habermann B. Tumor cell-platelet interaction in metastatic disease. Haemostasis 2001; **31** (Suppl 1): 55–8.

39. Poggi A, Rossi C, Beviglia L et al. Platelet-tumor cell interactions. In: Joseph M, ed. The Handbook of Immunopharmacology. (Academic Press: London, 1995)151–65.

40. Al-Mondhiry H. Beta-thromboglobulin and platelet factor 4 in patients with cancer. Correlation with the stage of disease and the effect of

chemotherapy. Am J Hematol 1983; **14**:105–11.

41. Grignani G, Falanga A, Pacchiarini L et al. Human breast and colon carcinomas express cysteine proteinase activities with pro-aggregating and pro-coagulant properties. Int J Cancer 1988; **42**:554–7.

42. Lampugnani MG, Donati MB. Thrombin stimulates arachidonate metabolism in murine tumor cells. Int J Cancer 1987; **39**:367–72.

43. Lampugnani MG, Pedenovi M, Niewiarowski A et al. Effects of dimethyl sulfoxide (DMSO) on microfilament organization, cellular adhesion, and growth of cultured mouse B16 melanoma cells. Exp Cell Res 1987; **172**:385–96.

44. Pinedo HM, Verheul HMW, D'Amato AJ et al. Involvement of platelets in tumor angiogenesis? Lancet, 1998; **352**:1775–7.

45. Coussen LM, Werb Z. Inflammation and cancer. Nature 2002; **420**:860–7.

46. Aeed, PA, Nakajima M, Welch DR. The role of polymorphonuclear leukocytes (PMN) on the growth and metastatic potential of 13762NF mammary adenocarcinoma cells. Int J Cancer 1988; **42**:748–59.

47. Starkey, JR, Liggitt HD, Jones W et al. Influence of migratory blood cells on the attachment of tumor cells to vascular endothelium. Int J Cancer 1984; **34**:535–43.

48. Welch, DR, Schissel DJ, Howrey RP et al. Tumor-elicited polymorphonuclear cells, in contrast to 'normal' circulating polymorphonuclear cells, stimulate invasive and metastatic potentials of rat mammary adenocarcinoma cells. Proc Natl Acad Sci USA 1989; **86**: 5859–63.

49. Wu QD, Wang JH, Condron C et al. Human neutrophils facilitate tumor cell transendothelial migration. Am J Physiol Cell Physiol 2001; **280**:814–22.

50. Falanga A, Marchetti M, Evangelista V et al. Neutrophil activation and hemostatic changes in healthy donors given granulocyte-colony stimulating factor. Blood 1999; **93**:2506–14.

51. Semeraro N, Colucci M. Tissue factor in health and disease. Thromb Haemost 1997; **78**:759–64.

52. Lorenzet R, Peri G, Locati D et al. Generation of procoagulant activity by mononuclear phagocytes: a possible mechanism contributing to blood clotting activation within malignant tissue. Blood 1983; **62**:2721–3.

53. Mussoni L, Donati MB. Expression of plasminogen activator as a marker of stimulation in tumor-associated macrophages. Haemostasis 1988; **18**:66–71.

54. Gordon SG. Tumor cell procoagulants and their role in malignant disease. Semin Thromb Hemost 1992; **18**:424–33.

55. Falanga A, Rickels FR. Pathophysiology of the thrombophilic state in the cancer patients. Semin Thromb Hemost 1999; **25**:173–82.

56. Van de Water L, Tracy PB, Aronson D et al. Tumor cell generation of thrombin via prothrombinase assembly. Cancer Res 1985; **45**:5521–5.

57. Hettasch JM, Bandarenko N, Burchette JL et al. Tissue transglutaminase expression in human breast cancer. Lab Invest 1997; **75**:637–45.

58. Andoh D, Kubota T, Takada M et al. Tissue factor activity in leukemia cells. Special reference to disseminated intravascular coagulation. Cancer 1987; **59**:748–54.

59. Nemerson Y. The tissue factor pathway of blood coagulation. Semin Hematol 1992; **29**:170–6.

60. Rickles FR, Falanga A. Molecular basis for the relationship between thrombosis and cancer. Thromb Res 2001; **102**:V215–24.

61. Zhang, Y, Deng Y, Luther T et al. Tissue factor controls the balance of angiogenic and antiangiogenic properties of tumor cells in mice. J Clin Invest 1994; **94**:1320–7.

62. Shoji M, Hancock WW, Abe K et al. Activation of coagulation and angiogenesis in cancer. Immuno-histochemical localization in situ of clotting proteins and VEGF in human cancers. Am J Pathol 1998; **152**:399–411.

63. Abe K, Shoji M, Chen J et al. Regulation of vascular endothelial growth factor production and angiogenesis by the cytoplasmic tail of tissue factor. Proc Natl Acad Sci USA 1999; **96**:8663–8.

64. Falanga A, Gordon SG. Isolation and characterization of cancer pro-coagulant: a cysteine proteinase from malignant tissue. Biochemistry 1985; **24**:5558–67.

65. Gordon SG, Mourad AM. The site of activation of factor X by cancer procoagulant. Blood Coagul Fibrinolysis 1991; **2**:735–9.

66. Mielicki WP, Gordon SG. Three-stage chromogenic assay for the analysis of activation properties of factor X by cancer procoagulant. Blood Coagul Fibrinolysis 1993; **4**:441–6.

67. Donati MB, Gambacorti Passerini C, Casali B et al. Cancer procoag-ulant in human tumor cells: evidence from melanoma patients. Cancer Res 1986; **46**:6471–4.

68. Gordon SG, Hashiba U, Poole MA et al. Cysteine proteinase procoag-ulant from amnion-chorion. Blood 1985; **66**:1261–5.

69. Falanga A, Consonni R, Marchetti M et al. Cancer procoagulant and tissue factor are differently modu-lated by all-*trans*-retinoic acid (ATRA) in acute promyelocytic leukemia cells. Blood 1998; **92**:143–51.

70. Donati MB, Falanga A, Consonni R et al. Cancer procoagulant in acute non-lymphoid leukemia: relation-ship of enzyme detection to disease activity. Thromb Haemost 1990; **64**:11–6.

71. Gordon SG, Cross BA. An enzyme-linked immunosorbent assay for cancer procoagulant and its poten-tial as new tumor marker. Cancer Res 1990; **50**:6229–34.

72. Gordon SG, Benson B. Analysis of serum cancer procoagulant activi-ty: its possible use as a tumor marker. Thromb Res 1989; **56**:431–4.

73. Edwards RL, Silver J, Rickles FR. Human tumor procoagulants: Registry of the Subcommittee on Haemostasis and Malignancy of the Scientific and Standardization Committee, International Society of Thrombosis and Haemostasis. Thromb Haemost 1993; **63**: 205–13.

74. Koyama T, Hirosawa S, Kawamata N et al. All-*trans*-retinoic acid upregulates thrombomodulin and downregulates tissue factor expression in acute promyelocytic leukemia cells: distinct expression of thrombomodulin and tissue fac-tor in human leukemic cells. Blood 1994; **84**:3001–9.

75. De Stefano V, Teofili L, Sica S et al. Effect of all-*trans*-retinoic acid on procoagulant and fibrinolytic activi-ties of cultured blast cells from patients with acute promyelocytic leukemia. Blood 1995; **86**: 3535–41.

76. Falanga A, Alessio MG, Donati MB et al. A new procoagulant in acute leukemia. Blood 1988; **71**:870–5.

77. Alessio MG, Falanga A, Consonni R et al. Cancer procoagulant in acute lymphoblastic leukemia. Eur J Haematol 1990; **445**:78–81.

78. Falanga A, Consonni R, Marchetti M et al. Cancer procoagulant in the human promyelocytic cell line NB4 and its modulation by retinoic acid. Leukemia 1994; **8**:156–9.

79. Falanga A, Toma S, Marchetti M et al. Effect of all-*trans*-retinoic acid on the hypercoagulable state of patients with breast cancer. Am J Hematol 2002; **70**:9–15.

80. Balducci D, Marchetti M, Suardi S et al. All-*trans*-retinoic acid (ATRA) reduces procoagulant activity (PCA) and induces apoptosis in human breast cancer cells. Thromb Haemost 2001; Supp: July OC904.

81. Binder BR. Physiology and pathophysiology of the fibrinolytic system. Fibrinolysis 1995; **9**:3–8.

82. Bell WR. The fibrinolytic system in neoplasia. Semin Thromb Hemost 1996; **22**:459–78.

83. McMahon GA, Petitclerc E, Stefansson S et al. Plasminogen activator inhibitor-1 regulates tumor growth and angiogenesis. J Biol Chem 2001; **276**:33964–8.

84. Kwaan HC, Keer HN. Fibrinolysis and cancer. Semin Thromb Hemost 1990; **16**:230–5.

85. Stephens R, Alitalo R, Tapiovaara H et al. Production of an active urokinase by leukemia cells. A novel distinction from cell lines of solid tumors. Leuk Res 1988; **12**:419–22.

86. Hajjar KA. Cellular receptors in the regulation of plasmin generation. Thromb Haemost 1995; **74**:294–301.

87. Rocha E, Pàramo JA, Fernàndez FJ et al. Clotting activation and impairment of fibrinolysis in malignancy. Thromb Res 189; **54**:699–707.

88. Harbeck N, Schmitt M, Kates RE et al. Clinical utility of urokinase-type plasminogen activator and plasminogen activator inhibitor-1 determination in primary breast cancer tissue for individualized therapy concepts. Clin Breast Cancer 2002; **3**:196–200.

89. Grignani G, Maiolo A. Cytokines and hemostasis. Haematologica 2000; **85**:967–72.

90. Brown LF, Detmas M, Claffey K et al. Vascular permeability factor/vascular endothelial growth factor: a multifunctional angiogenesis factor. In: Goldberg ID, Rosen EM, eds. Regulation of Angiogenesis. (Birkhauser: Basel, 1998)233–69.

91. Clauss M, Gerlach M, Gerlach H et al. Vascular permeability factor: a tumor-derived polypeptide that induces endothelial cell and monocyte procoagulant activity, and promotes monocyte migration. J Exp Med 1990; **172**:1535–45.

92. Shoji M, Abe K, Nawroth PP et al. Molecular mechanisms linking thrombosis and angiogenesis in cancer. Trends Cardiovasc Med 1997; **7**:52–9.

93. Falanga A. Mechanisms of hypercoagulation in malignancy and during chemotherapy. Haemostasis 1998: **28**(Suppl 3): 50–60.

94. Levine MN, Gent M, Hirsh J et al. The thrombogenic effect of anticancer drug therapy in women with stage II breast cancer. N Engl J Med 1988; **318**:404–7.

95. Saphner T, Tormey DC, Gray R. Venous and arterial thrombosis in patients who received adjuvant therapy for breast cancer. J Clin Oncol 1991; **9**:286–94.

96. Levine MN, Gent M, Hirsh J et al. Double-blind randomised trial of very-low-dose warfarin for prevention of thromboembolism in stage IV breast cancer. Lancet 1994; **343**:886–9.

97. Barbui T, Finazzi G, Grassi A et al. Thrombosis in cancer patients treated with hematopoietic growth factors—a meta-analysis. Thromb Haemost 1996; **75**:368–71.

98. Bertomeu MC, Gallo S, Lauri D et al. Chemotherapy enhances endothelial cell reactivity to platelets. Clin Expl Metastasis 1990; 8:511–18.

99. Nicolson GL, Custead SE. Effects of chemotherapeutic drugs on platelet and metastatic tumor cell–endothelial cell interactions as a model for assessing vascular endothelial integrity. Cancer Res 1985; 45:331–6.

100. Sporn LA, Rubin P, Marder VJ et al. Irradiation induces release of von Willebrand protein from endothelial cells in culture. Blood 1984; 64:567–70.

101. Poggi A, Kornblitt L, Delaini F et al. Delayed hypercoagulability after a single dose of Adriamycin to normal rats. Thromb Res 1979; 16:639–50.

102. Walsh J, Wheeler HR, Geczy CL. Modulation of tissue factor on human monocytes by cisplatin and Adriamycin. Br J Haematol 1992; 81:480–8.

103. Harper PL, Jarvis J, Jennings I et al. Changes in the natural anticoagulants following bone marrow transplantation. Bone Marrow Transplant 1990; 5:39–42.

104. Ruiz MA, Marugan I, Estelles A et al. The influence of chemotherapy on plasma coagulation and fibrinolytic systems in lung cancer patients. Cancer 1989; 63:643–8.

105. Zurborn KH, Gram J, Glander K et al. Influence of cytostatic treatment on the coagulation system and fibrinolysis in patients with non-Hodgkin's lymphomas and acute leukemias. Eur J Haematol 1991; 47:55–9.

106. Fukutomi T, Adachi I, Watanabe T. Effects of combined tamoxifen and medroxyprogesterone treatment on coagulation–fibrinolytic systems in patients with advanced breast cancer. Acta Oncol 1993; 32:573–4.

107. Japan Advanced Breast Cancer Study Group and Japan Clinical Oncology Group. Effects of chemoendocrine therapy on the coagulation–fibrinolytic systems in patients with advanced breast cancer. Jpn J Cancer Res 1993; 84:455–61.

108. Wang J, Weiss I, Svoboda K et al. Thrombogenic role of cells undergoing apoptosis. Br J Haematol 2001; 115:382–91.

109. Zhu J, Guo WM, Yao YY et al. Tissue factors on acute promyelocytic leukemia and endothelial cells are differently regulated by retinoic acid, arsenic trioxide and chemotherapeutic agents. Leukemia 1999; 13:1062–70.

110. Marchetti M, Barbui T, Falanga A. All-trans-retinoic acid (ATRA) counteracts the adhesion of the human promyelocytic leukemia (APL) NB4 cells to the endothelium. Thrombosis and Haemostasis, Supplement June 1997: 551.

3

Platelets and cancer

Abraham Klepfish, Ami Schattner, Gilles Lugassy, and
Simon Karpatkin

Introduction

Armand Trousseau was probably the first to recognize, almost 140 years
ago, the linkage between cancer and thromboembolism, when he noted
a high incidence of thrombophlebitis in patients with gastrointestinal
malignancy. The bilateral mode of the link between thrombosis and cancer was appreciated by Billroth: he reported that tumor cells may be
part of blood thrombi and suggested that the distant embolization of
blood vessels is a possible mechanism of metastasis. Ninety years later,
Gasic and co-workers were the first to show the direct requirement of
platelets for experimental tumor metastasis. Since then, a remarkable
amount of information has accumulated on different aspects of
platelet–tumor interaction. The presence of cancer may affect the
platelets quantitatively (causing either thrombocytopenia or thrombocytosis) and/or qualitatively (causing platelet activation). In turn, platelets
are involved by a variety of mechanisms in the progression of neoplasms, mostly during the different stages of tumor metastasis. In this
chapter, we will review the pathophysiological mechanisms involved in
the tumor–platelet interaction and describe some of its clinical and therapeutic aspects.

Thrombocytosis and thrombocytopenia in cancer patients

Alterations in platelet number and function can occur in patients with
cancer (hematological malignancies and the consequences of
chemo/radiotherapy are excluded from this discussion). Such alterations
have diverse and intriguing underlying pathophysiological mechanisms.
Their recognition and study is important since it may aid in diagnosis
and reveal important pathogenetic mechanisms, although their impact

31

on the patient's prognosis remains limited in most cases. Five clinical syndromes involving platelets in cancer will be discussed: reactive thrombocytosis, disseminated intravascular coagulation (DIC), myeloph-thisis, immune thrombocytopenia, and thrombotic thrombocutopenic purpura (TTP)/hemolytic uremic syndrome (HUS).

Thrombocytosis

A platelet count higher than 500 000/μl is a common accompaniment of cancer and is referred to as reactive thrombocytosis. Of patients with malignancies, 30–60% have thrombocytosis, making it one of the most common hematological abnormalities in this group of patients.[1,2] In a large survey of patients in the Johns Hopkins Hospital in the 1960s, neoplasms (other than myeloproliferative disorders) were responsible for 38% of the cases of thrombocytosis.[3] Platelet counts of up to 1 345 000/μl were encountered, although most patients had values of less than 1×10^6/μl (29/31 patients). The neoplasms most commonly represented in this series were adenocarcinoma of the gastrointestinal tract (stomach and colorectal cancer) and lung cancer, although practically any tumor may be associated with thrombocytosis, including malignant lymphoma. The association between thrombocytosis and malignancy were later confirmed by a number of investigators.[4-8] When other causes of reactive thrombocytosis can be excluded, this finding may suggest a diagnosis of malignancy. However, its implications are limited, since, in reactive thrombocytosis, tests of platelet function (including platelet-aggregation studies) are generally normal, and patients do not experience increased incidence of hemorrhage or thromboembolism even when the platelet count exceeds 1×10^6/μl.[9]

The mechanisms underlying the development of thrombocytosis in patients with malignancy are probably cytokine-mediated. Hollen et al[10] reported that patients with malignant tumors associated with thrombocytosis had high serum levels of interleukin-6 (IL-6). IL-6 stimulates thrombopoiesis by enhancing thrombopoietin (TPO) mRNA expression in cancer cells in vitro and increasing TPO plasma levels.[11] The profile of cytokines mediating thrombocytosis may vary with the tumor, and often several cytokines are produced. For example, whereas hepatic tumors may autonomously overproduce TPO,[12] in other tumors a variety of cytokines (mostly IL-6, IL-11, and stem cell factor [SCF]) may mediate the enhanced thrombopoiesis.[13]

The prognostic impact of thrombocytosis in cancer patients is also diverse. Although it may sometimes predict a survival benefit, as was recently demonstrated in patients with periampullary adenocarcinoma treated by surgery,[14] the opposite is true for the majority of reports in other cancers, such as breast, gastric and renal-cell carcinomas.[15-17] Of interest is the finding that in patients suspected to have lung cancer (versus a noncancerous lung lesion), the presence of thrombocytosis is correlated with having a malignancy.[18]

Disseminated intravascular coagulopathy (DIC)

Thrombocytopenia occurs in 4–11% of untreated cancer patients.[19–21] Among the many etiologies of thrombocytopenia in cancer patients, DIC is the most commonly encountered pathogenetic mechanism and has been reported in as many as 15%.[22] Although it may manifest only as asymptomatic laboratory abnormality, warranting the term 'low-grade' or compensated DIC, this represents one part of a disease continuum. Patients may therefore lapse from one end of the spectrum into another, and develop fulminant DIC with systemic thrombohemorrhagic disorder and end-organ damage. Myriads of coagulation mediators are expressed or released by tumor cells.[23] These include procoagulant activity—in particular, tissue factor, plasminogen activators, and vascular permeability factor (VPF; also VEGF)—which appears to be the initiating event in the DIC cascade.[24] Lymphomas and adenocarcinomas of the lung, breast, gastrointestinal tract, and kidney—especially when metastatic—and promyelocytic leukemia have a special propensity to initiate the cascade, leading to the generation of large amounts of thrombin, fibrin deposition in the microvasculature, and possible thrombocytopenia as part of the consumption coagulopathy syndrome. An additional common laboratory feature of DIC is fibrinolytic activation with fibrinogen or fibrin degradation. This is characterized by increases in blood levels of D-dimer and fibrinogen degradation products (FDP) that have a very high predictive value for DIC.[25] Nevertheless, these changes are most often clinically silent. Hemorrhage occurs in about one in 10 cancer patients. Roughly half of these cases result from thrombocytopenia due to chemotherapy, and one-third of patients bleed due to direct tumor invasion. Only about 10% of all bleeds in cancer are the result of DIC.[26] Thrombosis in cancer has likewise a multifactorial pathogenesis.[27] DIC is uncommonly responsible, though it is often associated with,[28] and can be diagnosed as, a cluster of laboratory abnormalities in patients with cancer-associated thrombophilia.

Myelophthisis

A second potential cause of thrombocytopenia in the cancer patient that is not due to chemotherapy is metastatic bone-marrow involvement. Various cancers, notably adenocarcinoma of the prostate and breast cancer as well as malignant lymphoma and other hematological malignancies, may invade the bone marrow.[29] Bone metastases may also be associated. As a result, failure in the production of blood elements may include thrombocytopenia, and, rarely, thrombocytopenia is the only cytopenia caused by marrow infiltration by tumor cells.[30] In fact, a platelet count under 100 000/μl, together with bone pain, serum lactic dehydrogenase over 500 IU/liter, and a typical blood smear, strongly correlates with bone-marrow metastasis.[31] Examination of the peripheral blood smear shows a leukoerythroblastic response,[30] which is characterized by the presence of teardrop and nucleated red blood cells, a shift to the left in the white blood cells (presence of early myeloid forms), and large, bizarre-shaped platelets. These cases are readily diagnosed by the examination of a bone-marrow aspiration and biopsy.[32] Their prognosis is governed by that of the underlying tumor, which is often widely disseminated.

Immune thrombocytopenia

Thrombocytopenia in cancer may also be due to increased platelet destruction by immune mechanisms. The clinical picture resembles that of chronic immune thrombocytopenic purpura (ITP), which is mediated by antibodies produced as part of chronic lymphatic leukemia (CLL), lymphoma, and—uncommonly—solid tumors (secondary autoimmune thrombocytopenia).[30,33,34]

Occasionally, immune thrombocytopenia may be the presenting manifestation of the tumor.[35–37] Most published cases merely report on the association between cancer and an ITP-like illness, inferring the presence of tumor-related antiplatelet antibodies. In just a few cases, a study of the platelet-associated antibodies suggests that they are directed against either platelet glycoprotein (GP) IIb/IIIa or GP Ib/IX.[38,39] In that, they are similar to idiopathic ITP.[40] The antiplatelet antibodies may sometimes be monoclonal immunoglobulins,[41] especially in patients with non-Hodgkin's lymphoma. Another open question is the role of antibody-mediated inhibition of thrombopoiesis by binding to megakaryocytes, which is rarely documented in patients with tumors.[42]

Thrombotic microangiopathy

Finally, thrombotic microangiopathy, manifesting as thrombotic thrombocytopenic purpura (TTP)/hemolytic uremic syndrome (HUS), can occur in the cancer patient. Most of the cases reported occur in patients with adenocarcinoma (88% in one series), gastric cancer being the most common type.[43] However, chemotherapy with mitomycin C or many other anticancer drugs (including bleomycin, cisplatin, and gemcitabine) may also cause a similar syndrome.[44] A high cumulative dose of the drug appears to be a significant risk factor, increasing the risk of thrombotic microangiopathy.[43,45] A variety of other drugs given for comorbid conditions may also cause TTP.[40] In addition, the syndrome is a well-recognized complication of bone-marrow transplantation, particularly in the allogeneic setting.[46] The distinction between cancer-associated and anticancer chemotherapy-associated TTP/HUS may be difficult. Furthermore, DIC may coexist in these patients, and this may confuse the diagnosis. The initiating event in the varied forms of thrombotic microangiopathy in the cancer patient seems to be endothelial cell injury.[47] It is postulated that extensive occlusive hyaline thrombi formed in the small arterial vessels (arterioles and capillaries) lead to platelet consumption and thrombocytopenia (but, as opposed to DIC, there is no consumption of coagulation factors in TTP/HUS), together with red blood-cell fragmentation and microangiopathic hemolytic anemia. Tissue ischemia is another important outcome, leading primarily to renal and neurological dysfunction. An additional abnormality is the presence of ultralarge multimers of von Willebrand factor (vWF) due to antibody-mediated inhibition of vWF-cleaving protease.[48] These multimers bind platelet membrane-adhesive glycoproteins, resulting in further activation of GP IIb/IIIa.

Thrombotic microangiopathy in the cancer patient differs from most other thrombocytopenic syndromes in this group by its being a severe progressive illness that mandates rapid recognition and intervention.[47] The anemia and thrombocytopenia are usually severe and out of proportion to what is usually found with cancer or chemotherapy. In addition, the identification of Coombs-negative hemolytic process, prevalence of characteristic schistocytes in the peripheral blood smear, and ongoing end-organ damage are highly suggestive. Plasma exchange is the most important component of therapy, whatever the etiology. However, 70–80% of cancer patients may not respond, versus about 20% or less in 'classic' TTP.[44] In nonresponders, immunoadsorption with plasma perfusion over a staphylococcal protein A column that removes immune complexes[49] has been reported to be effective.

Platelets, cancer metastasis, and cancer growth

The pathogenesis of cancer metastasis is a complex, sequential cascade of events, involving detachment of the metastasizing malignant cells at the primary tumor site, intravasation, survival in the circulation, adhesion to vascular-wall components at the new site, invasion of the vessel wall, growth, neovascularization (neoangiogenesis), and, possibly, secondary metastasis formation.

Gasic et al[50] were the first to show the requirement of platelets for experimental hematogenous metastasis (tail-vein injection of tumor cells and quantization of pulmonary metastases thus caused): induction of severe thrombocytopenia prior to tumor-cell injection almost completely abolished the ability of tumor cells to cause pulmonary metastasis in the experimental animals. This ability can be restored with human platelets.[51]

The following mechanisms—probably in combination—may provide an explanation for this phenomenon:

(1) Platelet–tumor cell adhesion and activation are one mechanism.
(2) Activated platelets generate thrombin on their surface, and this can stimulate platelet–tumor and platelet and tumor cell–endothelial cell adhesion, as well as tumor growth and metastasis.
(3) Platelets binding to tumor cells induce the prolongation of tumor-cell survival in the circulation.
(4) Platelet–tumor emboli induce downstream ischemic endothelial damage, leading to the increase of the adhesive properties of the endothelium.
(5) Activated platelets in close contact with tumor cells secrete substances capable of increasing the permeability of the vessel wall, thus facilitating tumor-cell invasion.
(6) Platelet-derived growth factors may support tumor growth at the metastatic site.
(7) Platelets are a source of angiogenesis-promoting factors, providing the new metastatic tumor with neoangiogenesis ability.

Platelet–tumor cell adhesion and activation

The early data on the requirement of platelets for experimental hematogenous metastasis and the ability of tumor cells to aggregate platelets,[50,52] as well as the correlation shown between the ability of some tumor cells to aggregate platelets in vitro and their requirement for metastasis in vivo,[53] prompted attempts to inhibit experimental tumor metastasis with antiaggregating agents, such as prostacyclin (PGI2),[54] aspirin, and ticlopidine.[51] No inhibitory effect was demonstrated. Studies focused then on platelet adhesion. Tumor cells adhere to platelets in vitro, requiring platelet integrin GP IIb/IIIa ($\alpha_2 \beta_3$), fibronectin, vWF, and the RGDS domain of the adhesive proteins.[55] Monoclonal antibodies against vWF and GP IIb/IIIa remarkably inhibit experimental murine hematogenous metastasis.[55]

P-selectin, which is known to mediate leukocyte adhesion to vascular endothelium and platelets under flow conditions, has also been shown to be involved in the initial phase of adhesion of tumor cells to platelets under flow.[56] Tumor cells lacking P-selectin-mediated adhesion bind poorly to platelets under flow, despite extensive binding under static conditions.[57] P-selectin receptors have been demonstrated in some tumor-cell lines;[58,59] mucin-type glycoprotein, characteristic of many carcinomas, has been shown to act as P-selectin ligand;[59] and decreased tumor growth and metastasis has been shown in P-selectin-deficient mice.[60]

Effect of thrombin on platelet–tumor cell interaction and experimental pulmonary metastasis in vivo

Tumors may activate platelets via several mediators, such as adenosine diphosphate (ADP), but thrombin, the most potent physiological activator of platelets, is probably the most important among them. Tumor cells cause thrombin generation by producing tumor-associated tissue factor (TF), which is not usually expressed on normal epithelial cells and may be further upregulated in hypoxic states, such as within tumor tissue.[61] Thrombin activates platelets, leading to overexpression of GP IIb/IIIa, vWF, P-selectin and other adhesive molecules, such as fibronectin (Fn). Therefore, it is not surprising that thrombin-pretreated platelets enhance the adhesion of tumor cells to them.[55] However, thrombin treatment of tumor cells (human colon carcinoma, murine melanoma, and several other cell lines) also increases platelet–tumor cell adhesion.[62,63] Several melanoma cell lines show enhanced binding to platelets and to the adhesive ligands Fn and vWF by a 'GP IIb/IIIa-like' receptor.[64,65] The presence of and the requirement for thrombin-enhanced binding to platelets[66] and pulmonary metastasis[67] of protease-activated thrombin receptor (PAR-1) have been shown recently.

Thrombin enhances not only in vitro binding of tumor cells to platelets, but also in vivo experimental pulmonary metastasis: both injecting thrombin (at a dose not reducing the platelet count) together with tumor cells and pretreatment of tumor cells with thrombin caused a dramatic increase in pulmonary metastasis.[62]

The effect of thrombin on experimental pulmonary metastasis of tumor cells is not limited to the enhancement of platelet–tumor cell adhesion. Thrombin-activated tumor cells enhance their adhesion to endothelial cells.[68] Activation of PAR-1 by thrombin PAR-1 activation peptide (TRAP) in at least two cell lines (melanoma and colon carcinoma) increases pulmonary metastasis despite having no effect of enhancing adhesion to platelets.[66] Activation of PAR-1 was also shown to promote cell growth in NIH3T3 cells[69] and cell invasion in breast cancer in an experimental model.[70]

Other platelet–tumor interactions

Several additional mechanisms involving platelet–tumor cell interaction promote the malignant process.

Platelets adhering to tumor cells entering the circulation may prolong otherwise very short tumor-cell survival in the blood vessels,[71] possibly by protecting the tumor cells from lysis by natural killer cells.[72] Platelet–tumor cell emboli (which may also contain leukocytes) induce downstream ischemic endothelial damage, which exposes the subendothelial matrix rich in adhesive molecules (that is, Fn, Vn, Ln, vWF, and TSP) for binding of mutually activated tumor cells and platelets.[73]

Platelets contain, and activated platelets release, growth factors involved in tumor growth and metastasis. Platelet-derived growth factor (PDGF) was shown to support certain tumors' (Ewing sarcoma and brain tumors) growth and metastasis.[74,75] Platelets may also serve as a source of VEGF,[76] one of the most potent known factors supporting angiogenesis, which is essential for tumor growth and development. The expression of VEGF has been recently linked to adverse prognosis in certain cancers (such as, gastrointestinal and non-small-cell lung) and has even been shown to be a marker of success in chemotherapy for metastatic cancer.[77–79] VEGF also causes increase of vascular-wall permeability,[80] possibly facilitating tumor-cell migration.

Anticancer and antimetastatic therapy based on principles of platelet–tumor interaction: is it a real option?

Since a convincing amount of experimental and clinical data confirm the hypothesis that interaction between tumor cells and platelets supports the dissemination and growth of metastasizing malignant cells, it seems reasonable to look for anticancer and antimetastatic therapy targeting one or more of the mechanisms involved.

Aspirin and related compounds

Clinical evidence of a protective role of aspirin against the risk of colorectal cancer has been building up since the end of the 1980s, with numerous epidemiological (case–control and cohort) studies indicating that long-term use of aspirin is associated with a reduced risk (relative risk of 0.71–0.84) of colorectal cancer.[81] Recently, two large randomized studies, using the recurrence rate of precancerous colon adenomas as a surrogate (for cancer) endpoint, showed a protective effect of aspirin in patients with previous adenomas[82] and previous history of colon cancer.[83] Despite the clearly protective effect of aspirin, adenomas developed in some patients in the aspirin group. For that reason, aspirin cannot be viewed as a replacement for surveillance colonoscopy. In fact, a cost-effectiveness estimate of aspirin chemoprevention suggested its inferiority to surveillance colonoscopy as a prevention policy for colon cancer.[84]

More scanty and mostly epidemiological positive data in the same direction exist for other common cancers, such as breast,[85] stomach and esophagus,[81,86] lung (especially in tobacco users),[87,88] and pancreas.[89] Some controversy exists, since some studies showed no protective effect in the tumors analyzed, such as in ovarian carcinoma and even in otherwise well-established colon cancer in a population-based study.[90]

Aspirin inhibits platelet aggregation by inhibiting cyclooxygenase (COX), which is also overexpressed in a large number of human cancers and cancer-cell lines.[91] The understanding of the mechanisms of this protective effect of aspirin is incomplete, and it may not be platelet-dependent only, and may even not be COX-dependent, despite the overexpression of COX in tumors,[91] which may be associated with poor prognosis.[92] Several other pathways, each providing a partial explanation for the effect, have been demonstrated. Some of them are possibly related to tumor-cell proliferation, differentiation, and apoptosis: aspirin induces differentiation in murine erythroleukemia cells,[93] inhibits proliferation, and promotes apoptosis (probably downregulating *BCL2* expression) in a human colon cancer-cell line.[94]

Other pathways may decrease the metastatic potential: aspirin inhibits proliferation of vascular smooth muscle cells by involving transforming growth factor β (TGF-β) (an antiangiogenesis activity)[95] and inhibits hepatocyte growth factor (HGF)-induced invasiveness of HepG2 human hepatoma cells through ERK (extracellular signal-regulated kinase)1/2.[96]

Finally, aspirin and related compounds may increase host immune anticancer function: a selective COX-2 inhibitor, rofecoxib, contributes to the restoration of monocyte function in cancer patients.[97]

Heparin and thrombin inhibitors

Since thrombosis is associated with cancer and requires curative and preventive treatment, numerous studies using heparin—both low-molecular-weight (LMWH) and unfractionated (UFH)—exist. Using meta-analysis, many of them suggest a survival advantage for patients treated with LMWH not explained by the differences in fatal pulmonary embolism.[98,99] A controlled study specifically designed to analyze the antitumor effect of heparin (382 patients with advanced cancer and no thrombotic complications) showed no effect on early mortality, but the late (17-month) mortality rate was decreased, suggesting a so-far unexplained long-term anticancer effect of LMWH.[100] Recently, selected cancers have been shown to respond to a thrombin inhibitor, hirudin.[101] Anti-tissue factor antibodies show an antimetastatic activity in an animal model, but no clinical data are currently available.[102]

Whether the anticancer effect of heparin and antithrombins is induced in part by affecting platelet-related mechanisms is currently unknown, but several observations suggest this possibility. It is clear that heparin inhibits the generation of thrombin, a major factor in platelet–cancer cell interaction (see above). In addition, heparin blocks P-selectin-mediated interactions of endogenous platelets with sialylated fucosylated mucins on circulating carcinoma cells, interfering with P-selectin-mediated platelet coating of tumor cells during the initial phase of the metastatic process, and leading to a reduced tumor-cell survival and inhibition of metastasis.[103]

Novel therapeutic approaches targeting VEGF and other angiogenesis and mitogenesis platelet-associated molecules

It is a widely accepted axiom that formation of a new vascular network (neoangiogenesis) is essential for tumor growth and metastasis. Platelets interacting with tumor cells contain a large store of angiogenic and mitogenic factors (as described briefly above). Therefore, inhibiting angiogenesis is a potentially effective approach to cancer therapy, offering, at least theoretically, relative selectivity for tumors, since the endothelial cells of the new vascular networks in tumors are responding to angiogenic stimuli produced by the tumor, but are themselves genetically normal. Endothelium in normal tissue, by contrast, is usually quiescent.

Therefore, several classes of agents, recently reviewed by Shepherd and Sridhar,[104] target different steps and molecules involved in angiogenesis, VEGF and its receptor (VEFGR) being probably the most attractive among them. These include bevacizumab, a monoclonal anti-VEGF antibody, which has shown initial preclinical and clinical activity in colorectal cancer,[105] and several 'code-named' molecules, currently in early stages of clinical trials. Antisense oligonucleotides were shown to have in vitro activity.[106] Of interest is the inhibition of VEGF- and PDGF-mediated angiogenic and metastatic activity in experimental systems, as demonstrated with imatinib (STI-571), a novel BCR–ABL protein tyrosine kinase and Kit receptor tyrosine kinase inhibitor.[107] Other agents targeting molecules, such as matrix metalloproteinases, are also under investigation. No comparative clinical studies demonstrating a significant survival advantage for those agents are currently available.

Conclusions

The elucidation of the role of platelets in cancer started with the observation of a relationship between thrombosis and cancer, and has now evolved into an important area of cancer-associated basic and clinical research. Platelets may respond to the presence of cancer either by increasing their count (thrombocytosis) or by decreasing it (thrombocytopenia), both with important clinical implications. Platelets participate in tumor progression by contributing to the metastatic cascade, by generating and responding to thrombin, by protecting tumor cells from immune surveillance, and by regulating tumor invasion and angiogenesis. This wide range of cancer-promoting mechanisms provides an extensive area for targeted therapeutic interventions. Some of them, such as aspirin for cancer prevention and probably LMWH, are at the stage of proven clinical efficacy. Others, such as VEGF-targeting molecules, are currently under investigation. We hope that expanding the understanding of the complex process of platelet–cancer interaction will lead to further progress in developing novel effective and selective agents for better control of cancer growth and metastasis.

References

1. Sun NCJ, McAfee WM, Hum GJ et al. Hemostatic abnormalities in malignancy, a prospective study of 108 patients. Am J Clin Pathol 1979; **71**:10–16.

2. Rickles FR, Edwards RL. Activation of blood coagulation in cancer. Trousseau's syndrome revisited. Blood 1983; **62**:14–31.

3. Levin J, Conley CL. Thrombocytosis associated with malignant disease. Arch Intern Med 1964; **114**:497–500.

4. Harker LA, Finch CA. Thrombokinetics in man. J Clin Invest 1969; **48**:963–96.

5. Silvis SE, Turkbas N, Doscherholmen A. Thrombocytosis in patients with lung cancer. JAMA 1970; **211**:1852–5.

6. Tranum BL, Haut A. Thrombocytosis: platelet kinetics in neoplasia. J Lab Clin Med 1974; **84**:615–61.

7. Ginsburg AD. Platelet function in patients with high platelet counts. Ann Intern Med 1975; **82**:506–11.

8. Chahinian AP, Pajak TF, Holland JF et al. Diffuse malignant mesothelioma. Prospective evaluation of 69 patients. Ann Intern Med 1982; **96**:746–74 .

9. Leung LLK. Hemorrhagic disorders. In: Dale DC, Federman DD, eds. Scientific American Medicine. (WebMD: New York, 1999) Vol 2, 13:1–21.

10. Hollen CW, Henthorn J, Koziol JA et al. Elevated serum interleukin-6 levels in patients with reactive thrombocytosis. Br J Haematol 1991; **19**:286–290.

11. Kaser A, Brandacher G, Steuree W et al. Interleukin-6 stimulates thrombopoiesis through thrombopoietin: role in inflammatory thrombocytosis. Blood 2002; **98**:2720–5.

12. Komura E, Matsumura T, Kato T et al. Thrombopoietin in patients with hepatoblastoma. Stem Cells 1998; **16**:329–33.

13. Hsu HC, Tsai WH, Jiang ML et al. Circulating levels of thrombopoietic and inflammatory cytokines in patients with clonal and reactive thrombocytosis. J Lab Clin Med 1999; **134**:392–7.

14. Schwarz RE, Keny H. Preoperative platelet count predicts survival after resection of periampullary adenocarcinoma. Hepatogastroenterology 2001; **48**:1493–8.

15. Taucher S, Salat A, Gnant M et al. Impact of pretreatment thrombocytosis on survival in primary breast cancer. Thromb Haemost 2003; **89**:1098–1106.

16. Ikeda M, Furukawa H, Imamura H et al. Poor prognosis associated with thrombocytosis in patients with gastric cancer. Ann Surg Oncol 2002; **9**:287–91.

17. O'Keefe SC, Marshall FF, Issa MM et al. Thrombocytosis is associated with a significant increase in the cancer specific death rate after radical nephrectomy. J Urol 2002; **168**:1378–80.

18. Pedersen LM, Milman N. Diagnostic significance of platelet count and other blood analyses in patients with lung cancer. Oncol Rep 2003; **10**:213–6.

19. Kies MS, Kwaan HC. Thromboembolism in cancer patients. In: Kwaan MC, Bowie EJW, eds. Thrombosis. (WB Saunders: Philadelphia, 1982)176–7.

20. Hagedorn AB, Bowie EJW, Elveback LR et al. Coagulation abnormalities in patients with inoperable lung cancer. Mayo Clin Proc 1974; **49**:649–53.

21. Edwards RL, Rickles FR, Moritz TE et al. Abnormalities of blood coagulation tests in patients with cancer. Am J Clin Pathol 1987; **88**:596–602.

22. Bick RL. Disseminated intravascular coagulation: objective clinical and laboratory diagnosis, treatment, and assessment of therapeutic response. Semin Thromb Hemost 1996; **22**:69–88.

23. Nand S, Messmore H. Hemostasis in malignancy. Am J Hematol 1990; **35**:45–55.

24. Dvorak HF, Van De Water L, Bitzer AM et al. Procoagulant activity associated with plasma membrane vesicles shed by cultured tumor cells. Cancer Res 1983; **43**:4434–42.

25. Carr JM, McKinney M, McDonagh J. Diagnosis of disseminated intravascular coagulation: role of D-dimer. Am J Clin Pathol 1989; **91**:280–7.

26. Belt RJ, Leite C, Haas CD et al. Incidence of hemorrhagic complications in patients with cancer. JAMA 1978; **239**:2571–4.

27. Francis JL, Biggerstaff J, Amirkhosravi A. Hemostasis and malignancy. Semin Thromb Hemost 1998; **24**:93–109.

28. Schattner A, Klepfish A, Huszar M et al. Two patients with arterial thromboembolism among 311 patients with pancreatic cancer. Am J Med Sci 2002; **324**:335–8.

29. Papac RJ. Bone marrow metastases. A review. Cancer 1994; **74**:2403–13.

30. Rutherford CJ, Frenkel EP. Thrombocytopenia. Issues in diagnosis and therapy. Med Clin North Am 1994; **78**:555–76.

31. Chernow B, Wallner SF. Variables predictive of bone marrow metastasis. Cancer 1978; **42**:2373–8.

32. Wong KF, Chan JK, Ma SK. Solid tumors with initial presentation in the bone marrow—a clinicopathologic study of 25 adult cases. Hematol Oncol 1993; **11**:35–42.

33. Kim HD, Boggs DR. A syndrome resembling idiopathic thrombocytopenic purpura in 10 patients with diverse forms of cancer. Am J Med 1979; **67**:371–7.

34. Schwartz KA, Slichter SJ, Harker LA. Immune-mediated platelet destruction and thrombocytopenia in patients with solid tumours. Br J Haematol 1982; **51**:17–24.

35. Porrata LF, Alberts S, Hook C et al. Idiopathic thrombocytopenic purpura associated with breast cancer: a case report and review of the current literature. Am J Clin Oncol 1999; **22**:411–13.

36. Murphy WG, Allan NC, Perry DJ et al. Hodgkin's disease presenting as idiopathic thrombocytopenic purpura. Postgrad Med J 1984; **60**:614–15.

37. Bachmeyer C, Audouin J, Bouillot JL et al. Immune thrombocytopenic purpura as the presenting feature of gastric MALT lymphoma. Am J Gastroenterol 2000; **95**:1599–1600.

38. Kobayashi H, Kitano K, Ishida F et al. Aplastic anemia and idiopathic thrombocytopenic purpura with antibody to platelet glycoprotein IIb/IIIa following resection of malignant thymoma. Acta Haematol 1993; **90**:42–5.

39. Nobuoka A, Sakamaki S, Kogawa K et al. A case of malignant lymphoma producing autoantibody against platelet glycoprotein Ib. Int J Hematol 1999; **70**:200–6.

40. McMillan R. The pathogenesis of chronic immune (idiopathic) thrombocytopenic purpura. Semin Hematol 2000; **37**(Suppl 1):5–9.

41. Veenhoven WA, Thomas-van der Schans GS, Nieweg HO. Monoclonal immunoglobulins with affinity for platelets and their relationship to malignant lymphoma. Cancer 1982; **49**:40–2.

42. Lugassy G. Non-Hodgkin's lymphoma presenting with amegakaryocytic thrombocytopenic purpura. Ann Hematol 1996; **73**:41–2.

43. Lesesne JB, Rothschild N, Erickson B et al. Cancer-associated hemolytic–uremic syndrome: analysis of 85 cases from a national registry. J Clin Oncol 1989; **7**:781–9.

44. Kwaan HC, Gordon LI. Thrombotic microangiopathy in the cancer patient. Acta Hematol 2001; **106**:52–6.

45. Wu DC, Liu JM, Chen YM et al. Mitomycin-C induced hemolytic uremic syndrome: a case report and literature review. Jpn J Clin Oncol 1997; **27**:115–18.

46. Schriber JR, Herzig GP. Transplantation-associated TTP and HUS. Semin Hematol 1997; **34**:126–33.

47. Gordon LI, Kwaan HC. Thrombotic microangiopathy manifesting as thrombotic thrombocytopenic purpura/hemolytic uremic syndrome in the cancer patient. Semin Thromb Hemost 1999; **25**:217–21.

48. Tsai H-M, Chun-Yet Lian E. Antibodies to von Willebrand factor-cleaving protease in acute thrombotic thrombocytopenic purpura. N Engl J Med 1998; **339**:1585–94.

49. Snyder HW Jr, Mittelman A, Oral A et al. Treatment of cancer chemotherapy-associated thrombotic thrombocytopenic purpura/hemolytic uremic syndrome by protein A immunoadsorption of plasma. Cancer 1993; **71**:1882–92.

50. Gasic GJ, Gasic TB, Stewart CC. Antimetastatic effects associated with platelet reduction. Proc Natl Acad Sci USA 1968; **61**:46–52.

51. Karpatkin S, Pearlstein E, Ambrogio C et al. Role of adhesive proteins in platelet interaction in vitro and metastasis formation in vivo. J Clin Invest 1988; **81**: 1012–19.

52. Gasic GJ, Gasic TB, Galanti N et al. Platelet tumor cell interaction in mice. The role of platelets in the spread of malignant disease. Int J Cancer 1973; **11**:704–18.

53. Pearlstein E, Salk PL, Yogeeswaran G et al. Correlation between spontaneous metastatic potential, platelet aggregation activity of cell surface extracts, and cell surface sialylation in ten metastatic-variant derivatives of a rat renal carcinoma cell line. Proc Natl Acad Sci USA 1980; **77**:4336–9.

54. Karpatkin S, Ambrogio C, Pearlstein E. Lack of effect of PGI2 on the development of pulmonary metastases in mice following intravenous injection of CT26 colon carcinoma, Lewis lung carcinoma or B16 amelanotic melanoma cells. Cancer Res 1984; **44**:3880–3.

55. Nierodzik ML, Klepfish A, Karpatkin S. Role of platelet integrin GPIIb–GPIIIa, fibronectin, von Willebrand factor, and thrombin in platelet–tumor interaction in vitro and metastasis in vivo. Thromb Hemost 1995; **74**:282–90.

56. Dardic R, Savion N, Kaufmann Y et al. Thrombin promotes platelet-mediated melanoma cell adhesion to endothelial cells under flow conditions: role of platelet glycoproteins P-selectin and GPIIbIIIa. Br J Cancer 1998; **77**:2069–75.

57. McCarty OJT, Mousa SA, Bray PF et al. Immobilized platelets support human colon carcinoma cell tethering, rolling and firm adhesion under dynamic flow conditions. Blood 2000; **96**:1789–97.

58. Aigner S, Ramos CL, Hafezi-Moghadam A et al. CD24 mediates rolling of breast carcinoma cells on P-selectin. FASEB J 1998; **12**: 1241-51

59. Aigner S, Sthoeger Z, Fogel MEW et al. CD24, a mucine-type glyco-protein, is a ligand for P-selectin on human tumor cells. Blood 1997; **89**:3385-95

60. Kim YJ, Borsig L, Varki NM et al. P-selectin deficiency attenuates tumor growth and metastasis. Proc Natl Acad Sci USA 1998; **95**: 9325-30.

61. Falanga A, Ofosu FA, Delaini F et al. The hypercoagulable state in cancer patients: evidence for impaired thrombin inhibition. Blood Coagul Fibrinolysis 1994; **5**:19-23.

62. Nierodzik ML, Plotkin A, Kajumo F et al. Thrombin stimulates tumor-platelet adhesion in vitro and metastasis in vivo. J Clin Invest 1991; **87**:229-36.

63. Nierodzik ML, Kajumo F, Karpatkin S. Effect of thrombin treatment of tumor cells on adhesion of tumor cells to platelets in vitro and metas-tasis in vivo. Cancer Res 1992; **52**:3267-72.

64. Cheresh DA, Spiro RS. Biosynthetic and functional proper-ties of an arg-gly-asp-directed receptor involved in human melanoma cell attachment to vit-ronectin, fibrinogen and von Willebrand factor. J Biol Chem 1987; **262**:17703-11.

65. Trikha M, Timar J, Lundy SK et al. The high affinity alpha2-beta3 inte-grin is involved in invasion of human melanoma cells. Cancer Res 1997; **57**:2522-8.

66. Nierodzik ML, Bain MR, Liu L-X et al. Presence of seven transmem-brane domains thrombin receptor on human tumor cells: effect of activation on tumor adhesion to platelets and tumor tyrosine phos-phorylation. Br J Haematol 1996; **92**:452-7.

67. Nierodzik ML, Chen K, Takeshita K et al. Protease-activated receptor 1 (PAR-1) is required and rate-limiting for thrombin-enhanced experimen-tal pulmonary metastasis. Blood 1998; **92**:3694-700.

68. Klepfish A, Greco MA, Karpatkin S. Thrombin stimulates melanoma tumor cell binding to endothelial cells and subendothelial matrix. Int J Cancer 1993; **53**:978-82.

69. Martin CB, Mahon GM, Klinger MB et al. The thrombin receptor, PAR-1, causes transformation by activation of Rho-mediated signal-ing pathways. Oncogene 2001: **20**:1953-63.

70. Even-Ram S, Maoz M, Pokroy E et al. Tumor cell invasion is promoted by activation of protease activated receptor-1 in cooperation with the alphav-beta5 integrin. J Biol Chem 2001; **276**:10952-62.

71. Jones JD, Wallace AC, Fraser EF. Sequence of events in experimen-tal metastasis of Walker 256 tumor: light, immunofluorescent and elec-tron microscopic observations. J Natl Cancer Inst 1971; **46**: 493-504.

72. Nieswandt B, Hafner M, Echtenacher B et al. Lysis of tumor cells by natural killer cells in mice is impeded by platelets. Cancer Res 1999; **59**:1295-1300.

73. Warren BA. The microinjury hypoth-esis and metastasis. In: Honn KV, Sloane BF, eds. Hemostatic Mechanisms and Metastasis. (Nijhoff: Boston, MA, 1984)56.

74. Uren A, Merchant MS, Sun CJ et al. Beta-platelet-derived growth factor receptor mediates motility and growth of Ewing's sarcoma cells. Oncogene 2003; **22**: 2334-42.

75. Guo P, Hu B, Gu W et al. Platelet-derived growth factor-B enhances glioma angiogenesis by stimulating vascular endothelial growth factor expression in tumor endothelia and by promoting pericyte recruitment. Am J Pathol 2003; **162**:1083–93.

76. Mohle R, Green D, Moore MAS et al. Constitutive production and thrombin-induced release of VEGF by human megakaryocytes and platelets. Proc Natl Acad Sci USA 1997; **94**:663–8.

77. Chim KF, Greenman J, Reusch P et al. Vascular endothelial growth factor and soluble Tie-2 receptor in colorectal cancer: association with disease recurrence. Eur J Surg Oncol 2003; **29**:497–505.

78. Li Q, Dong X, Gu W et al. Clinical significance of co-expression of VEGF-C and VEGFR-3 in non-small cell lung cancer. Chin Med J (Engl) 2003; **116**:727–30.

79. Lissoni P, Rovelli F, Malugani F et al. Changes in circulating VEGF levels in relation to clinical response during chemotherapy for metastatic cancer. Int J Biol Markers 2003; **18**:152–5.

80. Bates DO, Harper SJ. Regulation of vascular permeability by vascular endothelial growth factors. Vascul Pharmacol 2002; **39**:225–37.

81. Bosetti C, Gallus S, La Vecchia C. Aspirin and cancer risk: an update to 2001. Eur J Cancer Prev 2002; **11**:535–42.

82. Baron JA, Cole BF, Sandler RS et al. A randomized trial of aspirin to prevent colorectal adenomas. N Engl J Med 2003; **348**:891–9.

83. Sandler RS, Halabi S, Baron JA et al. A randomized trial of aspirin to prevent colorectal adenomas in patients with previous colorectal cancer. N Engl J Med 2003; **348**:883–90.

84. Suleiman S, Rex DK, Sonnenberg A. Chemoprevention of colorectal cancer by aspirin: a cost-effectiveness analysis. Gastroenterology 2002; **122**:230–3

85. Johnson TW, Anderson KE, Lozovich D et al. Association of aspirin and non-steroidal anti-inflammatory drug use with breast cancer. Cancer Epidemiol Biomark Prev 2002; **11**:1586–91.

86. Corley DA, Kerlikowske K, Verma R et al. Protective association of aspirin/NSAIDs and esophageal cancer: a systematic review and meta-analysis. Gastroenterology 2003; **124**:246–8.

87. Moysich KB, Menezes RJ, Ronsani A et al. Regular aspirin use and lung cancer risk. BMC Cancer 2002; **2**:31.

88. Harris RE, Beebe-Donk J, Schuller HM. Chemoprevention of lung cancer by non-steroidal anti-inflammatory drugs among cigarette smokers. Oncol Rep 2002; **9**:693–5.

89. Anderson KE, Johnson TW, Lozovich D et al. Association between nonsteroidal anti-inflammatory drug use and the incidence of pancreatic cancer. J Natl Cancer Inst 2002; **94**:1168–71.

90. Friis S, Sorensen HT, McLaughlin JK et al. A population-based cohort study of the risk of colorectal and other cancers among users of low-dose aspirin. Br J Cancer 2003; **88**:684–8.

91. Hussain T, Gupta S, Mukhtar H. Cyclooxygenase-2 and prostate carcinogenesis. Cancer Lett 2003; **191**:125–35.

92. Lim SC. Role of COX-2, VEGF and cyclin D1 in mammary infiltrating duct carcinoma. Oncol Rep 2003; **10**:1241–9.

93. Ebisuzaki K. Aspirin and methysulfonylmethane (MSM): a search for common mechanisms, with implications for cancer prevention. Anticancer Res 2003; **23**:453–8.

94. Yu HG, Huang JA, Yang YN et al. The effects of acetylsalicylic acid on

proliferation, apoptosis, and invasion of cyclooxygenase-2-negative colon cancer cells. Eur J Clin Invest 2002; **32**:793–4.

95. Redondo S, Santos-Gallego CG, Ganado P et al. Acetylsalicylic acid inhibits cell proliferation by involving transforming growth factor-beta. Circulation 2003; **107**:626–9.

96. Abiru S, Nakao K, Ichikawa T et al. Aspirin and NS 398 inhibit hepatocyte growth factor-induced invasiveness of human hepatoma cells. Hepatology 2002; **35**: 1117–24.

97. Lang S, Lauffer L, Clausen C et al. Impaired monocyte function in cancer patients: restoration with cyclooxygenase-2 inhibitor. FASEB J 2003; **17**:286–8.

98. Siragusa S, Cosmi B, Piovella F et al. Low-molecular-weight heparins and unfractionated heparin in the treatment of patients with acute venous thromboembolism: results of meta-analysis. Am J Med 1996; **100**:269–77.

99. Hettiarachchi RJ, Smorenburg SM, Ginsberg J et al. Do heparins do more than just treat thrombosis? The influence of heparins on cancer spread. Thromb Haemost 1999; **82**:947–52.

100. Kakkar AK, Kadziola Z, Williamson RCN et al. Low molecular heparin therapy and survival in advanced cancer. Blood 2002; **100**: 557 (abst).

101. Walz DA, Fenton JW. The role of thrombin in tumor cell metastasis. Invasion Metastasis 1994–95; **14**: 303–8.

102. Francis JL, Amirkhosravi A. Effect of antihemostatic agents on experimental tumor dissemination. Semin Thromb Hemost 2002; **28**:29–38.

103. Varki NM, Varki A. Heparin inhibition of selectin-mediated interactions during the hematogenous phase of carcinoma metastasis: rationale for clinical studies in humans. Semin Thromb Hemost 2002; **28**:53–66.

104. Shepherd FA, Sridhar SS. Angiogenesis inhibitors under study for the treatment of lung cancer. Lung Cancer 2003; **41**(Suppl 1): S63–72.

105. Fernando NH, Hurwitz HI. Inhibition of vascular endothelial growth factor in the treatment of colorectal cancer. Semin Oncol 2003; **30**(3 Suppl 6):39–50.

106. Smyth AP, Rook SL, Detmar M et al. Antisense oligonucleotides inhibit vascular endothelial growth factor/vascular permeability factor expression in normal human epidermal keratinocytes. J Invest Dermatol 1997; **108**:523–6.

107. Buchdunger E, O'Reilly T, Wood G. Pharmacology of imatinib (STI571). Eur J Cancer 2002; **38**(Suppl 5): S28–36.

4

The role of blood clotting in tumor metastasis: A case for tissue factor

Maria Benedetta Donati and Roberto Lorenzet

Introduction

The association between human cancer and the clotting system has been recognized for more than a century, even if many aspects of this interaction still await clarification. This association has been evaluated from two viewpoints and with a dual meaning: on one hand, significant hemostatic abnormalities and thrombotic and hemorragic complications have been observed in cancer patients; hemostatic complications are indeed a common cause of death in cancer patients; among the underlying mechanisms, many tumor cells possess strong procoagulant activities that promote the local activation of the coagulation system (for a review, see Donati and Falanga[1]); on the other hand, tumor-mediated activation of the coagulation cascade has been implicated in both the formation of tumor stroma and the promotion of hematogenous metastases.

Most solid tumors contain fibrinogen-derived material, which is important in the formation of tumor stroma, since fibrin matrices promote the migration of several cell types (transformed cells, macrophages, and fibroblasts).[2,3] Moreover, in hematogenous metastasis, activation of the coagulation system has been implicated, since, following entry into the circulation, tumor cells must be arrested in the microvasculature of a target organ prior to metastasis growth. The formation of platelet/ fibrin/tumor cell aggregates may be causally related to endothelial adhesion and metastatic potential (for a review, see Donati and Evangelista[4]); from studies in experimental models, it can be concluded that, whatever modality is applied to reduce the clotting potential of the host (acting on fibrinogen itself, or blocking thrombin generation or platelet activation), intravenously injected tumor cells will be kept longer in circulation and will then be more susceptible to destruction by the reticuloendothelial system.[5] In this review, we shall focus on the role of the coagulation system in tumor metastases with special emphasis, on a pivotal system of clotting activation, the tissue factor:factor VII complex.

The blood-clotting scheme and cancer procoagulants

The ultimate function of the coagulation pathway is the conversion of soluble circulating fibrinogen to insoluble fibrin. Tissue factor (TF), a 47-kDa membrane glycoprotein closely associated with phospholipids, is the in vivo trigger of this pathway. The TF molecule consists of three domains: a 21-residue intracellular region, a single, 23-residue trans-membrane domain, and a 219-residue extracellular domain. The latter functions as receptor and cofactor for coagulation factor VII (FVII) and its active form FVIIa.[6] The resulting TF:FVIIa complex activates factors IX and X, which are then responsible for the generation of thrombin, which, in turn, cleaves fibrinogen to fibrin.[7] An oversimplified scheme of the clotting cascade is reported in Figure 4.1. Since the activation process is remarkably fast, TF segregation from cells in direct contact with the bloodstream has to be constantly ensured. Accordingly, immunohisto-

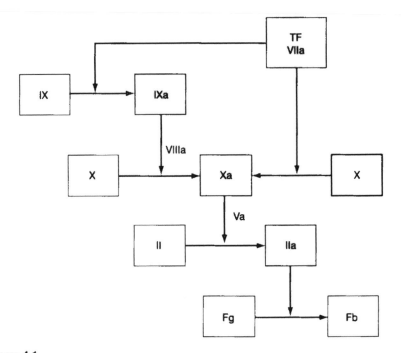

Figure 4.1

Oversimplified scheme of the blood-clotting cascade, underlying the central role of the tissue factor/factor VII complex. The grey squares represents enzymatically active molecules.

chemical studies have localized TF in capsules surrounding organs, in cells of epithelial surfaces, and, more generally, at tissue barriers between the body and the environment.[8] This pattern is consistent with the hypothesis that TF can be considered as a 'hemostatic envelope', whose function is to minimize blood loss following vessel damage.

Although monocytes and endothelial cells under normal conditions do not express TF antigen or activity, these cells, upon appropriate stimulation, can be induced to synthesize and express TF on their membranes. The number of relevant agents for TF synthesis in endothelial cells and monocytes is constantly increasing.[9]

TF gene expression is regulated mainly at the level of transcription.[10] The presence of regulatory elements, putative binding sites for various transcription factors in the promoter region of human TF, has been identified. In unstimulated monocytes and endothelial cells, c-Rel/p65 heterodimers, components of the NFκB transacting factor family, are retained in the cytoplasm by the binding of the inhibitor IκBα. When these cells are exposed to lipopolysaccharide (LPS) or inflammatory cytokines, IκBα is phosphorylated and degraded, and c-Rel/p65 heterodimers migrate to the nucleus, where they bind to the κB site in the TF promoter, inducing TF gene transcriptional activation.[11] This mechanism is schematically represented in Figure 4.2. Agents known to modulate TF expression in these cells exert their action through this pathway.[12,13]

Unlike endothelial cells and monocytes, tumor cells express intrinsic procoagulant properties without the need for exposure to any inducing agent. Since the first observation that cancer tissues shorten the clotting time of normal recalcified plasma,[14] further investigations have characterized the different procoagulant activity of various tumor cells. The main procoagulant activity of a wide variety of tumor cells has been ascribed to TF associated with cell membranes.[15] Notably, tumor cells could shed TF-rich plasma membrane vesicles, thus contributing, during hematogenous dissemination, to the well-known tumor-associated thrombophilia.

In addition to tumor cells, TF may also be expressed in malignancy by tumor-infiltrating and circulating monocytes. We have shown that both circulating monocytes and tumor-associated macrophages from the V2 rabbit carcinoma express higher TF activity than those from control animals.[16] Moreover, both peripheral blood monocytes cultured from cancer patients and tumor-associated macrophages harvested from some experimental tumors express markedly increased amounts of TF.[17,18]

Studies in malignant tumors have shown that tumor cells may also express a FVII-independent procoagulant activity. This molecule, named cancer procoagulant (CP), is a cysteine proteinase with direct FX-activating activity that is expressed by some experimental and

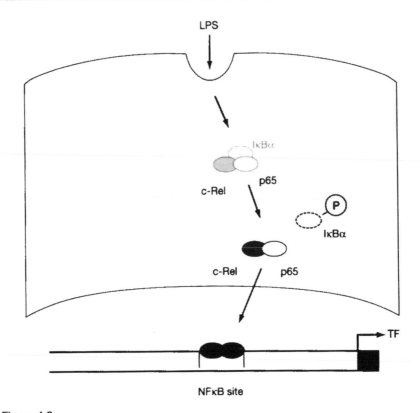

Figure 4.2

Schematic overview of events occurring at the level of the LPS response element of the TF gene promoter, following stimulation with one of the classical inducers, LPS. Binding of LPS to its receptor on the cell membrane leads to IκBα phosphorylation and proteolysis. The released c-Rel/p65 complex translocates to the nucleus and binds the NF κB-like site, causing transcription of TF mRNA.

human tumor cells.[19,20] CP is confined to the malignant phenotype and, in murine tumors, is associated with the metastatic potential of tumor cells. CP appears to be a novel vitamin K-dependent activity, since, both in murine and in human tumors, it is depressed by treatment with warfarin or a vitamin K-deficient diet.[21,22]

Increased CP levels have been reported in different types of advanced solid tumors and in acute promyelocytic leukemia, where they correlate with the stage of the disease and the response to chemotherapy.[23–25] Antibodies to CP also block the metastatic seeding of lung colonies in vivo and decrease the viability of tumor cells in vitro.[26]

Less studied, but of potential importance in tumor procoagulant activity, is the cell-surface trypsin-like protease hepsin. This molecule, which is capable of activating FVII, has been found to be overexpressed in several tumors, and has been proposed as a candidate in the invasive process of tumor cells.[27]

TF and tumor metastasis

Metastasis is a multifactorial process, and intravascular activation of coagulation has long been proposed to be one of the key factors favoring metastatization. Numerous attempts have been made to correlate the procoagulant activity of tumor cells, and particularly TF, with the metastatic process.

Several years ago, assuming that cancer-cell procoagulant activity could influence metastasis formation by promoting fibrin deposition around tumors, we studied the procoagulant activity of various tumor-cell sublines with different metastatic capacity derived from a murine fibrosarcoma.[28] Although all the cells tested expressed a TF-like activity, the cells with the highest metastatic potential were those whose TF expression was lower, suggesting a possible role of tumor-cell TF at the site of the primary tumor in promoting fibrin deposition and lower cell escape into the blood circulation. Later, in a study performed on 85 different tumor specimens with an anti-TF IgG antibody for immunohistochemical localization of TF antigen, TF expression did not appear to correlate with malignant transformation in the majority of specimens of solid tumors.[29] The authors concluded that the presence or absence of TF antigen in a tumor cannot absolutely define the risk of thrombosis.

However, evidence for a role of TF in the metastatic process has repeatedly been proposed and is supported by an increasing number of studies. Constitutive TF expression is reported as a characteristic feature of numerous malignant tumors. Kataoka et al, examining human colorectal carcinoma cell lines, found higher cellular TF activity in the metastatic sublines than in the parent line.[30] Later, Shigemori et al detected TF in the tumors of 57% of colorectal cancer patients, and its expression significantly increased to 88% in metastatic tumors.[31] Similarly, TF expression was reported to be a significant and independent risk factor for hepatic metastasis in human colorectal carcinoma.[32] Cells from non-small-cell lung-cancer patients with metastasis stain stronger for TF than those from patients with no metastasis.[33] Highly metastatic human melanoma cells express TF levels 1000 times higher than nonmetastatic melanoma cells.[34] In breast cancer, expression of TF in tumor stroma correlates with progression to invasive cancer,[35] and tumor TF expression was proposed as an independent prognostic indicator for overall survival.[36] In addition, expression of TF in glioma cell lines and glioma surgical specimens correlates with the histological grade of malignancy.[37] Finally, transfection of a TF-expressing vector in a human pancreatic adenocarcinoma cell line enhanced in vitro invasion and primary tumor growth in immunodeficient mice.[38]

Mechanisms of tumor metastasis modulation by TF

Binding of FVIIa to TF mediates cell signaling and induces gene expression, an effect which may be important in various cellular processes other than triggering blood coagulation;[39] therefore, the role of procoagulant activity in the metastatic enhancement by TF has been extensively debated. A selective inhibition of the procoagulant activity of TF by treatment of severe combined immunodeficient (SCID) mice with anti-TF monoclonal antibodies abolished prolonged adherence of metastatic melanoma cells in the vasculature and inhibited pulmonary metastasis.[40] Similarly, blocking the coagulation pathway at the level of TF, FXa, or thrombin inhibited hematogenous M24met metastasis in SCID mice,[41] and desulfatohirudin, a highly specific thrombin inhibitor, reduced murine melanoma experimental metastasis,[42] suggesting a role for one or more products of the coagulation cascade in the metastatic process. In addition, an emerging role for TF pathway inhibitor (TFPI) as an antimetastatic agent is presently being discussed.[43] More generally, metastasis inhibition by anticoagulant treatments stresses the importance of clotting activation in the invasive process.

The influence of TF on the metastatic process may, however, be more complex. Bromberg et al tested the metastatic potential of melanoma cell lines transfected by mutants in either the extracellular or cytoplasmic domains of the transmembrane TF molecule in a SCID mouse model.[44] A two-amino-acid substitution in the extracellular mutation downregulated the procoagulant activity of TF. Only mice injected with this mutant, and not those injected with the cytoplasmic domain mutant, developed metastasis, indicating that, at least in this experimental model, products of the coagulation pathway were not involved in the metastatic effect of TF. Using TF cDNA constructs in Chinese hamster ovary cells and injecting them in SCID mice, Mueller and Ruf demonstrated that TF supports metastasis by both undefined functions of the cytoplasmic domain and the proteolytic activity of the TF:FVIIa complex.[45] In a similar way, by site-specific mutagenesis, it was shown that, for the full metastatic effect of TF, phosphorylation of the cytoplasmic domain and formation of a complex with FVIIa by the extracellular domain are required.[46] The role of the cytoplasmic domain of TF was further studied by Ott et al, who, by means of a yeast two-hybrid system, identified an intracellular protein, actin-binding protein 280 (filamin 1), as ligand for the TF cytoplasmic domain.[47] The interaction with filamin 1, a cytoskeletal component, was enhanced by a Ser-to-Asp substitution, which mimics phosphorylation, in the TF domain, and abolished with Ala mutations, reducing cell spreading. These findings provide a molecular pathway in which, through alterations in the tumor-cell cytoskeleton, the TF cytoplasmic domain supports cell migration and adhesion.

TF, protease-activated receptors (PAR), and tumor metastasis

Since recent studies suggest that TF:FVIIa can activate the protease-activated receptors (PAR)-1 and -2 directly, as well as an unidentified PAR,[48] several attempts to investigate the involvement of PARs in the metastatic process were carried out. Bromberg et al[49] studied a human melanoma cell line, SIT1, with low metastatic potential, low endogenous levels of TF, and negligible levels of PARs. Transfection of this line with human cDNA resulted in an increase in the metastatic potential of the cells that was not accompanied by enhanced levels of PARs. However, PAR-1, whose overexpression is insufficient to induce metastasis in cells with low TF expression, enhanced the metastatic potential of cells with high TF expression. A possible synergy between TF and PAR-1 in promoting metastasis was suggested. A direct role of PAR-1 in the pathological process of breast cancer has also been proposed: PAR-1 has been shown to be preferentially expressed in highly metastatic human breast-carcinoma cell lines and breast-carcinoma biopsy specimens.[50] A PAR-1 antisense cDNA markedly limited the invasion of the metastatic cells in culture.

Unexpectedly, Kamath et al reported that activation of PAR-1 with thrombin markedly inhibited invasion and migration of the highly invasive and highly PAR-1-expressing MDAMB231 breast-cancer cell line.[51] Since PAR-1, the thrombin G-protein coupled receptor, has been proposed also as a target of the TF:FVIIa complex,[48] the role of the latter remains to be elucidated.

TF and angiogenesis

Angiogenesis is a multifactorial process of de novo vessel formation required for invasive tumor growth and metastasis. In 1996, Carmeliet et al reported a markedly defective vessel formation of yolk-sac vessels in TF knockout mice embryos followed by massive hemorrhaging of embryonic blood, thus suggesting a role of TF in fetal angiogenesis.[52] Abnormal vascular development in the yolk sac of TF-null mouse embryos could be rescued by human TF lacking the cytoplasmic domain, suggesting that embryogenesis requires the extracellular protease activity of the TF:VIIa complex.[53] In 1994, Zhang et al transfected Meth-A sarcoma cells to overexpress or underexpress TF.[54] In vivo, cells overexpressing TF grew more rapidly and formed larger and more vascularized tumor than control cells. In addition, cells overexpressing TF released more mitogenic activity for endothelial cells in parallel with enhanced transcription of vascular endothelial cell growth factor (VEGF), and diminished transcription of the antiangiogenic molecule thrombospondin-2, indicating that the capability of the tumor to induce a supporting neovasculature is dependent upon TF expression by tumor cells. Anticoagulation of the experimental animals with warfarin or pretreatment of the cells with hirudin had comparable results, suggesting that coagulation was not involved.

A positive correlation between angiogenesis and levels of TF expression was found in human prostate carcinoma[55] and in non-small-cell lung carcinoma.[56] TF and VEGF were found to colocalize in human tumor cells from patients with breast cancer,[57] lung cancer,[58] and non-small-cell lung carcinoma.[56] Later, Abe et al reported a significant correlation between TF and VEGF in 13 human malignant melanoma cell lines.[59] By means of transfection of a full-length TF, an extracellular domain mutant with diminished function for activation of FX, or a cytoplasmic deletion mutant in a low TF and VEGF cell-line producer, they showed that the full-length transfectant produced increased levels of TF and VEGF, that the extracellular mutant transfectant induced the same levels of VEGF mRNA, and that the cytoplamic mutant transfectant induced TF, but not VEGF, indicating that the cytoplasmic domain is the one which plays a role, and that FVIIa/FX interactions are not required. Different findings showing that FVIIa leads to VEGF synthesis in TF-expressing human lung fibroblasts, and that this effect is mostly dependent on the proteolytic activity of the TF:FVIIa complex, were later reported by others.[60]

In 1990, Clauss et al observed induction of monocyte and endothelial cell TF by Meth-A-derived VEGF.[61] A logical speculation would be that VEGF produced by tumor cells could be responsible for the TF expression of tumor-associated endothelial cells found by Contrino et al.[57] From different pieces of evidence, it can be concluded that the effects of TF expression on angiogenetic processes may further contribute to the complex TF modulation of tumor metastasis.

Conclusions

Both intravascular and cell-mediated activation of clotting promote cancer metastasis and growth, as documented in experimental models and some clinical studies. Tumor-cell procoagulant activities have been extensively investigated in this context. The expression of TF, the principal cellular activator of the coagulation cascade, can be considered a hallmark of cancer progression.

The procoagulant functions of TF that lead to thrombin generation are critically important to support metastasis, in part through the generation of fibrin, which allows prolonged arrest of tumor cells in target organs. In addition, the coagulation initiation complex, that is, TF:FVIIa, generates autocrine cell signaling through protease-activated receptors. Cooperation of the TF cytoplasmic domain with protease signaling may explain the different contributions of TF to metastasis and angiogenesis.

The pieces of evidence collected in this survey may offer a rational basis to test currently developed inhibitors of TF in a combined modality approach to control tumor metastasis.

Acknowledgments

Part of the authors' work reviewed in this survey was supported by the Italian Ministry of Health (ICS 120.4/RF99.11, ISS Convenzione N: 1AI/F3).

References

1. Donati MB, Falanga A. Pathogenetic mechanisms of thrombosis in malignancy. Acta Haematol 2001; **106**:18–24.

2. Costantini V, Zacharski LR. Fibrin and cancer. Thromb Haemost 1993; **69**:406–14.

3. Dejana E, Languino LR, Polentarutti N et al. Interaction between fibrinogen and cultured endothelial cells. Induction of migration and specific binding. J Clin Invest 1985; **75**:11–18.

4. Donati MB, Evangelista V. Platelets and tumor. In: Gresele P, Page CP, Fuster V et al, eds. Platelets in Thrombotic and Non-thrombotic Disorders. (Cambridge University Press: Cambridge, 2002)824–36.

5. Donati MB. Cancer and thrombosis: from phlegmasia alba dolens to transgenic mice. Thromb Haemost 1995; **74**:278–81.

6. Nemerson Y. Tissue factor and hemostasis. Blood 1988; **71**:1–8.

7. Østerud B, Rapaport SI. Activation of factor IX by the reaction product of tissue factor and factor VII: additional pathway for initiating blood coagulation. Proc Natl Acad Sci USA 1977; **74**:5260–4.

8. Drake TA, Morrissey JH, Edgington TS. Selective cellular expression of tissue factor in human tissues. Implications for disorders of hemostasis and thrombosis. Am J Pathol 1989; **134**:1087–97.

9. Lorenzet R, Napoleone E, Celi A et al. Cell–cell interaction and tissue factor expression. Blood Coagul Fibrinolysis 1998; **9**(Suppl 1): S49–59.

10. Edgington TS, Mackman N, Brand K et al. The structural biology of expression and function of tissue factor. Thromb Haemost 1991; **66**:67–79.

11. Oeth P, Parry GCN, Mackman N. Regulation of the tissue factor gene in human monocytic cells. Role of AP-1, NF-kB/Rel, and Sp1 proteins in uninduced and lipopolysaccharide-induced expression. Arterioscler Thromb Vasc Biol 1997; **17**:365–74.

12. Napoleone E, Di Santo A, Camera M et al. Angiotensin-converting enzyme inhibitors downregulate tissue factor synthesis in monocytes. Circ Res 2000; **86**:139–43.

13. Napoleone E, Di Santo A, Bastone A et al. The long pentraxin PTX3 upregulates tissue factor expression in human endothelial cells: a novel link between vascular inflammation and clotting activation. Arterioscl Thromb Vasc Biol 2002; **22**:782–7.

14. O'Meara RAQ. Coagulative properties of cancers. Ir J Med Sci 1958; **394**:474–9.

15. Dvorak HF, Van DeWater L, Bitzer AM et al. Procoagulant activity associated with plasma membrane vesicles shed by cultured tumor cells. Cancer Res 1983; **43**:4434–42.

16. Lorenzet R, Peri G, Locati D et al. Generation of procoagulant activity by mononuclear phagocytes: a possible mechanism contributing to blood clotting activation within malignant tissues. Blood 1983; **62**:271–3.

17. Morgan D, Edwards RL, Rickles FR. Monocyte procoagulant activity as a peripheral marker of clotting activation in cancer patients. Haemostasis 1988; **18**:55–65.

18. Semeraro N, Colucci M. Tissue factor in health and disease. Thromb Haemost 1997; **78**:759–64.

19. Falanga A, Alessio MG, Donati MB, et al. A new procoagulant in acute leukemia. Blood 1988; **71**: 870–5.

20. Falanga A, Gordon SG. Isolation and characterization of cancer procoagulant: a cysteine proteinase from malignant tissue. Biochemistry 1985; **24**:5558–67.

21. Colucci M, Delaini F, De Bellis Vitti G et al. Warfarin inhibits both procoagulant activity and metastatic capacity of Lewis lung carcinoma cells. Role of vitamin K deficiency. Biochem Pharmacol 1983; **32**:1689–91.

22. Roncaglioni MC, D'Alessandro AP, Casali B et al. Gamma-glutamyl carboxylase activity in experimental tumor tissues: a biochemical basis for vitamin K dependence of cancer procoagulant. Haemostasis 1986; **16**:235–9.

23. Donati MB, Falanga A, Consonni R et al. Cancer procoagulant in acute non-lymphoid leukemia: relationship of enzyme detection to disease activity. Thromb Haemost 1990; **64**:11–16.

24. Barbui T, Finazzi G, Falanga A. The impact of all-*trans*-retinoic acid on the coagulopathy of acute promyelocytic leukemia. Blood 1998; **91**:3093–102.

25. Donati MB, Gambacorti Passerini C, Casali B et al. Cancer procoagulant in human tumor cells: evidence from melanoma patients. Cancer Res 1986; **46**:6471–4.

26. Gordon SG, Mielicki WP. Cancer procoagulant: a factor X activator, tumor marker and growth factor from malignant tissue. Blood Coagul Fibrinolysis 1997; **8**:73–86.

27. Sampson MT, Kakkar AK. Coagulation proteases and human cancer. Biochem Soc Trans 2002; **30**:201–7.

28. Colucci M, Giavazzi R, Alessandri G et al. Procoagulant activity of sarcoma sublines with different metastatic potential. Blood 1981; **57**:733–5.

29. Callander NS, Varki N, Rao LV. Immunohistochemical identification of tissue factor in solid tumors. Cancer 1992; **70**:1194–1201.

30. Kataoka H, Uchino H, Asada Y et al. Analysis of tissue factor and tissue factor pathway inhibitor expression in human colorectal carcinoma cell lines and metastatic sublines to the liver. Int J Cancer 1997; **72**:878–84.

31. Shigemori C, Wada H, Matsumoto K et al. Tissue factor expression and metastatic potential of colorectal cancer. Thromb Haemost 1998; 80:894–8.

32. Seto S, Onodera H, Kaido T et al. Tissue factor expression in human colorectal carcinoma: correlation with hepatic metastasis and impact on prognosis. Cancer 2000; 88:295–301.

33. Sawada M, Miyake S, Ohdama S et al. Expression of tissue factor in non-small-cell lung cancers and its relationship to metastasis. Br J Cancer 1999; 79:472–7.

34. Mueller BM, Reisfeld RA, Edgington TS et al. Expression of tissue factor by melanoma cells promotes efficient hematogenous metastasis. Proc Natl Acad Sci USA 1992; 89:11832–6.

35. Vrana JA, Stang MT, Grande JP et al. Expression of tissue factor in tumor stroma correlates with progression to invasive human breast cancer: paracrine regulation by carcinoma cell-derived members of the transforming growth factor beta family. Cancer Res 1996; 56: 5063–70.

36. Ueno T, Toi M, Koike M et al. Tissue factor expression in breast cancer tissues: its correlation with prognosis and plasma concentration. Br J Cancer 2000; 83: 164–70.

37. Hamada K, Kuratsu J, Saitoh Y et al. Expression of tissue factor correlates with grade of malignancy in human glioma. Cancer 1996; 77:1877–83.

38. Kakkar AK, Chinswangwatanakul V, Lemoine NR et al. Role of tissue factor expression on tumour cell invasion and growth of experimental pancreatic adenocarcinoma. Br J Surg 1999; 86:890–4.

39. Prydz H, Camerer E, Rottingen JA et al. Cellular consequences of the initiation of blood coagulation. Thromb Haemost 1999; 82: 183–92.

40. Mueller BM, Reisfeld RA, Edgington TS et al. Expression of tissue factor by melanoma cells promotes efficient hematogenous metastasis. Proc Natl Acad Sci USA 1992; 89:1183–6.

41. Fischer EG, Ruf W, Mueller BM. Tissue factor-initiated thrombin generation activates the signaling thrombin receptor on malignant melanoma cells. Cancer Res 1995; 55:1629–32.

42. Esumi N, Fan D, Fidler IJ. Inhibition of murine melanoma experimental metastasis by recombinant de-sulfatohirudin, a highly specific thrombin inhibitor. Cancer Res 1991; 51:4549–56.

43. Lorenzet R, Donati MB. Blood clotting activation, angiogenesis and tumor metastasis: any role for TFPI? Thromb Haemost 2002; 87:928–9.

44. Bromberg ME, Konigsberg WH, Madison JF et al. Tissue factor promotes melanoma metastasis by a pathway independent of blood coagulation. Proc Natl Acad Sci USA 1995; 92:8205–9.

45. Mueller BM, Ruf W. Requirement for binding of catalytically active factor VIIa in tissue factor-dependent experimental metastasis. J Clin Invest 1998; 101:1372–8.

46. Bromberg ME, Sundaram R, Homer RJ et al. Role of tissue factor in metastasis: functions of the cytoplasmic and extracellular domains of the molecule. Thromb Haemost 1999; 82:88–92.

47. Ott I, Fischer EG, Miyagi Y et al. A role for tissue factor in cell adhesion and migration mediated by interaction with actin-binding protein 280. J Cell Biol 1998; 140: 1241–53.

48. Ruf W, Mueller BM. Tissue factor signaling. Thromb Haemost 1999; 82:175–82.

49. Bromberg ME, Bailly MA, Konigsberg WH. Role of protease-activated receptor 1 in tumor metastasis promoted by tissue factor. Thromb Haemost 2000; **86**: 1210–14.

50. Even-Ram S, Uziely B, Cohen P et al. Thrombin receptor overexpression in malignant and physiological invasion processes. Nat Med 1998; **4**:909–14.

51. Kamath L, Meydani A, Foss F et al. Signaling from protease-activated receptor-1 inhibits migration and invasion of breast cancer cells. Cancer Res 2001; **61**:5933–40.

52. Carmeliet P, Mackman N, Moons L et al. Role of tissue factor in embryonic blood vessel development. Nature 1996; **383**:73–75.

53. Parry GC, Mackman N. Mouse embryogenesis requires the tissue factor extracellular domain but not the cytoplasmic domain. J Clin Invest 2000; **105**:1547–54.

54. Zhang Y, Deng Y, Luther T et al. Tissue factor controls the balance of angiogenic and antiangiogenic properties of tumor cells in mice. J Clin Invest 1994; **94**:1320–7.

55. Abdulkadir SA, Carvalhal GF, Kaleem Z et al. Tissue factor expression and angiogenesis in human prostate carcinoma. Hum Pathol 2000; **31**:443–7.

56. Koomagi R, Volm M. Tissue-factor expression in human non-small-cell lung carcinoma measured by immunohistochemistry: correlation between tissue factor and angiogenesis. Int J Cancer 1998; **79**: 19–22.

57. Contrino J, Hair G, Kreutzer DL et al. In situ detection of tissue factor in vascular endothelial cells: correlation with the malignant phenotype of human breast disease. Nat Med 1996; **2**:209–15.

58. Shoji M, Hancock WW, Abe K et al. Activation of coagulation and angiogenesis in cancer: immunohistochemical localization in situ of clotting proteins and vascular endothelial growth factor in human cancer. Am J Pathol 1998; **152**:399–411.

59. Abe K, Shoji M, Chen J et al. Regulation of vascular endothelial growth factor production and angiogenesis by the cytoplasmic tail of tissue factor. Proc Natl Acad Sci USA 1999; **96**:8663–8.

60. Ollivier V, Chabbat J, Herbert JM et al. Vascular endothelial growth factor production by fibroblasts in response to factor VIIa binding to tissue factor involves thrombin and factor Xa. Arterioscler Thromb Vasc Biol 2000; **20**:1374–81.

61. Clauss M, Gerlach M, Gerlach H et al. Vascular permeability factor: a tumor-derived polypeptide that induces endothelial cell and monocyte procoagulant activity, and promotes monocyte migration. J Exp Med 1990; **172**:1535–45.

5

The fibrinolytic system in cancer

Gilles Lugassy and Abraham Klepfish

The fibrinolytic (plasminogen–plasmin proteolytic enzyme) system is responsible for the lysis of fibrin clots, and is also involved in collagen degradation and angiogenesis. The fibrinolytic system is a fundamental component in the pathogenesis of neoplasia and tumor metastasis.

Basic mechanisms in fibrinolysis

The central enzyme of the fibrinolytic system is plasminogen, a precursor of the serine protease plasmin, a very powerful enzyme which cleaves the fibrin network, and releases fibrin degradation products (FDP), such as fragments D and E and D-dimer. Plasmin also cleaves fibrinogen and releases FDP: the fragments X and Y. The two most important activators of plasminogen are tissue plasminogen activator (t-PA) and urokinase-type plasminogen activator (u-PA).

Fibrinolysis inhibitors

Under physiological conditions, plasmin is inactivated by α_2-antiplasmin, while plasminogen activator inhibitor (PAI-1) is an active specific inhibitor of both t-PA and u-PA. Other inhibitors of the fibrinolytic system include thrombin-activated fibrinolysis inhibitor (TAFI), α_2-macroglobulin, and PAI 3.

Fibrin and cancer

The early observation, by electron microscopy and immunofluorescence, of fibrin deposition within, or adjacent to, malignant tumors in several experimental and human neoplasms was supportive, but not conclusive, of a direct role of fibrin in the progression of malignancy, since fibrin deposition may also occur in other inflammatory and systemic disorders, or be an artifact due to tumor manipulation.[1] The use of monoclonal antibodies and the analysis of electron-microscopic patterns have demonstrated that fibrin is an integral component of the tested tumors.[2]

Fibrin has been ascribed a dual role in tumor growth and spread. On the one hand, fibrin may enhance metastatic emboli by providing attachment sites for malignant cells to migrate along. The fibrin strands can also be a barrier to inflammatory cells, protecting neoplastic cells from being recognized and destroyed by competent cells of the host defense mechanisms. On the other hand, fibrin strands can form a rigid barrier that encapsulates the tumor and prevents its dissemination.[3] The recent generation of viable mouse lines with specific deficits in hemostatic factors has shed new light on the possible role of fibrin/fibrinogen in the progression and spread of some experimental tumors. Using fibrinogen-deficient mice, Palumbo et al[4] have demonstrated that fibrinogen does play a pivotal role in two transplantable murine tumor cell lines, Lewis lung carcinoma and B16-BL6 melanoma, and is a determinant of their metastatic potential. These authors have shown that fibrinogen is not strictly required for hematogenous metastasis and does not play a critical role in the growth of established metastasis. However, fibrinogen may increase the metastatic potential of circulating tumor cells, by enhancing the sustained adherence and survival of individual tumor cell emboli in the vessels of the target organs.

Fibrinolytic activities of cancer cells

The elevated levels of plasminogen activators (PA) demonstrated in many tumor tissues have led to the hypothesis that overexpression of PA could be involved in tumor-cell invasion. During tumor invasion and metastasis, tumor cells cross host cellular and extracellular matrix barriers by attachment to, and interaction with, components of the basement membrane and the extracellular matrix, and by local proteolysis. Penetrating tumor cells focus proteolytic activity to the cell surface through receptors for serine protease, plasmin, and u-PA. After binding to its receptor (u-PAR), the u-PA released by the surrounding tumor, or by stroma cells, converts inactive plasminogen into plasmin, a serine protease that disintegrates the extracellular matrix and facilitates tumor-cell proliferation, invasion, and metastasis.[5]

This hypothesis has been supported by several experimental results. Overexpression of u-PAR in breast-tumor cells has been shown to increase metastatic potential.[6] In small-cell lung cancer, low-molecular-weight urokinase was found in the foci of tumor cells adjacent to areas of necrosis.[7]

Several u-PA-secreting tumors are thought to mediate their invasiveness through u-PAR bond-surface u-PA: colon, prostate, glioblastoma, breast, and lung tumors, and gliblastoma.[8] In the lung-cancer model, preincubation of tumor-cell membranes with the fibrinolytic inhibitor PAI-1 reversed the u-PA-mediated invasion. Most authors agree, however, that tumor-cell invasiveness, focal proteolysis, and metastasis with secondary tumor growth are optimal when a critical balance is achieved between the protease u-PA, the cell-surface receptor u-PAR, and the inhibitor PAI-1.[9]

The exact mechanism by which this complex, tumor-cell-associated proteolytic system may confer a selective advantage to the malignant cell is still unclear. As u-PA is not dependent on fibrin for its ability to activate plasminogen, the tumor has an increased ability to generate plasmin, irrespective of local fibrin deposition, and thus contribute to the degradation of the basement membrane and the extracellular barriers.

Several conditions and factors may modify u-PA/u-PAR expression. Downregulation of u-PAR expression may be secondary to exposure to hormonal or antihormonal stimuli: tamoxifen downregulates u-PAR expression in a u-PAR-overexpressing breast-cancer cell line in vitro, leading to decreased invasive capacity of the tumor in vivo.[10] Another example is the increased u-PA expression of a prostate-carcinoma cell line upon stimulation with dihydrotestosterone.[11]

Activated factor VII is able to upregulate u-PAR expression in a pancreatic cancer cell line, causing increased invasiveness of the cancer cells. Upregulation of u-PAR could be successfully prevented when an anti-tissue-factor antibody was added.[12] These data suggest a role for the tissue-factor gene as a regulator of u-PAR gene expression.

u-PAR expression can also be stimulated by the epidermal growth factor receptor (EGFR). Expression of EGFR has been found to correlate with tumor-cell metastasis and survival.

A number of oncogenes are involved in the regulation of the plasminogen–plasmin proteolytic enzyme system. They include ras, jun, myc, fos, rel, and ets.[13] These oncogenes induce receptors on the membrane of malignant cells that facilitate local growth and metastatic migration of the cells.[14]

Clinical and prognostic significance of the plasminogen activator system in the cancer patient

A strong correlation has been found between overexpression of proteolytic factors and the clinical prognosis of many malignancies, including cancer of breast, gastrointestinal tract, lung, and the urological and gynecological systems.

Breast cancer

Proteolytic components have gained wide acceptance as biological factors of prognostic importance in breast cancer. Elevated levels of u-PA, u-PAR, and PAI-1 found in malignant tissue of breast-cancer patients indicate a higher risk of metastatic spread.

In a prospective study, Shiba et al[15] determined u-PA concentrations in the cytosol of 226 breast-cancer tissues by ELISA, using cytosol fractions prepared for steroid hormone assay. Patients with primary breast cancer containing high levels of u-PA had a significantly shorter disease-free survival period than patients with low levels of u-PA antigens during a 6-month follow-up period. A high level of u-PA was an independent risk factor for disease-free survival, independently of age, axillary node status, and estrogen-receptor status.

Other authors[16] found PAI-1 to be the second strongest prognostic factor after nodal status. In contrast, elevation of the other plasminogen activator inhibitor, PAI-2, could indicate a good prognosis if u-PA and PAI-1 were increased in parallel.[17]

It is not clear why the elevated tumor tissue content of PAI-1 indicates a poor prognosis for breast-cancer patients. Degradation of the tumor stroma could be prevented through interaction of PAI-1 with u-PA, allowing the formation of a new extracellular matrix. PAI-1 may also be involved in the modulation of u-PAR binding to the extracellular matrix components and interfere with cell attachment to the matrix. Tumor cells could then be alternatively attached to the extracellular matrix or detached from it.

PAI-2 acts on tumor cells in a different way than PAI-1: u-PA–PAI-2 complexes are cleaved upon binding to the u-PAR in tumor cells, and are not internalized. PAI-2 is also an important regulator of apoptosis through tumor necrosis factor (TNF) α-mediated processes.[18]

Several authors have recently shown that plasma D-dimer levels are viable markers of lymph-node and lymphovascular involvement in operable breast cancer. They also correlate with tumor volume, progression rate, and survival in patients with metastatic breast cancer.[19]

Cancers of the gastrointestinal tract

Elevated levels of both u-PA and PAI-1 have been constantly demonstrated in tumor tissues of esophageal,[20] gastric,[21] colorectal,[22] and pancreatic cancers.[23]

Elevated tissue levels of u-PA and PAI-1 are associated with a poorer prognosis in patients with completely resected gastric cancer. This represents the strongest prognostic factor in this group of patients, together with nodal status and WHO classification. These findings have been confirmed by many investigators as strong prognostic predictors of a shorter disease-free survival, higher frequency of metastatic spread, and greater failure of surgical or cytotoxic treatments.[24] Tissue concentrations of u-PA receptor and PAI-2 can be used to predict lymph-node involvement in patients with gastric cancer.[25]

In colorectal cancer, expression of u-PA, u-PAR, and PAI-1 and -2 constitutes an important predictor of overall survival and metastasis, independently of other major clinicopathological parameters.

Clinical studies of pancreatic cancer are few (possibly because of short patient survival). In vitro studies[23] have shown that urokinase is produced by most human pancreatic carcinoma cells. Andren-Sandberg et al[26] hypothesized that elevated plasma PAI-1 levels could cause thrombosis in pancreatic cancer patients. Kuramoto et al[27] proposed that t-PA could predict the endocrine responsiveness of human pancreatic carcinoma cells.

Lung cancer

The prognostic importance of fibrinolytic parameters has also been extensively studied in patients with carcinoma of the lung, mainly of the squamous-cell type. The combination of elevated u-PAR and PAI-1 levels is predictive of a shorter survival.[28] Increased levels of PAI-1 are associated with poor prognosis and shorter survival in adenocarcinoma of the lung. Data on large-cell lung cancer are more controversial: it seems that overexpression of u-PA, u-PAR, and PAI-1 is of no real significance for that type of lung cancer.

Urological malignancies

In a prospective study of 152 patients with kidney cancer, Hofmann et al[29] demonstrated that elevated u-PA, u-PAR, and PAI-1 are good predictors of metastatic spread and poor survival. The prognostic value of fibrinolytic activation markers in prostatic carcinoma is not well established. The conflicting results of several clinical studies may be due to the fact that normal prostatic tissue and fluid contain u-PA. The most recent clinical evaluations estimate that fibrinolytic parameters have no prognostic value in patients with prostatic cancer.[30,31]

Superficial bladder cancer

u-PA antigen expression is an important prognostic factor for SBC.[32] In a large review of fibrinolytic markers in SBC, Tsihilas et al emphasized good sensitivity to urinary FDP levels combined with urine cytology for the surveillance of that type of tumor.[33]

Ovarian cancer

There is strong clinical evidence that the fibrinolytic system is activated in ovarian cancer. Low levels of u-PA and PAI-1 in the primary tumor indicate a better prognosis in terms of prolonged survival.[34] Plasma levels of PAI-1 also have a prognostic significance, since they are correlated with a higher stage of the disease.[35] Similarly, elevated D-dimer levels are associated with shorter survival.[36]

Hematological malignancies

Interestingly enough, the fibrinolytic system has been given little attention in malignancies of the hematopoietic system. In polycythemia vera, investigators have found decreased levels of tissue plasminogen inhibitor antigen.[37] In a prospective clinical comparative study of the fibrinolytic system in different types of polycythemia, we have found no clear relation between thrombotic complications and fibrinolytic parameters, although elevated serum α_2-antiplasmin levels were associated with severe arterial thrombosis.[38]

The tumor-associated plasminogen activation system: a possible target for anticancer therapy

The therapeutic potential of drugs that could modify the fibrinolytic system and inhibit cancer growth and spread have not been evaluated as extensively as other anticoagulant therapies. Several methods have been tested either to enhance or inhibit the fibrinolytic system.[5,8,39] In a phase II study conducted at the University of Navarra,[40] intravenous urokinase was given in combination with chemotherapy to 12 patients with small-cell lung cancer. The response rate was compared with a group of 13 patients treated with chemotherapy alone. Overall response rates were similar in both arms, but complete response was more frequent within the urokinase group: 83% versus 53%. At 1 year, disease-free survival was also better in the combination group: 50% versus 30%.

Urokinase therapy alone or in combination with cytotoxic therapy has been found to be feasible in a few other tumors, such as breast, bladder, and stomach, with no definitive conclusions. Experimental methods have included the following:

- u-PA and u-PAR antisense oligodeoxynucleotide therapy[41]
- Disruption of u-PA with u-PAR
- PAI-1 and PAI-2 overexpression by transfection experiments.[42]

References

1. Bini A, Mes-Tejada R, Fenoglio JJ Jr et al. Immunohistochemical characterization of fibrin(ogen)-related antigens in human tissues using monoclonal antibodies. Lab Invest 1989; **60**:814–21.

2. Costantini V, Zacharski LR. Fibrin and cancer. Thromb Haemost 1993; **69**:406–14.

3. Bell WR. The fibrinolytic system in neoplasia. Semin Thromb Hemost 1996; **22**:459–78.

4. Palumbo JS, Kombrick KW, Drew AF et al. Fibrinogen is an important determinant of the metastatic potential of circulating tumor cells. Blood 2000; **96**:3302–9.

5. Schmitt M, Harbeck N, Thomssen C et al. Clinical impact of the plasminogen activation system in tumor invasion and metastasis: prognostic relevance and target for therapy. Thromb Haemost 1997; **78**: 285–96.

6. Xing RH, Rabbani SH. Overexpression of urokinase receptor in breast cancer cells results in increased tumor invasion, growth and metastasis. Int J Cancer 1996; **67**:423–9.

7. Wojtukiewicz MZ, Zacharski LR, Memoli VA et al. Abnormal regulation of coagulation/fibrinolysis in small cell carcinoma of the lung. Cancer 1990; **65**:480–5.

8. Korte W. Changes in the coagulation and fibrinolysis system in malignancy: their possible impact on future diagnostic and therapeutic procedures. Clin Chem Lab Med 2000; **38**:679–92.

9. Liu G, Shuman MA, Cohen RL. Co-expression of urokinase, urokinase receptor and PAI-1 is necessary for optimum invasiveness of cultured lung cells. Int J Cancer 1995; **60**: 501–6.

10. Xing RH, Mazar A, Henkin J et al. Prevention of breast cancer growth, invasion and metastasis by antiestrogen tamoxifen alone or in combination with urokinase inhibitor B-428. Cancer Res 1997; **57**:3585–93.

11. Pentyala SN, Whyard TC, Waltzer WC et al. Androgen induction of urokinase gene expression in LNCaP cells is dependent on their interaction with the extracellular matrix. Cancer Lett 1998; **130**: 121–6.

12. Tanigushi T, Kakkar AK, Tuddenham EG et al. Enhanced expression of urokinase receptor induced through the tissue factor–factor VIIa pathway in human pancreatic cancer. Cancer Res 1998; **58**:4461–7.

13. Zacharski LR, Wojtukiewicz MZ, Constantini V. Pathways of coagulation/fibrinolysis activation in malignancy. Semin Thromb Hemostas 1992; **18**:104–16.

14. Blasi F. Molecular mechanisms of protease-mediated tumor invasiveness. J Surg Oncol 1993; **3**:21–3.

15. Shiba E, Kim SJ, Tagushi T et al. A prospective study on the prognostic significance of urokinase-type plasminogen activator levels in breast cancer tissue. J Cancer Res Clin Oncol 1997; **123**: 555–9.

16. Foekens JA, Peters HA, Look MP et al. The urokinase system of plasminogen activation and prognosis in 2780 breast cancer patients. Cancer Res 2000; **60**:636–43.

17. Foekens JA, Buessecker F, Peters HA et al. Plasminogen activator inhibitor-2: prognostic relevance in 1012 patients with primary breast cancer. Cancer Res 1995; **55**:1423–7.

18. Ragno P, Montuori N, Rossi G. Urokinase type plasminogen activator/type 2 plasminogen activator inhibitor complexes are not internalized upon binding to the

urokinase type plasminogen activator receptor in THP-1 cells. Eur J Biochem 1995; **233**:514–9.

19. Dirix LY, Salgado R, Weytjens R et al. Plasma fibrin D-dimer levels correlate with tumor volume, progression rate and survival in patients with metastatic breast cancer. Br J Cancer 2002; **86**:389–95.

20. Hewin DF, Savage PB, Alderson D et al. Plasminogen activators in oesophageal carcinoma. Br J Surg 1996; **83**:1152–5.

21. Nekarda H, Schmitt M, Ulm K et al. Prognostic impact of urokinase-type plasminogen activator and its inhibitor PAI 1 in completely resected gastric cancer. Cancer Res 1994; **54**:2900–7.

22. Ganesh S, Sier CF, Griffioen G et al. Prognostic relevance of plasminogen activators and their inhibitors in colorectal cancer. Cancer Res 1994; **54**:4065–71.

23. Kakkar AK, Chinswangwatanakul V, Tebbutt S et al. A characterization of the coagulant and fibrinolytic profile of human pancreatic carcinoma cells. Haemostasis 1998; **28**:1–6.

24. Heiss MM, Babic R, Allgayer H. Tumor associated proteolysis and prognosis: new functional risk factors in gastric cancer defined by the urokinase-type plasminogen activator system. J Clin Oncol 1995; **13**:2084–93.

25. Ho CH, Chao Y, Lee SD et al. Diagnostic and prognostic values of plasma levels of fibrinolytic markers in gastric cancer. Thromb Res 1998; **91**:23–7.

26. Andren-Sandberg A, Lecander I, Martinsson G. Peaks in plasma PAI 1 concentration may explain thrombotic events in cases of pancreatic carcinoma. Cancer 1992; **69**:2884–7.

27. Karamoto M, Yamashita J, Ogova M. Tissue-type plasminogen activator predicts endocrine responsiveness of human pancreatic carcinoma cells. Cancer 1995; **75**:1263–72.

28. Pedersen H, Brunner N, Francis D et al. Prognostic impact of urokinase, urokinase receptor and type 1 plasminogen activator inhibitor in squamous and large cell lung cancer tissue. Cancer Res 1994; **54**:4671–5.

29. Hofmann R, Lehmer A, Buresch M et al. Clinical relevance of urokinase plasminogen activator, its receptor and its inhibitor in patients with renal cell carcinoma. Cancer 1996; **78**:487–92.

30. Lehmann K, Plas E, Gantshi K et al. Prognostic value of urokinase plasminogen activator for prostatic carcinoma. Urol Int 1994; **52**:159–61.

31. Van Veldhuizen PJ, Sadasivan R, Cherian R et al. Urokinase-type plasminogen activator expression in human prostate carcinomas. Am J Med Sci 1996; **312**:8–11.

32. Hasui Y, Marutsuka K, Asada Y et al. Prognostic value of urokinase type plasminogen activator in patients with superficial bladder cancer. Urology 1996; **47**:34–7.

33. Tsihlas J, Barton Grossman H. Superficial bladder cancer. New strategies in diagnosis and treatment. The utility of fibrin/fibrinogen degradation products in superficial bladder cancer. Urol Clin North Am 2000; **27**:39–45.

34. Kuhn W, Pache L, Schmalfeldt B et al. Urokinase (uPA) and PAI 1 predict survival in advanced ovarian cancer patients (FIGO III) after radical surgery and platinum based chemotherapy. Gynecol Oncol 1994; **55**:401–9.

35. Ho CH, Yuan CC, Liu SM. Diagnostic and prognostic values of plasma levels of fibrinolytic markers in ovarian cancers. Gynecol Oncol 1999; **75**:397–400.

36. Koh SC, Than KF, Razvi K et al. Hemostatic and fibrinolytic status in patients with ovarian cancer and benign ovarian cysts. Clin Appl Thromb Haemost 2001; 7:141–8.

37. Cohen AM, Gelvan A, Kadouri A et al. Tissue plasminogen activation levels in different types of polycythemia. Eur J Haematol 1990; 45:48–51.

38. Lugassy G, Filin I. Study of fibrinolytic parameters in different types of polycythemia. Am J Hematol 1999; 60:196–9.

39. Zacharski LR, Ornstein D, Gabbaza EC et al. Treatment of malignancy by activation of the plasminogen system. Semin Thromb Hemost 2002; 28:5–17.

40. Calvo FA, Hidalgo OF, Gonzales F et al. Urokinase combination chemotherapy in small cell lung cancer. A phase II study. Cancer 1992; 70:2624–30.

41. Li H, Lu H, Friscelli F et al. Adenovirus mediated delivery of a uPA/uPAR antagonist suppresses angiogenesis-dependent tumor growth and dissemination in mice. Gene Ther 1998; 5:1105–13.

42. Prans M, Wanterickx K, Collen D et al. Reduction of tumor cell migration and metastasis by adenoviral gene transfer of plasminogen activator inhibitors. Gene Ther 1999; 6:227–36.

6

Tumor angiogenesis and blood coagulation

Patricia M Fernandez, Steven R Patierno, and
Frederick R Rickles

Abbreviations

ABP-280	actin-binding protein 280 (thrombin-activated)
Ang-1	angiopoietin-1
bFGF	basic fibroblast growth factor
CAM	chick chorioallantoic membrane
egr-1	early growth response 1 gene
FAK	focal adhesion kinase
FBG	fibrinogen
FVa	activated factor V
FVII	factor VII
FVIIa	activated factor VII
FX	factor X
FXa	activated factor X
HBD	heparin-binding domain
HUVEC	human umbilical vein endothelial cell
MAPK	mitogen-activated protein kinase
MMP-2	matrix metalloproteinase 2
PAR	protease-activated receptor
PI3-K	phosphatidylinositol 3-kinase
PKC	protein kinase C
SCID	severe combined immunodeficient
TF	tissue factor
TFPI	tissue factor pathway inhibitor
TM	thrombomodulin
TNF-α	tumor necrosis factor-α
TSP	thrombospondin
VE-cadherin	vascular endothelial cadherin
VEC	vascular endothelial cell
VEGF/VPF	vascular endothelial growth factor/vascular permeability factor
VEGFR-2	vascular endothelial growth factor receptor 2
VTE	venous thromboembolism
XLF	cross-linked fibrin (thrombin-activated, factor XIIIa-mediated)

Introduction

Patients who present with idiopathic venous thromboembolism (VTE) frequently harbor an occult cancer that does not become clinically evident until months or even years later. Although Professor Armand Trousseau first recognized this link between coagulation and malignancy in 1865,[1] the mechanisms underlying this association have only recently started to unravel. The key mediator of this link is tissue factor (TF), the primary initiator of the coagulation cascade. Via both clotting-dependent and clotting-independent pathways, TF induces angiogenesis, the process of generating new blood vessels from pre-existing vessels, a process that is essential for tumor growth and metastasis. Other players downstream of TF activation that also induce angiogenesis include thrombin, protease-activated receptors (PARs), and fibrin, some of which are schematically represented in Figure 6.1. This chapter will dissect the coagulation cascade from TF activation through fibrin deposition, and will explore how key members of this cascade contribute directly and/or indirectly to tumor angiogenesis. While the principal goal of this chapter is to provide evidence supporting the hypothesis that tumor angiogenesis is the central link between blood coagulation and tumorigenesis, tumor growth may be promoted by coagulation products via pathways other than those related to angiogenesis. Fields of experimental oncology and thrombosis are being bridged to develop novel approaches that may hold promise for the treatment of cancer.

Tissue factor (TF)

TF structure and function

TF is a 47-kDa transmembrane receptor that initiates the coagulation cascade.[2] It comprises a 219-amino-acid extracellular domain, a 23-amino-acid hydrophobic transmembrane domain, and a 21-amino-acid intracellular tail that contains three putative serine phosphorylation sites. Under normal physiological conditions, TF serves a protective role by being localized to extravascular tissues not in direct contact with blood, such as the subendothelial layers of vessel walls. Exposure of these cells to blood follows vascular injury and results in the activation of TF receptor function via binding of its cognate ligand, factor VII (FVII), which circulates freely in the bloodstream.[3] TF promotes the activation of FVII to FVIIa, and the TF:FVIIa complex initiates the coagulation cascade.[2] Factor X (FX) is activated by the TF:FVIIa complex and forms part of the prothrombinase complex that proteolytically converts the zymogen prothrombin to the reactive serine protease thrombin. Thrombin induces clot formation by cleaving fibrinogen (FBG), activating platelets, and

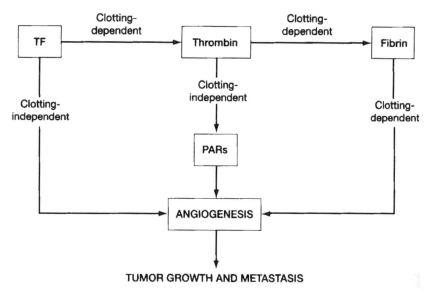

Figure 6.1

Coagulation cascade, angiogenesis, and tumor growth and metastasis. The coagulation cascade is linked to tumor growth and metastasis via its induction of angiogenesis. Both clotting-dependent and -independent mechanisms induce angiogenesis. Tissue factor (TF) induces non-clotting-dependent mechanisms via phosphorylation of its cytoplasmic tail and subsequent signal transduction cascades. TF induces angiogenesis via clotting-dependent mechanisms by downstream generation of the serine protease thrombin. Thrombin also induces angiogenesis via clotting-independent and -dependent mechanisms. Clotting-independent mechanisms are thought to be mediated via proteolytic cleavage of the protease-activated receptors (PARs) and subsequent activation of G-protein-coupled signal transduction cascades that induce angiogenesis-related genes. Clotting-dependent mechanisms are medi-ated via fibrin deposition and platelet activation. Fibrin induces angiogenesis via clot formation. Cross-linked fibrin matrices provide provisional, proangiogenic matrices that facilitate endothe-lial infiltration and tubule formation. Degradation of the fibrin matrix exposes cryptic sites that facilitate endothelial cell adhesion and migration. Byproducts of fibrinolysis can also elicit proangiogenic effects.

mediating feedback amplification of various earlier steps in clotting, ulti-mately leading to the deposition of fibrin. Thrombin also mediates a number of additional cellular responses, including angiogenesis, by cleaving PARs that are linked to various signaling cascades.

Several mechanisms control activation of the coagulation cascade. TF pathway inhibitor (TFPI), a Kunitz-type serine proteinase inhibitor, forms a quarternary complex with TF, FVIIa, and FXa on the cell membrane that prevents the release of FXa to the prothrombinase complex.[4] The inhibitory activity of TFPI can be increased if bound to thrombospondin (TSP).[5] The inactive TF:FVIIa:FXa:TFPI complex can be translocated into membrane caveolae, thereby downregulating cell-surface proteolysis.[6,7] TF receptors can also be expressed in an encrypted or inactive state on the cell surface, thus necessitating de-encryption before being activated by FVII/FVIIa.[8–12] Membrane phospholipid symmetry and charge play a key role in the encryption status of TF receptors.[13] In addition, cooperation between agonists such as vascular endothelial growth factor (VEGF) and tumor necrosis factor α (TNF-α) also regulates TF procoagulant activity.[14] It has been postulated that aberrant TF expression, in addition to dysregulation of mechanisms controlling TF procoagulant activity, contributes to the systemic hypercoagulability inherent in many cancer patients.

Aberrant TF expression in tumors

During pathological conditions such as inflammation and cancer, TF is inappropriately expressed on the surface of endothelial cells, monocytes, macrophages, fibroblasts, and tumor cells. Since TF shares homology with members of the cytokine receptor superfamily, cytokines and growth factors[15] prevalent in many inflammatory and malignant conditions induce its expression.[16] Inappropriate expression of TF alters the behavior of cells. Cancer cells transfected with TF cDNA exhibit a more malignant phenotype both in vitro and in vivo than parent cell lines do.[17,18] Aberrant TF expression has been detected in many different types of human tumors,[19] including glioma,[20,21] breast cancer,[22,23] non-small-cell lung cancer,[24,25] leukemia,[26] colon cancer,[27–30] and pancreatic cancer,[31,32] but not in corresponding normal tissues. Elevated TF expression in tumors has been correlated with unfavorable prognostic indicators, such as increased angiogenesis, advanced stages of disease, and the multidrug-resistant phenotype,[33] that contribute to poorer survival rates in cancer patients. Using quantitative reverse-transcription polymerase chain reaction (RT-PCR) methodology, Guan and colleagues quantified TF expression levels in 34 human glioma specimens and detected strong TF expression in 90%, 58%, 43%, and 20% of the grade IV, grade III, grade II, and grade I cases, respectively.[20] The increased TF-positivity in the higher tumor grades correlated directly with increased vascular density in the corresponding specimens. Using immunohistochemical techniques, Nakasaki and colleagues analyzed the expression of TF, VEGF, and microvessel density in 100 colorectal cancer specimens and found TF expression to be correlated directly with VEGF expression, clinical stage of colorectal cancer, Dukes classification, and angiogenesis.[27] TF was expressed in 81.3%, 84.6%, 52.6%, 45.5%, and 41.1% of tumors from patients in clinical stages IV, IIIB, IIIA, II, and I, respectively. Similar correlations between TF expression, VEGF expression, and microvessel density have also been found in non-small-cell lung cancers.[25] In situ analysis of TF expression in seven malignant and 10 benign breast tumors localized TF exclusively to the vascular endothelial cells (VECs) and tumor cells of the malignant phenotype.[23] Therefore, TF expression in malignant tumors appears to correlate with other poor prognostic factors.

TF and angiogenesis

TF plays a critical role in both physiological and pathological angiogenesis. Murine knockout experiments reveal that TF deficiency causes embryonic lethality by day 10.5 due to impaired vascular integrity and abnormal development of the yolk sac.[34-36] Similar histopathology associated with lethality occurs with VEGF-deficient embryos,[37,38] suggesting that TF and VEGF regulate similar functions. Strong correlations between TF, VEGF, and angiogenesis are most evident in pathological conditions.

In order for a tumor to progress from an occult focus to a malignant lesion, it must develop a vascular supply by inducing the sprouting of new blood vessels from pre-existing vessels in a process called angiogenesis. The switch to an angiogenic phenotype requires a shift in balance between endogenous pro- and antiangiogenic factors that regulate vessel growth and development. Aberrant expression of TF in tumors contributes to the angiogenic phenotype, in part by upregulating the expression of the proangiogenic protein VEGF and downregulating the expression of the antiangiogenic protein thrombospondin (TSP).[39,40] High microvessel density and elevated VEGF expression level are more common in TF-positive than TF-negative colorectal tumors.[27] TF and VEGF have also been found to be colocalized on tumor cells of human lung- and breast-cancer specimens.[41] Analysis of several human breast cancer[41] and melanoma[42] cell lines revealed a significant correlation between the synthesis of VEGF and TF in vitro. Subcutaneous inoculation of a high TF- and VEGF-producing melanoma cell line (RPMI-7951) into severe combined immunodeficient (SCID) mice yielded highly vascular tumors in vivo.[42] Similar experiments with a low TF- and VEGF-producing cell line (WM-115) produced relatively avascular tumors in vivo. However, when a low TF- and VEGF-producing melanoma cell line (HT144) that had been transfected with full-length TF cDNA was used in these experiments, vascular tumors grew that expressed high levels of both TF and VEGF. These studies support the hypothesis that TF regulates VEGF synthesis and contributes to tumor angiogenesis.

TF and VEGF participate in a vicious cycle of clot formation and tumor growth. Not only does TF induce VEGF, but the converse also holds true, since VEGF, in turn, upregulates the expression of TF on endothelial cells by activating the early growth response 1 (egr-1) gene.[43] Using specific low-molecular-weight inhibitors, Blum and colleagues investigated signaling cascades that regulated TF expression in human umbilical vein endothelial cells (HUVECs) and elucidated a mechanism that triggers differential activation of TF on endothelial cells during physiological (versus pathological) conditions.[44] Under physiological conditions, Blum and colleagues postulate that plasma components, such as growth factors, continuously activate the phosphatidylinositol 3-kinase (PI3-K)–Akt signaling pathway that causes suppression of TF production in normal endothelial cells. Within tumors, PI3-K activity is diminished by poor perfusion conditions that limit access to plasma components. Decreased PI3-K activity concurrent with increased p38 and ERK-1/2 mitogen-activated protein kinase (MAPK) activity induce positive regulation of TF expression by VEGF in tumor-related endothelial cells.[44] Another recent study lends support to this novel mechanism. Kim and colleagues reported that angiopoietin-1 (Ang-1), an activator of intracellular PI3-K–Akt signaling, inhibits TNF-α- and VEGF-induced expression of TF in endothelial cells.[45]

Clotting-dependent and -independent pathways of TF-induced angiogenesis

We believe that TF contributes to tumor angiogenesis via both clotting-dependent and clotting-independent mechanisms.[46,47] Clotting-dependent pathways probably involve activation of the TF receptor via ligand binding, followed by downstream production of thrombin and ensuing clot formation. Clotting-independent pathways appear to involve phosphorylation of the cytoplasmic domain of the TF receptor and subsequent downstream signaling events that occur independently of thrombin production or clot formation, and possibly even independently of ligand activation (Figure 6.2).[40] Both pathways can directly and/or indirectly contribute to angiogenesis and tumor progression.

TF is classified as an 'immediate early gene'. Following cell activation, transcription factors bind to corresponding transcription binding sites located on the promoter region of the TF gene and rapidly induce its expression independently of clotting. Some transcription factors, including SP1, AP-1, and NFκB are involved in the regulation of both TF and VEGF, offering a potential mechanism for their colocalization and coregulation in many tumors. Since VEGF is characterized as one of the most potent regulators of angiogenesis, the direct association of TF with VEGF offers strong support for a link between TF and tumor angiogenesis. Differential signaling pathways may control TF-induced regulation of VEGF during physiological and pathological angiogenesis. Using human fibroblasts, Ollivier and colleagues reported that TF-induced production of VEGF required the binding of FVIIa to TF and subsequent generation of FXa and thrombin.[48,49] However, in some (but not all) malignant melanoma cell lines,[50] TF-mediated regulation of VEGF is regulated independently of clotting via activation of the cytoplasmic tail of TF, rather than via the ligand-binding extracellular domain.[42] The serine

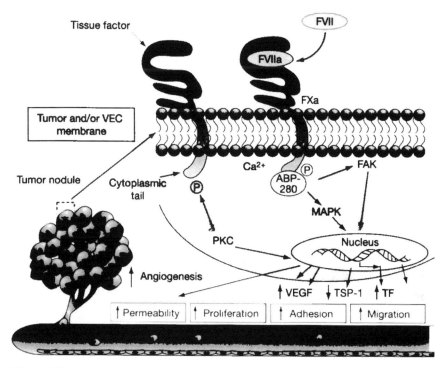

Figure 6.2

Tissue factor (TF) and angiogenesis: clotting-independent mechanisms. TF can induce angiogenesis via mechanisms that are independent of thrombin generation and fibrin deposition. These mechanisms are primarily mediated by the constitutive and aberrant expression of TF observed in many tumor cells and associated vascular endothelial cells (VECs). The serine residues on the cytoplasmic tail of the TF receptor can be phosphorylated by protein kinase C (PKC), independently of ligand binding. Phosphorylation of the receptor initiates downstream signaling cascades that result in the transcriptional activation or inactivation of different genes. Vascular endothelial growth factor (VEGF), a proangiogenic factor, is upregulated by TF activation, while thrombospondin-1 (TSP-1), an antiangiogenic factor, is downregulated by TF activation. VEGF, in turn, upregulates TF to continue the vicious cycle of tumor growth and clot formation. VEGF also increases the vascular permeability that leads to plasma protein leakage and the deposition of a fibrin-rich proangiogenic matrix around tumor cells and VECs. Increased VEGF and decreased TSP-1 induce the proliferation of endothelial cells that contributes to increased tumor angiogenesis. The binding of factor VII (FVII) to its cognate receptor TF results in the activation of FVII (FVIIa) and an increase in intracellular calcium (Ca^{2+}). Intracellular Ca^{2+} activates PKC, which, in turn, phosphorylates the cytoplasmic tail of the TF receptor. Ligand binding also promotes the attachment of actin-binding protein 280 (ABP-280) to the cytoplasmic tail, resulting in the assembly of actin filaments. This association regulates MAPK signaling and phosphorylation of focal adhesion kinases (FAKs) and downstream signaling cascades that promote the increased endothelial cell adhesion and migration essential for tumor angiogenesis.

residues on the cytoplasmic tail of the TF receptor can be phosphorylated by protein kinase C (PKC)-mediated mechanisms.[40,51]

The cytoplasmic tail of TF appears to regulate non-clotting-dependent mechanisms, including cytoskeletal reorganization, vascular remodeling, angiogenesis, and cellular metastasis. Following extracellular binding of the TF receptor, actin-binding protein 280 (ABP-280) is recruited to the cytoplasmic tail, where it participates in the assembly of actin filaments (Figure 6.2).[52] The C-terminus of ABP-280 associates with the cytoplasmic domain of TF, while its N-terminus interacts with the actin filaments. This association regulates MAPK signaling and phosphorylation of focal adhesion kinases (FAKs) that promote cell adhesion and migration. Mechanisms mediated by the cytoplasmic tail of TF are important for embryonic vessel development, tumor angiogenesis, and metastasis. An in vivo model of metastasis demonstrated that the cytoplasmic tail of TF is essential for metastasis.[53] In studies of transfected Chinese hamster ovary (CHO) cells, Mueller and Ruf concluded that the extracellular proteolytic activity of the TF receptor was also required for TF-dependent metastasis.[54] This mechanism may be mediated via ensuing PAR activation that leads to the phosphorylation of the serine residues in the cytoplasmic tail of the TF receptor.

Thrombin

Thrombin and angiogenesis: clotting-independent mechanism

Clotting-dependent mechanisms of TF-induced angiogenesis involve thrombin generation. The extrinsic coagulation cascade culminates in the proteolytic conversion of prothrombin to thrombin by the prothrombinase complex of FXa and factor Va (FVa) that assembles on phospholipid membranes (such as platelet, monocyte/macrophage, or tumor-cell membranes) in the presence of calcium ions. Thrombin is a highly active but short-lived serine protease that elicits a plethora of cellular effects within the arena of its production. Although thrombin is best known for its direct role in clot formation via platelet activation and fibrin deposition, it also regulates cellular behavior independently of clotting by activating G-protein-coupled PARs that orchestrate a network of signaling cascades (Figure 6.3).[55] Many of the effects elicited by thrombin facilitate tumor progression by promoting angiogenesis.[56] The two prothrombin fragments (F1 and 2) released upon thrombin activation may help control the angiogenic response by functioning as antiangiogenic factors in vivo.[57] Another negative feedback mechanism of thrombin activation involves binding with thrombomodulin (TM), a transmembrane glycoprotein that resides on the luminal surface of endothelial cells. When complexed with TM, thrombin activates the anticoagulant protein C instead of proteolytically cleaving FBG or PARs.[58]

Using various analogs of thrombin, Tsopanoglou and colleagues demonstrated that thrombin promotes angiogenesis in the chick

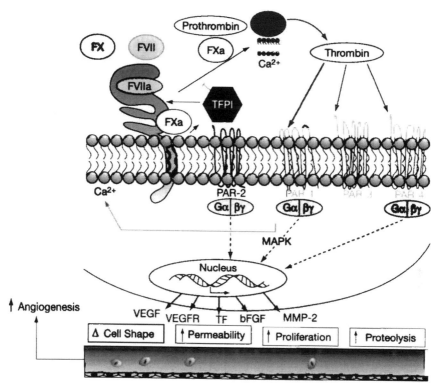

Figure 6.3

Thrombin and angiogenesis: clotting-independent mechanism. Tissue factor (TF) can induce angiogenesis via thrombin generation, independently of fibrin deposition and clot formation. Activation of the TF receptor occurs via binding of its cognate ligand, Factor VII (FVII). FVII is activated (FVIIa), and the TF:FVIIa complex, in turn, activates FX (FXa). If the tissue factor pathway inhibitor (TFPI) does not bind and inactivate the TF:FVIIa:FXa ternary complex, FXa dissociates from the complex and associates with another phospholipid membrane in the presence of Ca²⁺ and FVa to form the prothrombinase complex that proteolytically converts prothrombin to thrombin. Thrombin can induce angiogenesis independently of clot formation by cleaving the cell membrane-bound protease-activated receptors (PARs). Thrombin-generated cleavage of part of the N-terminal domain of the PARs exposes a neo-N-terminus that functions as a tethered ligand. This tethered ligand binds intramolecularly to the second transmembrane domain of this seven transmembrane G-protein coupled receptor. Thrombin cleaves PAR-1, PAR-3, and PAR-4, but not PAR-2. Other proteases, such as trypsin, tryptase, the TF:FVIIa complex, or FXa, can activate PAR-2. Activation of the PARs causes a conformational change that results in the exchange of bound GDP for GTP on associated G proteins. The G proteins comprise an α-subunit that contains the nucleotide binding site, and a βγ heterodimer. Tissue-specific expression of various G-protein subunits confers differential responses to thrombin. The specific signal transduction cascade induced by PAR activation is dependent on the type of G-protein subunit that is attached to the PAR. Signal transduction cascades, such as the MAPKs, can lead to the transcriptional activation of a number of genes that are involved in angiogenesis. Thrombin activation of PARs leads to the upregulation of many angiogenesis-related genes, including VEGF, VEGFRs, TF, bFGF, and MMP-2. These genes can lead to a number of pleiotropic responses, such as change in endothelial cell shape, increased vascular permeability, increased endothelial cell proliferation, and increased proteolysis, that all contribute to increased tumor angiogenesis.

chorioallantoic membrane (CAM) assay independently of its clotting activity.[59] Thrombin has also been shown to induce microvessel infiltration in vivo and promote PKC-dependent morphological differentiation of HUVECs in vitro.[60]

Thrombin contributes to a number of critical events in the angiogenic process. Under most physiological conditions, endothelial cells reside in a quiescent state. In response to vascular injury, thrombin activates the proliferation and migration of endothelial cells for promotion of wound repair. In the context of a tumor microenvironment, these actions invoke the recruitment of new blood vessels into the developing tumor. Tumor cells frequently secrete the proangiogenic VEGF to attract new vessels. Thrombin stimulates the release of VEGF (and other growth factors) from the α-granules of platelets[61,62] and indirectly upregulates the transcription of VEGF in vascular smooth muscle cells by inducing the production of reactive oxygen species (ROS) and subsequent expression of the hypoxia-inducible factor 1α (HIF-1α) transcription factor. The HIF-1 complex binds to the VEGF gene and induces its transcription.[63] Thrombin also directly upregulates VEGF expression via PAR activation. Treatment of human FS4 fibroblasts, DU145 human prostate cancer cells, and CHRF-288 megakaryocytes with 0.5 U/ml thrombin caused a significant upregulation and stabilization of VEGF mRNA in these cells that resulted in increased synthesis and secretion of the VEGF protein.[64] Studies with specific kinase inhibitors revealed that PI3-K and serine/threonine kinase pathways, but not the MAPK pathway, mediated these effects via thrombin activation of PAR-1. Different tissues may utilize alternate mechanisms, since thrombin-induced upregulation of VEGF is inhibited by a MAPK inhibitor (PD98059) in lung fibroblasts.[49]

Studies with three human glioma cell lines (U-87 MG, U-251 MG, and U-105 MG) also confirmed the ability of thrombin to upregulate VEGF expression via its cognate receptor, although specific signal transduction mechanisms were not reported.[65] Immunohistochemistry and in situ hybridization detection of VEGF and prothrombin expression, respectively, in human glioma specimens were used to demonstrate a direct correlation between the two, suggesting potential autocrine regulation of angiogenesis in glioma tumors via thrombin production.[65] Herbert and colleagues reported autocrine regulation of endothelial cell growth via thrombin-induced secretion of basic fibroblast growth factor (bFGF).[66] In addition, thrombin has been shown to upregulate angiopoietin-2 (Ang-2), the proangiogenic factor that antagonizes the blood vessel-stabilizing effects of Ang-1.[67] In vitro studies have shown that thrombin induces DNA synthesis in endothelial cells.[68] When endothelial cells were treated with both thrombin and VEGF, a synergistic induction of mitogenic activity occurred. Tsopanoglou and Maragoudakis suggested that these results were due to the ability of thrombin to upregulate expression of the VEGF receptors Flt-1 and KDR in endothelial cells via protein kinase (PKC) and MAPK signaling mechanisms.[68]

Thrombin promotes reversible rounding of endothelial cells and increases vascular permeability,[69] which results in plasma protein leakage and the development of a provisional proangiogenic matrix.[55] The mechanisms underlying thrombin-induced endothelial barrier dysfunction usually commence with the induction of inositol 1,4,5-trisphosphate (IP_3), which leads to the release of intracellular Ca^{2+} stores and the activation of the p42/44 MAPK signaling pathway.[70-72] Keogh and colleagues proposed that proline-rich kinase 2 (Pyk2), a non-receptor tyrosine kinase member of the focal adhesion kinase family, is phosphorylated by thrombin activation of PAR-1 and serves as a bridge between Ca^{2+} mobilization and MAPK activation.[73] Their studies suggest that Pyk2 activation is independent of PKC, PI3-K, and Src kinases.[73]

Angiogenesis not only involves activation of endothelial cells, but also requires invasion of the endothelial cells through their basement membrane and migration to distal sites. In vitro studies have demonstrated that thrombin contributes to each of these events. Thrombin decreases adhesion of endothelial cells to basement membrane proteins via cAMP, making them more mobile. Thrombin also mobilizes adhesion molecules to the endothelial surface (such as P-selectin) that facilitate platelet and tumor-cell adhesion. As demonstrated with a Boyden chamber invasion assay, immobilized thrombin functions as a chemoattractant to endothelial cells by inducing their migration and invasion towards high concentrations of the serine protease, as might exist at a site of injury or within a tumor microenvironment. Endothelial cells attach to thrombin via the angiogenic $\alpha_v\beta_3$ integrin, which is upregulated by thrombin. This attachment provides endothelial cells with survival signals during their anchorage-independent migration.[56] Thrombin also facilitates invasion through the basement membrane by activating the collagen type IV degrading enzyme, gelatinase A, also known as matrix metalloproteinase 2 (MMP-2).[74] Interestingly, both $\alpha_v\beta_3$ and MMP-2 functionally coexist on the surface of angiogenic capillaries.[75]

Thrombin dramatically increases the growth and metastatic potential of tumor cells, although these effects may be attributed in part to its proangiogenic effects.[68,76] By mobilizing adhesion molecules, such as the $\alpha_{IIb}\beta_3$ integrin,[77-79] P-selectin,[80,81] and CD40 ligand,[82] to the cell surface, thrombin enhances adhesion between tumor cells, platelets, endothelial cells, and the extracellular matrix, and contributes to tumor progression. Thrombin also triggers the release of growth factors,[83] chemokines, and extracellular proteins[84] that promote the proliferation and migration of tumor cells. The prometastatic activity of thrombin has been demonstrated in vivo with experimental pulmonary metastasis models that showed dramatic increase of lung metastases with thrombin-treated tumor cells compared with untreated tumor cells.[78,85,86] The principal thrombin receptor, PAR-1, has been implicated in the promotion of these effects.[87] Most of the cellular effects elicited by thrombin are mediated through the activation and subsequent signal transduction cascades of members of the PAR family, suggesting that proteolytic activity of thrombin is essential for the mediation of these events.

Thrombin receptors: PARs

PARs are a unique family of seven-transmembrane-domain G-protein-coupled receptors that carry their own activating ligand. Four members of the PAR family have been identified: PAR-1, PAR-2, PAR-3, and PAR-4. PAR-1 has the greatest influence on vascular development since knockout (–/–) experiments have revealed an embryonic lethality rate of 50% in PAR-1$^{-/-}$ mice.[88-90] In contrast, PAR-2$^{-/-}$ and PAR-3$^{-/-}$ mice developed relatively normally, suggesting potential redundancy in their function.[89,91] The phenotype of PAR-4$^{-/-}$ mice has not yet been reported. The expression of one or more of these receptors varies between different cell types and species. Human platelets express PAR-1 and PAR-4, while mouse platelets express PAR-3 and PAR-4. Human endothelial cells express PAR-1, PAR-2, and possibly PAR-3, but not PAR-4.

PAR expression and cancer

PAR-1 is the predominant thrombin receptor, and its expression has been correlated with the malignant phenotype. Using both breast cancer cell lines and breast cancer specimens, Even-Ram and colleagues found a direct correlation between elevated PAR expression and invasive potential.[76] Whereas normal or premalignant breast specimens lacked detectable PAR-1 expression, infiltrating ductal carcinomas expressed very high levels. Transfection of the metastatic MDA-435 breast cancer cell line with PAR-1 antisense cDNA significantly reduced its invasive potential, as evaluated by Boyden chamber invasion assay.[76]

Both thrombin and trypsin are common proteases secreted by malignant cells that are thought to contribute to their metastatic potential. Analysis has been accomplished of their corresponding receptors, PAR-1 and PAR-2, respectively, in situ in a variety of different cell types, both within and outside the tumor microenvironment. Expression of PAR-1 and PAR-2 was identified in tumor cells, endothelial cells, vascular smooth muscle cells, smooth muscle actin (SMA)-positive stromal fibroblasts, mast cells, and macrophages within the metastatic tumor microenvironment.[92] Although PAR-1 and PAR-2 expression has been observed in normal endothelial cells, vascular smooth muscle cells, and mast cells, the receptors have not been detected in normal/benign epithelial cells or stromal fibroblasts surrounding normal tissues. These results suggest that the tumor microenvironment is conducive to PAR-mediated gene induction, offering potential mechanisms for metastasis promoted by thrombin.

PAR activation

As indicated above, PAR-1, PAR-3, and PAR-4 are activated by thrombin, while PAR-2 is activated by proteases other than thrombin, including trypsin, tryptase, the TF:FVIIa complex, and FXa. FXa can also activate PAR-1, but with significantly delayed kinetics compared with thrombin cleavage.[93] Thrombin activates PAR-1 by attaching to and cleaving the N-terminal domain of the receptor between the Arg41 and Ser42 residues (R41–S42), exposing a new N-terminus. The neo-N-terminal domain functions as a tethered ligand that swings over and docks intramolecularly to its own receptor at the second transmembrane domain via the residues [42]SFLLRN[47] (for PAR-1). This event triggers the activation of the receptor and subsequent G-protein-mediated signal transduction cascades that result in the gene expression and pleiotropic effects elicited by thrombin.[55,94] Although PAR-2 is not activated by thrombin, the newly exposed N-terminus from PAR-1 can bind intermolecularly to a neighboring PAR-2 receptor and transactivate that receptor.[95] Unlike PAR-1 and PAR-3, PAR-4 lacks hirudin-like sequences ([50]DKYEPF[56] in PAR-1) that bind to the anion-binding exosite-1 of thrombin and facilitate receptor cleavage.[96] PAR-4 utilizes PAR-1 or PAR-3 as a coreceptor to localize thrombin to the cell surface for proteolytic cleavage and receptor activation. In a recent study, Cleary and colleagues reported that PAR-4 interacts directly with the active site of thrombin via the amino acids [44]PAPR[47], resulting in receptor cleavage between the R47 and G48 peptide bond that produces the [48]GYPGQV[53] tethered ligand.[97] Lower concentrations of thrombin are required to activate PAR-1 than PAR-4 because the hirudin-like sequence of PAR-1 optimizes thrombin binding. The key mechanism activating these receptors is not the cleavage of the N-terminus by a protease, but rather the intra- or intermolecular activation of the receptor with the newly exposed tethered ligand. Peptides that mimic the neo-N-terminus can bind and activate specific PAR receptors even in the presence of an uncleaved extracellular domain. PAR-3 has evolved as a cofactor to PAR-4 that does not mediate its own signaling.[55,98]

PAR-mediated signal transduction cascades

Proteolytic cleavage and activation of the PAR receptor(s) cue the cell to external injury, as evidenced by activation of the coagulation cascade, and trigger a host of cellular responses via different G-protein-coupled signaling cascades.[55,69] Intramolecular binding of the tethered ligand to the receptor results in a conformational change that causes the exchange of bound GDP for GTP on associated G proteins. The G proteins are heterodimeric complexes comprising an α subunit that contains the nucleotide-binding site, and a βγ heterodimer. Tissue-specific expression of various G-protein subunit families confers differential responses to thrombin. The $G_{12/13}α$-, $G_qα$-, and/or $G_iα$-subunit families can be linked to PARs. Different G-protein subunits link receptor activation with a host of intracellular signaling effectors, including protein kinase C, phospholipase Cβ and A_2, MAPK, adenylate cyclases, tyrosine kinase, and PI3-K. Activation or inhibition of these signaling cascades results in the pleiotropic effects elicited by thrombin independently of fibrin deposition and clot formation.

Since thrombin functions as a proteolytic enzyme rather than as a ligand for the PARs, a single thrombin molecule can activate more than one receptor. Cleavage of the receptor is irreversible. After signaling through its coupled G proteins, PARs are uncoupled and internalized via a phosphorylation-dependent mechanism for degradation in lysozymes. In endothelial cells and fibroblasts, but not megakaryocytes, new PARs can be shunted to the cell surface from intracellular stores in response to additional thrombin stimulation, accounting for dose-dependent effects.[55]

Fibrin

Fibrin and angiogenesis: clotting-dependent mechanisms

Thrombin is an effective activator of angiogenesis via both clotting-independent and clotting-dependent mechanisms. Whereas clotting-independent mechanisms are believed to be mediated by PAR activation and ensuing signal transduction cascades, clotting-dependent mechanisms involve platelet activation and fibrin deposition (Figure 6.4). Tumor vessels are inherently leaky as a consequence of the hyperpermeable effects of VEGF/VPF. In spite of its rather large molecular weight, the plasma protein fibrinogen (FBG) is capable of leaking into the extravascular tissue. FBG then binds to specific receptors on inflammatory and tumor cells in the tumor microenvironment and is cleaved by thrombin generated in the local tumor microenvironment. This fibrin can be found within the vascular endothelium of neoangiogenic vessels in the tumor,[23] bound to inflammatory cells or tumor cells, or deposited around tumor cells as a provisional scaffold that facilitates further angiogenesis.[99]

When thrombin is generated, it converts soluble FBG to insoluble fibrin by cleaving fibrinopeptides A and B (FPA and FPB) to yield fibrin monomers that become cross-linked into a fibrin matrix. Earlier studies observed that plasma levels of FPA in cancer patients varied proportionally to tumor growth and regression.[100–104] The turnover rate of plasma FBG was also reported to be higher in cancer patients.[105] The relationship of fibrin deposition to invasivity of tumors is controversial. A number

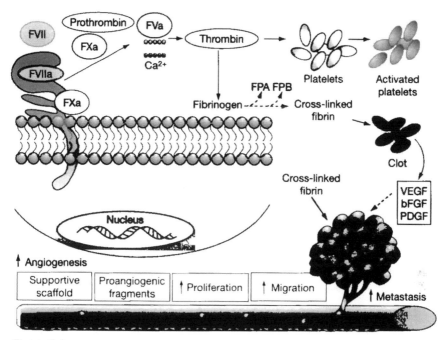

Figure 6.4.

Fibrin and angiogenesis: clotting-dependent mechanisms. Tissue factor (TF) can also induce angiogenesis by clotting-dependent mechanisms via thrombin generation and fibrin deposition. Generation of thrombin from the prothrombinase complex results in an active serine protease that cleaves fibrinopeptides A and B (FPA and FPB) from the fibrinogen (FBG) molecule, resulting in the eventual conversion of soluble FBG to cross-linked fibrin (XLF). Elevated levels of plasma FPA have been correlated with tumor growth and progression. Thrombin also activates platelets. Deposition of activated platelets with XLF forms the clot. Clot formation and dissolution contribute to tumor growth and angiogenesis. Activated platelets release a number of proangiogenic factors from their α-granules, including VEGF, basic fibroblast growth factor (bFGF), and platelet-derived growth factor (PDGF), that contribute to increased tumor and endothelial cell proliferation and migration. VEGF induces a plasma protein leakage that results in an extravascular XLF matrix around tumor cells. This matrix serves as a supportive scaffold that facilitates endothelial cell migration and tubule formation. The fibrinolytic degradation of the fibrin matrix also contributes to angiogenesis, since degradation results in the exposure of proangiogenic cryptic sites that facilitate cell adhesion and migration, and the release of small proangiogenic fragments and sequestered growth factors.

of investigators have reported that different types of solid tumors, including, brain,[106] lung,[41] and prostate,[107] are characterized by deposits of cross-linked fibrin (XLF).[108] Other investigators have suggested that still other tumor types, such as colon cancer,[109] lymphoma,[110] mesothelioma[111] and, in some studies, breast cancer,[112] contain FBG, but not XLF, within the tumor stroma. Furthermore, there is disagreement about a classification schema in which breast cancer was characterized with this latter group, since other investigators have identified XLF within the angiogenic vessels of invasive breast cancer specimens, but not within the vessels of benign tumors.[23]

FBG degradation products

Components of the coagulation and fibrinolytic systems work in opposition to maintain hemostatic balance between clot formation and clot dissolution. The fibrinolytic enzyme plasmin degrades the fibrin matrix into a number of small fragments, including D-dimer and fibrin fragments D and E.[113,114] Plasmin can also directly cleave FBG to yield similar low-molecular-weight fragments, including fragments D and E and the Bβ1–42 peptide.[113,115] Several of these biologically active fragments elicit pro- or antiangiogenic effects that contribute to wound-healing and tumorigenesis. Fibrin fragment E stimulates angiogenesis in vitro in the tubule-forming assay[113] and in vivo in the chick chorioallantoic membrane (CAM) assay.[116] An earlier study suggested that fibrin fragment E contributed to tumorigenesis, since use of an antibody directed against this fragment produced tumor regression and long-term survival in an in vivo tumor model.[117] FBG fragment E, however, can produce opposite effects—this fragment inhibits angiogenesis in vitro in endothelial migration and tubule-forming assays, with quantifiable effects comparable to those elicited by the endogenous antiangiogenic peptide endostatin.[113]

The prognostic significance of plasma-fibrin D-dimer levels was evaluated in cancer patients. Patients with advanced stages of colorectal,[118] lung,[119] and breast[120] cancers were observed to express elevated levels of plasma D-dimer. A recent study evaluated the validity of plasma D-dimer levels as a tumor marker in breast-cancer patients by quantifying D-dimer in plasma samples from cohorts of operable breast-cancer patients, metastatic breast-cancer patients, and healthy female volunteers.[121] This study found positive correlations between elevated plasma D-dimer levels and FBG levels, numbers of metastatic sites, tumor load, progression kinetics, and survival. Angiogenic factors, such as serum VEGF, serum interleukin-6 (IL-6), and calculated VEGF load in platelets, were also positively correlated with plasma D-dimer levels in this study.

FBG and adhesion molecules

Cleavage and degradation of FBG and fibrin expose cryptic sites in the molecules that facilitate adhesion to cell-surface receptors.[114] As predicted by the German pathologist Rudolf Virchow in his classic treatise on the pathogenesis of thrombosis, components of the blood contribute to the development of clots in cancer patients.[122] Different cellular components within or outside the bloodstream, including leukocytes,[123] platelets,[124] endothelial cells,[125] fibroblasts,[126] keratinocytes,[127] smooth muscle cells,[128] and tumor cells,[129] specifically bind fibrin matrices via both integrin and nonintegrin cell-surface adhesion molecules. Fibrin bridges cell–matrix interactions essential for physiological and pathological events, including inflammation, hemostasis, wound-healing, and tumor angiogenesis,[124] which is accomplished via multifunctional domains within FBG. The human FBG molecule contains Arg-Gly-Asp (RGD) sequences located at Aα95–98 (RGDF) and Aα572–575 (RGDS) that mediate specific binding to cell-surface integrins such as $\alpha_v\beta_3$ and $\alpha_5\beta_1$.[130] Non-integrin-mediated binding occurs through other functional binding regions, including the intercellular adhesion molecule 1 (ICAM-1) binding sites at γ117–133,[131] heparin-binding domains (HBD) on the N-terminal Bβ chain[132,133] that bind cell-surface heparin sulfate proteoglycans,[133] and platelet recognition sites at γ400–411 that promote platelet spreading.[134–136] Fibrin also interacts with vascular endothelial-cadherin (VE-cadherin) via exposure of its N-terminal β15–42 epitope[137,138] after cleavage of FPB.[139] Recent studies suggest that binding of endothelial cells to fibrin via VE-cadherin may be necessary for capillary tube formation.[140]

The fibrin matrix that develops around tumors provides a provisional proangiogenic scaffold that not only supports vessel formation, but also stimulates endothelial cell proliferation and migration.[141] Endothelial cells express different adhesion molecules on their surface based on the extracellular matrices they encounter. During wound-healing, the fibrin matrix provokes an angiogenic response by upregulating the expression of $\alpha_v\beta_3$ receptors that facilitate endothelial invasion[142] and tube formation.[143] The $\alpha_v\beta_3$ integrins provide survival signals to endothelial cells during their interaction with fibrin. In vitro studies have shown that $\alpha_v\beta_3$ mRNA of human dermal microvascular cells is more stable in fibrin gels than collagen gels.[144] When the collagen-rich matrix from mature granulation tissue replaces the fibrin clot in a wound, the integrin expression changes on the endothelial cells, signaling completion of repair and the end of the angiogenic state. Dvorak and colleagues characterized tumors as 'wounds that do not heal' because the continuous deposition of fibrin around tumors evoked by VEGF-induced vessel leakiness creates a persistent proangiogenic environment.[99,145,146]

Fibrin matrix and growth factors

The fibrin matrix not only functions as a multifunctional scaffold that promotes matrix–cell interactions essential for neovascularization, but also serves as a storehouse for proangiogenic growth factors. Growth factors such as bFGF and VEGF possess HBDs that mediate attachment to the fibrin matrix. Insulin-like growth factor I (IGF-I) is also sequestered in fibrin matrices via its association with IGF-binding protein 3 (IGFBP-3), which binds directly to fibrin. Within the fibrin matrix, the sequestered growth factors are protected from proteolytic degradation.[147] When the extracellular matrix is degraded by proteolytic enzymes during the invasion of endothelial and tumor cells, the sequestered growth factors are released from the matrix and become available to bind cognate receptors on the invading cells. Receptor activation promotes cell proliferation and migration that contribute to tumor angiogenesis and progression.[148,149] In vitro studies demonstrated that fibrin matrices stimulate the synthesis and secretion of the proangiogenic factor interleukin-8 (IL-8) from tumorigenic oral and pharyngeal cell lines (SCC-25 and FADU, respectively), but not from nontumorigenic oral epithelial cells (PP cells).[150] Other matrices such as collagen failed to induce IL-8, suggesting a specific response to the fibrin matrix.

In vitro studies suggest that fibrin can indirectly induce its own deposition by activating the coagulation cascade via induction of TF expression on neighboring endothelial cells. When HUVECs were cocultured with physiologically relevant concentrations of fibrin (1 mg/ml), TF expression was induced up to 150-fold.[151] This response required direct contact between fibrin and the endothelial cells since transwell studies that separated the two components failed to produce significant TF induction.

FBG-deficient mice

Although FBG plays a role in tumor angiogenesis and progression, studies with FBG-deficient mice have revealed that FBG is not required for these events to occur. When FBG-deficient mice were given subcutaneous injections of either B16–BL6 melanoma or Lewis lung carcinoma cells, palpable tumors developed comparable to tumors grown in control mice.[152] Although lack of FBG did not impair the growth and angiogenesis of the primary tumor, it did significantly reduce the metastatic potential of these cells in both experimental and spontaneous metastasis assays.[152,153] FBG deficiency may have contributed to diminished lung metastases by decreasing the adhesion and stability of the metastatic foci.[153] The thrombin inhibitor hirudin further decreased the metastatic potential in FBG-deficient mice, suggesting that nonclotting properties of thrombin (unrelated to FBG cleavage), such as PAR activation, contribute to metastasis.

Therapeutic applications

TF-targeted cancer therapy

Selective expression of TF on vascular endothelial cells and tumor cells of malignant, but not benign, tumors makes TF an ideal target for directed cancer therapeutics. Using a number of different approaches, several in vivo studies have demonstrated that TF-targeted cancer therapies can be efficacious.[154–158] Hu and Garen designed an immunoconjugate (icon) molecule that consisted of a mutated mouse FVII and the Fc effector domain of an IgG1 Ig.[156] After the icon was encoded in a replication-competent vector, it was injected into human prostate cancer and human melanoma xenograft tumors grown in SCID mice. The icon selectively localized to TF-expressing tumor cells and caused a cytolytic immune response against the Fc domain of the icon that resulted in significant tumor debulking. Nilsson and colleagues used antibody-mediated targeting of TF to the oncofetal extradomain B (ED-B) of fibronectin, expressed by blood vessels of malignant, but not benign, tissues, to induce thrombosis selectively at the tumor site.[154] This approach also produced significant tumor debulking, although residual tissue grew back in some of the mice. However, since this treatment produced low toxicity, higher treatment doses may improve efficacy. Although TF-targeted therapeutics have been evaluated only in animal models, they represent a novel strategy that holds significant promise for treating cancer patients.

Thrombotic complications of antiangiogenic agents

Since it is believed that all tumors require angiogenesis to grow and metastasize, targeting tumor vasculature with antiangiogenic agents has developed into a novel strategy for treating many cancers. Unlike standard chemotherapeutic agents that primarily elicit cytotoxic effects, antiangiogenic agents elicit fewer toxic side effects. As such, both animal studies and clinical trials have demonstrated that antiangiogenic agents are more effective when combined with standard chemotherapeutic agents. An alarming observation that has recently been reported in a number of clinical trials in which patients were treated with both antiangiogenic agents and standard chemotherapy is the unexpectedly high incidence of both arterial and venous thrombosis.[159–163] This serious complication has been observed with promising antiangiogenic agents such as SU5416,[162,163] the potent inhibitor of the vascular endothelial growth factor receptor 2 (VEGFR-2), and thalidomide,[159–161,164–167] a drug enjoying resurgent interest due to its ability to inhibit angiogenesis in multiple myeloma and other cancers. Although a prospective evaluation of VTE in cancer patients treated with these agents has not been published, VTE rates as high as 40% have been reported in some of these case series. It is plausible that what is occurring is synergism between these VEC-active agents and chemotherapy drugs that are toxic to VECs. Indeed, virtually all chemotherapeutic agents injected intravenously stimulate increased thrombin generation.[104] That the increase in thrombin generation observed in chemotherapy-treated patients is mediated largely by intravascular events is supported by the finding that this increase can be prevented by immediate pretreatment with intravenous unfractionated heparin.[104]

Therefore, adding anticoagulants to these combination therapies may help prevent some of these thrombotic complications.[160] Further stimulation for the addition of anticoagulants to cancer treatment regimens comes from recent experimental studies[168-171] and meta-analyses of various clinical trials.[172] These studies suggest that anticoagulants, such as low-molecular-weight heparins (LMWH), may possess antiangiogenic and/or antithrombotic effects that may help prolong patient survival. If the results of the current prospective, randomized, controlled trials of anticoagulant drugs in cancer support the findings of these earlier studies, then combination regimens of standard chemotherapeutics with anticoagulants may provide added benefit for control of tumor growth, while avoiding serious thrombotic complications.

Concluding remarks

Angiogenesis may be the central link between the coagulation cascade and tumorigenesis. Key players in the coagulation cascade, including TF, thrombin, and fibrin, induce angiogenesis via clotting-independent and/or clotting-dependent mechanisms. Targeting therapeutic modalities to one or more of these proteins may add to the armamentarium of novel approaches to controlling cancer, reducing the incidence of VTE, and thereby improving overall patient survival and quality of life.

Acknowledgment

This work was supported in part by a grant from Pharmacia Corporation.

References

1. Trousseau A. Phlegmasia alba dolens. In: Clinique medicale de l'Hôtel-Dieu de Paris, 2nd edn. (Baillière: Paris, 1865)654–712.

2. Morrissey J. Tissue factor: an enzyme cofactor and a true receptor. Thromb Haemost 2001; 86: 66–74.

3. Nemerson Y, Repke D. Tissue factor accelerates the activation of coagulation factor VII: the role of a bifunctional coagulation cofactor. Thromb Res 1985; 40:351–8.

4. Bajaj MS, Birktoft JJ, Steer SA et al. Structure and biology of tissue factor pathway inhibitor. Thromb Haemost 2001; 86:959–72.

5. Mast AE, Stadanlick JE, Lockett JM et al. Tissue factor pathway inhibitor binds to platelet thrombospondin-1. J Biol Chem 2000; 275:31715–21.

6. Shin JS, Abraham SN. Cell biology. Caveolae—not just crators in the cellular landscape. Science 2001; **293**:1447–8.

7. Sevinsky JR, Rao LV, Ruf W. Ligand-induced protease receptor translocation into caveolae: a mechanism for regulating cell surface proteolysis of the tissue factor-dependent coagulation pathway. J Cell Biol 1996; **133**: 293–304.

8. Carson SD, Bromberg ME. Tissue factor encryption/de-encryption is not altered in the absence of the cytoplasmic domain. Thromb Haemost 2000; **84**:657–63.

9. Wolberg AS, Monroe DM, Roberts HR et al. Tissue factor de-encryption: ionophore treatment induces changes in tissue factor activity by phosphatidylserine-dependent and -independent mechanisms. Blood Coagul Fibrinolysis 1999; **10**: 201–10.

10. Rao LV, Pendurthi UR. Tissue factor on cells. Blood Coagul Fibrinolysis 1998; **9**(Suppl 1): S27–35.

11. Nemerson Y, Giesen PL. Some thoughts about localization and expression of tissue factor. Blood Coagul Fibrinolysis 1998; **9**(Suppl 1): S45–7.

12. Bach RR. Mechanism of tissue factor activation on cells. Blood Coagul Fibrinolysis 1998; **9**(Suppl 1): S37–43.

13. Carson SD. Manifestation of cryptic fibroblast tissue factor occurs at detergent concentrations which dissolve the plasma membrane. Blood Coagul Fibrinolysis 1996; **7**:303–13.

14. Camera M, Giesen PL, Fallon J et al. Cooperation between VEGF and TNF-alpha is necessary for exposure of active tissue factor on the surface of human endothelial cells. Arterioscler Thromb Vasc Biol 1999; **19**:531–7.

15. Edgington TS, Mackman N, Brand K et al. The structural biology of expression and function of tissue factor. Thromb Haemost 1991; **66**:67–79.

16. Peppelenbosch MP, Versteeg HH. Cell biology of tissue factor, an unusual member of the cytokine receptor family. Trends Cardiovasc Med 2001; **11**:335–9.

17. Mueller BM, Reisfeld RA, Edgington TS et al. Expression of tissue factor by melanoma cells promotes efficient hematogenous metastasis. Proc Natl Acad Sci USA 1992; **89**:11832–6.

18. Kakkar AK, Chinswangwatanakul V, Lemoine NR et al. Role of tissue factor expression on tumour cell invasion and growth of experimental pancreatic adenocarcinoma. Br J Surg 1999; **86**:890–4.

19. Rickles F, Levine M, Dvorak H. Abnormalities of hemostasis in malignancy. In: Colman R, Hirsh J, Marder V et al, eds. Hemostasis and Thrombosis, 4th edn. (Lippincott Williams & Wilkins: Philadelphia, 2001)1131–52.

20. Guan M, Jin J, Su B et al. Tissue factor expression and angiogenesis in human gliomas. Clin Biochem 2002; **35**:321–5.

21. Guan M, Su B, Lu Y. Quantitative reverse transcription–PCR measurement of tissue factor mRNA in glioma. Mol Biotechnol 2002; **20**:123–9.

22. Ueno T, Toi M, Koike M et al. Tissue factor expression in breast cancer tissues: its correlation with prognosis and plasma concentration. Br J Cancer 2000; **83**:164–70.

23. Contrino J, Hair G, Kreutzer DL et al. In situ detection of tissue factor in vascular endothelial cells: correlation with the malignant phenotype of human breast disease. Nat Med 1996; **2**:209–15.

24. Sawada M, Miyake S, Ohdama S et al. Expression of tissue factor in non-small-cell lung cancers and its relationship to metastasis. Br J Cancer 1999; 79:472–7.

25. Koomagi R, Volm M. Tissue-factor expression in human non-small-cell lung carcinoma measured by immunohistochemistry: correlation between tissue factor and angiogenesis. Int J Cancer 1998; 79:19–22.

26. Hair GA, Padula S, Zeff R et al. Tissue factor expression in human leukemic cells. Leuk Res 1996; 20:1–11.

27. Nakasaki T, Wada H, Shigemori C et al. Expression of tissue factor and vascular endothelial growth factor is associated with angiogenesis in colorectal cancer. Am J Hematol 2002; 69:247–54.

28. Shigemori C, Wada H, Matsumoto K et al. Tissue factor expression and metastatic potential of colorectal cancer. Thromb Haemost 1998; 80:894–8.

29. Seto S, Onodera H, Kaido T et al. Tissue factor expression in human colorectal carcinoma: correlation with hepatic metastasis and impact on prognosis. Cancer 2000; 88: 295–301.

30. Kataoka H, Uchino H, Asada Y et al. Analysis of tissue factor and tissue factor pathway inhibitor expression in human colorectal carcinoma cell lines and metastatic sublines to the liver. Int J Cancer 1997; 72:878–84.

31. Ueda C, Hirohata Y, Kihara Y et al. Pancreatic cancer complicated by disseminated intravascular coagulation associated with production of tissue factor. J Gastroenterol 2001; 36:848–50.

32. Kakkar AK, Lemoine NR, Scully MF et al. Tissue factor expression correlates with histological grade in human pancreatic cancer. Br J Surg 1995; 82:1101–4.

33. Lwaleed BA, Cooper AJ. Tissue factor expression and multidrug resistance in cancer: two aspects of a common cellular response to a hostile milieu. Med Hypotheses 2000; 55:470–3.

34. Toomey JR, Kratzer KE, Lasky NM et al. Targeted disruption of the murine tissue factor gene results in embryonic lethality. Blood 1996; 88:1583–7.

35. Bugge TH, Xiao Q, Kombrinck KW et al. Fatal embryonic bleeding events in mice lacking tissue factor, the cell-associated initiator of blood coagulation. Proc Natl Acad Sci USA 1996; 93:6258–63.

36. Carmeliet P, Mackman N, Moons L et al. Role of tissue factor in embryonic blood vessel development. Nature 1996; 383:73–5.

37. Ferrara N, Carver-Moore K, Chen H et al. Heterozygous embryonic lethality induced by targeted inactivation of the VEGF gene. Nature 1996; 380:439–42.

38. Carmeliet P, Ferreira V, Breier G et al. Abnormal blood vessel development and lethality in embryos lacking a single VEGF allele. Nature 1996; 380:435–9.

39. Zhang Y, Deng Y, Luther T et al. Tissue factor controls the balance of angiogenic and antiangiogenic properties of tumor cells in mice. J Clin Invest 1994; 94:1320–7.

40. Shoji M, Abe K, Nawroth PP et al. Molecular mechanisms linking thrombosis and angiogenesis in cancer. Trends Cardiovasc Med 1997; 7:52–9.

41. Shoji M, Hancock WW, Abe K et al. Activation of coagulation and angiogenesis in cancer: immunohistochemical localization in situ of clotting proteins and vascular endothelial growth factor in human cancer. Am J Pathol 1998; 152: 399–411.

42. Abe K, Shoji M, Chen J et al. Regulation of vascular endothelial

growth factor production and angiogenesis by the cytoplasmic tail of tissue factor. Proc Natl Acad Sci USA 1999; **96**:8663–8.

43. Mechtcheriakova D, Wlachos A, Holzmuller H et al. Vascular endothelial growth factor-induced tissue factor expression in endothelial cells is mediated by EGR-1. Blood 1999; **93**:3811–23.

44. Blum S, Issbruker K, Willuweit A et al. An inhibitory role of phosphatidylinositol 3-kinase-signaling pathway in vascular endothelial growth factor-induced tissue factor expression. J Biol Chem 2001; **276**:33428–34.

45. Kim I, Oh JL, Ryu YS et al. Angiopoietin-1 negatively regulates expression and activity of tissue factor in endothelial cells. FASEB J 2002; **16**:126–8.

46. Rickles FR, Shoji M, Abe K. The role of the hemostatic system in tumor growth, metastasis, and angiogenesis: tissue factor is a bifunctional molecule capable of inducing both fibrin deposition and angiogenesis in cancer. Int J Hematol 2001; **73**:145–50.

47. Fernandez PM, Rickles FR. Tissue factor and angiogenesis in cancer. Curr Opin Hematol 2002; **9**:401–6.

48. Ollivier V, Bentolila S, Chabbat J et al. Tissue factor-dependent vascular endothelial growth factor production by human fibroblasts in response to activated factor VII. Blood 1998; **91**:2698–703.

49. Ollivier V, Chabbat J, Herbert JM et al. Vascular endothelial growth factor production by fibroblasts in response to factor VIIa binding to tissue factor involves thrombin and factor Xa. Arterioscler Thromb Vasc Biol 2000; **20**:1374–81.

50. Bromberg ME, Sundaram R, Homer RJ et al. Role of tissue factor in metastasis: functions of the cytoplasmic and extracellular

domains of the molecule. Thromb Haemost 1999; **82**:88–92.

51. Zioncheck TF, Roy S, Vehar GA. The cytoplasmic domain of tissue factor is phosphorylated by a protein kinase C-dependent mechanism. J Biol Chem 1992; **267**: 3561–4.

52. Ott I, Fischer EG, Miyagi Y et al. A role for tissue factor in cell adhesion and migration mediated by interaction with actin-binding protein 280. J Cell Biol 1998; **140**: 1241–53.

53. Bromberg ME, Konigsberg WH, Madison JF et al. Tissue factor promotes melanoma metastasis by a pathway independent of blood coagulation. Proc Natl Acad Sci USA 1995; **92**:8205–9.

54. Mueller BM, Ruf W. Requirement for binding of catalytically active factor VIIa in tissue factor-dependent experimental metastasis. J Clin Invest 1998; **101**:1372–8.

55. Coughlin SR. Thrombin signalling and protease-activated receptors. Nature 2000; **407**:258–64.

56. Maragoudakis ME, Tsopanoglou NE, Andriopoulou P. Mechanism of thrombin-induced angiogenesis. Biochem Soc Trans 2002; **30**: 173–7.

57. Rhim TY, Park CS, Kim E et al. Human prothrombin fragments 1 and 2 inhibit bFGF-induced BCE cell growth. Biochem Biophys Res Commun 1998; **252**:513–16.

58. Wang J, Zheng H, Ou X et al. Deficiency of microvascular thrombomodulin and upregulation of protease-activated receptor-1 in irradiated rat intestine: possible link between endothelial dysfunction and chronic radiation fibrosis. Am J Pathol 2002; **160**:2063–72.

59. Tsopanoglou NE, Pipili-Synetos E, Maragodakis ME. Thrombin promotes angiogenesis by a mechanism independent of fibrin

formation. Am J Physiol 1993; **264**:C1302–7.

60. Haralabopoulos GC, Grant DC, Kleinman HK et al. Thrombin promotes endothelial cell alignment in Matrigel in vitro and angiogenesis in vivo. Am J Physiol 1997; **273**:C239–45.

61. Mohle R, Green D, Moore MA et al. Constitutive production and thrombin-induced release of vascular endothelial growth factor by human megakaryocytes and platelets. Proc Natl Acad Sci USA 1997; **94**:663–8.

62. Maloney JP, Silliman CC, Ambruso DR et al. In vitro release of vascular endothelial growth factor during platelet aggregation. Am J Physiol 1998; **275**:H1054–61.

63. Richard DE, Vouret-Craviari V, Pouyssegur J. Angiogenesis and G-protein-coupled receptors: signals that bridge the gap. Oncogene 2001; **20**:1156–62.

64. Huang YQ, Li JJ, Hu L et al. Thrombin induces increased expression and secretion of VEGF from human FS4 fibroblasts, DU145 prostate cells and CHRF megakaryocytes. Thromb Haemost 2001; **86**:1094–8.

65. Yamahata H, Takeshima H, Kuratsu J et al. The role of thrombin in the neo-vascularization of malignant gliomas: an intrinsic modulator for the up-regulation of vascular endothelial growth factor. Int J Oncol 2002; **20**:921–8.

66. Herbert JM, Dupuy E, Laplace MC et al. Thrombin induces endothelial cell growth via both a proteolytic and a non-proteolytic pathway. Biochem J 1994; **303**:227–31.

67. Huang YQ, Li JJ, Hu L et al. Thrombin induces increased expression and secretion of angiopoietin-2 from human umbilical vein endothelial cells. Blood 2002; **99**:1646–50.

68. Tsopanoglou NE, Maragoudakis ME. On the mechanism of thrombin-induced angiogenesis. Potentiation of vascular endothelial growth factor activity on endothelial cells by up-regulation of its receptors. J Biol Chem 1999; **274**: 23969–76.

69. Bogatcheva NV, Garcia JG, Verin AD. Molecular mechanisms of thrombin-induced endothelial cell permeability. Biochemistry (Mosc) 2002; **67**:75–84.

70. Carter AJ, Eisert WG, Muller TH. Thrombin stimulates inositol phosphate accumulation and prostacyclin synthesis in human endothelial cells from umbilical vein but not from omentum. Thromb Haemost 1989; **61**:122–6.

71. Jaffe EA, Grulich J, Weksler BB et al. Correlation between thrombin-induced prostacyclin production and inositol triphosphate and cytosolic free calcium levels in cultured human endothelial cells. J Biol Chem 1987; **262**:8557–65.

72. Lum H, Aschner JL, Phillips PG et al. Time course of thrombin-induced increase in endothelial permeability: relationship to Ca^{2+}_i and inositol polyphosphates. Am J Physiol 1992; **263**:L219–25.

73. Keogh RJ, Houliston RA, Wheeler-Jones CP. Thrombin-stimulated Pyk2 phosphorylation in human endothelium is dependent on intracellular calcium and independent of protein kinase C and Src kinases. Biochem Biophys Res Commun 2002; **294**:1001–8.

74. Maragoudakis ME, Kraniti N, Giannopoulou E et al. Modulation of angiogenesis and progelatinase a by thrombin receptor mimetics and antagonists. Endothelium 2001; **8**:195–205.

75. Brooks PC, Strombald S, Sanders LC et al. Localization of matrix met-

alloproteinase MMP-2 to the surface of invasive cells by interaction with integrin alpha v beta 3. Cell 1996; **85**:683–93.

76. Even-Ram S, Uziely B, Cohen P et al. Thrombin receptor overexpression in malignant and physiological invasion processes. Nat Med 1998; **4**:909–14.

77. Wojtukiewicz MZ, Tang DG, Nelson KK et al. Thrombin enhances tumor cell adhesive and metastatic properties via increased alpha IIb beta 3 expression on the cell surface. Thromb Res 1992; **68**:233–45.

78. Wojtukiewicz MZ, Tang DG, Ciarelli JJ et al. Thrombin increases the metastatic potential of tumor cells. Int J Cancer 1993; **54**:793–806.

79. Hughes PE, Pfaff M. Integrin affinity modulation. Trends Cell Biol 1998; **8**:359–64.

80. Hattori R, Hamilton KK, Fugate RD et al. Stimulated secretion of endothelial von Willebrand factor is accompanied by rapid redistribution to the cell surface of the intracellular granule membrane protein GMP-140. J Biol Chem 1989; **264**:7768–71.

81. Stenberg PE, McEver RP, Shuman MA et al. A platelet alpha-granule membrane protein (GMP-140) is expressed on the plasma membrane after activation. J Cell Biol 1985; **101**:880–6.

82. Henn V, Slupsky JR, Grafe M et al. CD40 ligand on activated platelets triggers an inflammatory reaction of endothelial cells. Nature 1998; **391**:591–4.

83. Daniel TO, Gibbs VC, Milfay DF et al. Thrombin stimulates c-sis gene expression in microvascular endothelial cells. J Biol Chem 1986; **261**:9579–82.

84. Papadimitriou E, Manolopoulos VG, Hayman GT et al. Thrombin modulates vectorial secretion of extracellular matrix proteins in cultured endothelial cells. Am J Physiol 1997; **272**:C1112–22.

85. Nierodzik ML, Plotkin A, Kajumo F et al. Thrombin stimulates tumor-platelet adhesion in vitro and metastasis in vivo. J Clin Invest 1991; **87**:229–36.

86. Nierodzik ML, Kajumo F, Karpatkin S. Effect of thrombin treatment of tumor cells on adhesion of tumor cells to platelets in vitro and tumor metastasis in vivo. Cancer Res 1992; **52**:3267–72.

87. Nierodzik ML, Chen K, Takeshita K et al. Protease-activated receptor 1 (PAR-1) is required and rate-limiting for thrombin-enhanced experimental pulmonary metastasis. Blood 1998; **92**:3694–3700.

88. Darrow AL, Fung-Leung WP, Ye RD et al. Biological consequences of thrombin receptor deficiency in mice. Thromb Haemost 1996; **76**:860–6.

89. Damiano BP, Cheung WM, Santulli RJ et al. Cardiovascular responses mediated by protease-activated receptor-2 (PAR-2) and thrombin receptor (PAR-1) are distinguished in mice deficient in PAR-2 or PAR-1. J Pharmacol Exp Ther 1999; **288**:671–8.

90. Connolly AJ, Ishihara H, Kahn ML et al. Role of thrombin receptor in development and evidence for a second receptor. Nature 1996; **381**:516–9.

91. Kahn ML, Zheng YW, Huang W et al. A dual thrombin receptor system for platelet activation. Nature 1998; **394**:690–4.

92. D'Andrea MR, Derian CK, Santulli RJ et al. Differential expression of protease-activated receptors-1 and -2 in stromal fibroblasts of normal, benign, and malignant human tissues. Am J Pathol 2001; **158**:2031–41.

93. Riewald M, Kravchenko VV, Petrovan RJ et al. Gene induction

by coagulation factor Xa is mediated by activation of protease-activated receptor 1. Blood 2001; **97**:3109–16.

94. O'Brien PJ, Molino M, Kahn M et al. Protease activated receptors: theme and variations. Oncogene 2001; **20**:1570–81.

95. O'Brien PJ, Prevost N, Molino M et al. Thrombin responses in human endothelial cells. Contributions from receptors other than PAR1 include the transactivation of PAR2 by thrombin-cleaved PAR1. J Biol Chem 2000; **275**:13502–9.

96. Riewald M, Ruf W. Orchestration of coagulation protease signaling by tissue factor. Trends Cardiovasc Med 2002; **12**:149–54.

97. Cleary DB, Trumbo TA, Maurer MC. Protease-activated receptor 4-like peptides bind to thrombin through an optimized interaction with the enzyme active site surface. Arch Biochem Biophys 2002; **403**: 179–88.

98. Nakanishi-Matsui M, Zheng YW, Sulciner DJ et al. PAR3 is a cofactor for PAR4 activation by thrombin. Nature 2000; **404**: 609–13.

99. Nagy JA, Brown LF, Senger DR et al. Pathogenesis of tumor stroma generation: a critical role for leaky blood vessels and fibrin deposition. Biochim Biophys Acta 1989; **948**:305–26.

100. Myers TJ, Rickles FR, Barb C et al. Fibrinopeptide A in acute leukemia: relationship of activation of blood coagulation to disease activity. Blood 1981; **57**:518–25.

101. Edwards RL, Rickles FR, Cronlund M. Abnormalities of blood coagulation in patients with cancer. Mononuclear cell tissue factor generation. J Lab Clin Med 1981; **98**:917–28.

102. Edwards RL, Rickles FR, Moritz TE et al. Abnormalities of blood coagulation tests in patients with cancer. Am J Clin Pathol 1987; **88**: 596–602.

103. Rickles FR, Falanga A. Molecular basis for the relationship between thrombosis and cancer. Thromb Res 2001; **102**:V215–24.

104. Edwards RL, Klaus M, Matthews E et al. Heparin abolishes the chemotherapy-induced increase in plasma fibrinopeptide A levels. Am J Med 1990; **89**:25–8.

105. Yoda Y, Abe T. Fibrinopeptide A (FPA) level and fibrinogen kinetics in patients with malignant disease. Thromb Haemost 1981; **46**:706–9.

106. Bardos H, Molnar P, Csecsei G et al. Fibrin deposition in primary and metastatic human brain tumours. Blood Coagul Fibrinolysis 1996; **7**:536–48.

107. Wojtukiewicz MZ, Zacharski LR, Memoli VA et al. Fibrin formation on vessel walls in hyperplastic and malignant prostate tissues. Cancer 1991; **67**:1377–83.

108. Dvorak HF, Senger DR, Dvorak AM. Fibrin as a component of the tumor stroma: origins and biological significance. Cancer Metastasis Rev 1983; **2**:41–73.

109. Wojtukiewicz MZ, Zacharski LR, Memoli VA et al. Indirect activation of blood coagulation in colon cancer. Thromb Haemost 1989; **62**: 1062–6.

110. Costantini V, Zacharski LR, Memoli VA et al. Fibrinogen deposition and macrophage-associated fibrin formation in malignant and non-malignant lymphoid tissue. J Lab Clin Med 1992; **119**:124–31.

111. Wojtukiewicz MZ, Zacharski LR, Memoli VA et al. Absence of components of coagulation and fibrinolysis pathways in situ in mesothelioma. Thromb Res 1989; **55**:279–84.

112. Costantini V, Zacharski LR, Memoli VA et al. Fibrinogen deposition

without thrombin generation in primary human breast cancer tissue. Cancer Res 1991; **51**:349–53.

113. Bootle-Wilbraham CA, Tazzyman S, Marshall JM et al. Fibrinogen E-fragment inhibits the migration and tubule formation of human dermal microvascular endothelial cells in vitro. Cancer Res 2000; **60**: 4719–24.

114. Medved L, Tsurupa G, Yakovlev S. Conformational changes upon conversion of fibrinogen into fibrin. The mechanisms of exposure of cryptic sites. Ann NY Acad Sci 2001; **936**: 185–204.

115. Doolittle RF. Fibrinogen and fibrin. Sci Am 1981; **245**:126–35.

116. Thompson WD, Smith EB, Stirk CM et al. Angiogenic activity of fibrin degradation products is located in fibrin fragment E. J Pathol 1992; **168**:47–53.

117. Schlager SI, Dray S. Complete local tumor regression with antibody to fibrin fragment E. J Immunol 1975; **115**:976–81.

118. Oya M, Akiyama Y, Yanagida T et al. Plasma D-dimer level in patients with colorectal cancer: its role as a tumor marker. Surg Today 1998; **28**:373–8.

119. Taguchi O, Gabazza EC, Yasui H et al. Prognostic significance of plasma D-dimer levels in patients with lung cancer. Thorax 1997; **52**: 563–5.

120. Blackwell K, Haroon Z, Broadwater G et al. Plasma D-dimer levels in operable breast cancer patients correlate with clinical stage and axillary lymph node status. J Clin Oncol 2000; **18**:600–8.

121. Dirix LY, Salgado R, Weytjens R et al. Plasma fibrin D-dimer levels correlate with tumour volume, progression rate and survival in patients with metastatic breast cancer. Br J Cancer 2002; **86**: 389–95.

122. Virchow R. Abhaldungen zur Wissensdiaffichen Medicine. (Meidinger Sohn: Frankfurt,1856).

123. Altieri DC, Mannucci PM, Capitanio AM. Binding of fibrinogen to human monocytes. J Clin Invest 1986; **78**:968–76.

124. Degen JL, Drew AF, Palumbo JS et al. Genetic manipulation of fibrinogen and fibrinolysis in mice. Ann N Y Acad Sci 2001; **936**:276–90.

125. Dejana E, Languino LR, Polentarutti N et al. Interaction between fibrinogen and cultured endothelial cells. Induction of migration and specific binding. J Clin Invest 1985; **75**: 11–8.

126. Brown LF, Lanir N, McDonagh J et al. Fibroblast migration in fibrin gel matrices. Am J Pathol 1993; **142**: 273–83.

127. Donaldson DJ, Mahan JT, Amrani DL et al. Further studies on the interaction of migrating keratinocytes with fibrinogen. Cell Adhes Commun 1994; **2**:299-308.

128. Naito M, Funaki C, Hayashi T et al. Substrate-bound fibrinogen, fibrin and other cell attachment-promoting proteins as a scaffold for cultured vascular smooth muscle cells. Atherosclerosis 1992; **96**: 227–34.

129. Felding-Habermann B, Ruggeri ZM, Cheresh DA. Distinct biological consequences of integrin alpha v beta 3-mediated melanoma cell adhesion to fibrinogen and its plasmic fragments. J Biol Chem 1992; **267**:5070–7.

130. Henschen A, Lottspeich F, Kehl M et al. Covalent structure of fibrinogen. Ann NY Acad Sci 1983; **408**: 28–43.

131. Altieri DC, Duperray A, Plescia J et al. Structural recognition of a novel fibrinogen gamma chain sequence (117–133) by intercellular adhesion molecule-1 mediates leukocyte–endothelial interaction. J Biol Chem 1995; **270**:696–9.

132. Odrljin TM, Shainoff JR, Lawrence SO et al. Thrombin cleavage enhances exposure of a heparin binding domain in the N-terminus of the fibrin beta chain. Blood 1996; **88**:2050–61.

133. Odrljin TM, Francis CW, Sporn LA et al. Heparin-binding domain of fibrin mediates its binding to endothelial cells. Arterioscler thromb Vasc Biol 1996; **16**:1544–51.

134. Shattil SJ, Kashiwagi H, Pampori N. Integrin signaling: the platelet paradigm. Blood 1998; **91**:2645–57.

135. Phillips DR, Charo IF, Parise LV et al. The platelet membrane glyco-protein IIb–IIIa complex. Blood 1988; **71**:831–43.

136. Bennett JS, Vilaire G. Exposure of platelet fibrinogen receptors by ADP and epinephrine. J Clin Invest 1979; **64**:1393–1401.

137. Gorlatov S, Medved L. Interaction of fibrin(ogen) with the endothelial cell receptor VE-cadherin: mapping of the receptor-binding site in the NH$_2$-terminal portions of the fibrin beta chains. Biochemistry 2002; **41**:4107–16.

138. Bach TL, Barsigian C, Yaen CH et al. Endothelial cell VE-cadherin functions as a receptor for the beta15–42 sequence of fibrin. J Biol Chem 1998; **273**;30719–28.

139. Hantgan R, Simpson-Haidaris P, Francis C et al. Fibrinogen structure and physiology. In: Colman R, Hirsch J, Marder V et al, eds. Hemostasis and Thrombosis. Basic Principles and Clinical Practice, 4th edn. (Lippincott Williams & Wilkins: Philadelphia, 2001)203–32.

140. Martinez J, Ferber A, Bach TL et al. Interaction of fibrin with VE-cad-herin. Ann NY Acad Sci 2001; **936**:386–405.

141. van Hinsbergh VW, Collen A, Koolwijk P. Role of fibrin matrix in angiogenesis. Ann NY Acad Sci 2001; **936**:426–37.

142. Clark RA, Tonnesen MG, Gailit J et al. Transient functional expression of alpha V beta 3 on vascular cells during wound repair. Am J Pathol 1996; **148**:1407–21.

143. Dallabrida SM, De Sousa MA, Farrell DH. Expression of antisense to integrin subunit beta 3 inhibits microvascular endothelial cell capil-lary tube formation in fibrin. J Biol Chem 2000; **275**:32281–8.

144. Feng X, Clark RA, Galanakis D et al. Fibrin and collagen differentially regulate human dermal microvas-cular endothelial cell integrins: stabilization of alpha v beta 3 mRNA by fibrin 1. J Invest Dermatol 1999; **113**:913–99.

145. Dvorak HF, Harvey VS, Estrella P et al. Fibrin containing gels induce angiogenesis. Implications for tumor stroma generation and wound healing. Lab Invest 1987; **57**:673–86.

146. Dvorak HF. Tumors: wounds that do not heal. Similarities between tumor stroma generation and wound healing. N Engl J Med 1986; **315**:1650–9.

147. Sahni A, Baker CA, Sporn LA et al. Fibrinogen and fibrin protect fibro-blast growth factor-2 from pro-teolytic degradation. Thromb Haemost 2000; **83**:736–41.

148. Sahni A, Sporn LA, Francis CW. Potentiation of endothelial cell pro-liferation by fibrin(ogen)-bound fibroblast growth factor-2. J Biol Chem 1999; **274**:14936–41.

149. Sahni A, Francis CW. Vascular endothelial growth factor binds to fibrinogen and fibrin and stimulates endothelial cell proliferation. Blood 2000; **96**:3772–8.

150. Lalla RV, Goralnick SJ, Tanzer ML et al. Fibrin induces IL-8 expression from human oral squamous cell carcinoma cells. Oral Oncol 2001; **37**:234–42.

151. Contrino J, Goralnick S, Qi J et al. Fibrin induction of tissue factor

expression in human vascular endothelial cells. Circulation 1997; **96**:605–13.

152. Palumbo JS, Kombrinck KW, Drew AF et al. Fibrinogen is an important determinant of the metastatic potential of circulating tumor cells. Blood 2000; **96**:3302–9.

153. Palumbo JS, Degen JL. Fibrinogen and tumor cell metastasis. Haemostasis 2001; **31**(Suppl 1): 11–15.

154. Nilsson F, Kosmehl H, Zardi L et al. Targeted delivery of tissue factor to the ED-B domain of fibronectin, a marker of angiogenesis, mediates the infarction of solid tumors in mice. Cancer Res 2001; **61**: 711–16.

155. Hu Z, Sun Y, Garen A. Targeting tumor vasculature endothelial cells and tumor cells for immunotherapy of human melanoma in a mouse xenograft model. Proc Natl Acad Sci USA 1999; **96**:8161–6.

156. Hu Z, Garen A. Targeting tissue factor on tumor vascular endothelial cells and tumor cells for immunotherapy in mouse models of prostatic cancer. Proc Natl Acad Sci USA 2001; **98**:12180–5.

157. Huang X, Molema G, King S et al. Tumor infarction in mice by antibody-directed targeting of tissue factor to tumor vasculature. Science 1997; **275**:547–50.

158. Zhang Y, Deng Y, Wendt T et al. Intravenous somatic gene transfer with antisense tissue factor restores blood flow by reducing tumor necrosis factor-induced tissue factor expression and fibrin deposition in mouse meth-A sarcoma. J Clin Invest 1996; **97**: 2213–24.

159. Zangari M, Siegel E, Barlogie B et al. Thrombogenic activity of doxorubicin in myeloma patients receiving thalidomide: implications for therapy. Blood 2002; **100**: 1168–71.

160. Zangari M, Anaissie E, Barlogie B et al. Increased risk of deep-vein thrombosis in patients with multiple myeloma receiving thalidomide and chemotherapy. Blood 2001; **98**: 1614–15.

161. Osman K, Comenzo R, Rajkumar SV. Deep venous thrombosis and thalidomide therapy for multiple myeloma. N Engl J Med 2001; **344**:1951–2.

162. Marx GM, Steer CB, Harper P et al. Unexpected serious toxicity with chemotherapy and antiangiogenic combinations: time to take stock! J Clin Oncol 2002; **20**:1446–8.

163. Kuenen BC, Rosen L, Smit EF et al. Dose-finding and pharmacokinetic study of cisplatin, gemcitabine, and SU5416 in patients with solid tumors. J Clin Oncol 2002; **20**:1657–67 [Reply: 3042–3].

164. Cavo M, Zamagni E, Cellini C et al. Deep-vein thrombosis in patients with multiple myeloma receiving first-line thalidomide–dexamethasone therapy. Blood 2002; **100**: 2272–3.

165. Kaushal V, Kohli M, Zangari M et al. Endothelial dysfunction in antiangiogenesis-associated thrombosis. J Clin Oncol 2002; **20**:3042.

166. Escudier B, Lassau N, Leborgne S et al. Thalidomide and venous thrombosis. Ann Intern Med 2002; **136**:711.

167. Urbauer E, Kaufmann H, Nosslinger T et al. Thromboembolic events during treatment with thalidomide. Blood 2002; **99**: 4247–8.

168. Varki NM, Varki A. Heparin inhibition of selectin-mediated interactions during the hematogenous phase of carcinoma metastasis: rationale for clinical studies in humans. Semin Thromb Hemost 2002; **28**:53–66.

169. Collen A, Smorenburg SM, Peters E et al. Unfractionated and low molecular weight heparin affect fib-

rin structure and angiogenesis in vitro. Cancer Res 2000; **60**: 6196–200.

170. Mousa SA. Anticoagulants in thrombosis and cancer: the missing link. Semin Thromb Hemost 2002; **28**:45–52.

171. Norrby K, Ostergaard P. Basic-fibroblast-growth-factor-mediated de novo angiogeneis is more effec-

tively suppressed by low- molecular-weight than by high-molecular-weight heparin. Int J Microcirc Clin Exp 1996; **16**:8–15.

172. Hettiarachchi RJ, Smorenburg SM, Ginsberg J et al. Do heparins do more than just treat thrombosis? The influence of heparins on cancer spread. Thromb Haemost 1999; **82**:947–52.

7

Risk of cancer in patients presenting with venous thromboembolism

Andrea Piccioli and Paolo Prandoni

Introduction

The important relationship between cancer and venous thromboembolism (VTE) has been well recognized since Trousseau's time and has been confirmed and documented.[1] Cancer and VTE can be schematically reported as a bipolar item in which the two entities are strictly linked together by a two-way network of interconnections (Figure 7.1).

In fact, it has been clearly demonstrated that cancer patients experience a higher risk of developing a venous thromboembolic event than noncancer patients. Moreover, the most common situations that put cancer patients at risk of developing VTE are well defined and documented: immobilization due to poor physical condition or hospitalization, surgery, chemotherapy, or indwelling central venous lines.

There is also firm evidence of the increased risk of subsequent clinically overt malignancy during the follow-up of patients experiencing a venous thrombotic event, when compared to the general population, particularly patients experiencing idiopathic deep-vein thrombosis (DVT). Newly discovered malignancies during follow-up of these patients are

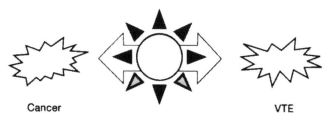

Cancer   VTE

Figure 7.1

Cancer and venous thromboembolism (VTE).

not limited to certain subtypes, but involve virtually all of the body systems.[2]

The present chapter focuses on the risk of cancer in patients presenting with VTE; it provides pathogenetic plausibility and speculates on the clinical implications, considering historical background, assessing present knowledge, and reflecting on future perspectives.

Historical background

The mid-nineteenth century was the period of important discoveries on the pathogenesis of thromboembolism, especially thanks to the pathophysiological finding of Rudolf Virchow on the causes of blood hypercoagulability. Accordingly, the interest of the scientific world was kept focused on the topic of hemostasis and thrombosis.

In this period, Armand Trousseau was the first to recognize a causal relationship between VTE and cancer.[3] As this author himself described, VTE may be a manifestation of occult malignancy as well as a complication of known cancer. In a lecture in Paris (1865), he stated: 'When you are in doubt about the nature of the disease of the stomach, when you hesitate between a chronic gastritis, a simple ulcer, and a carcinoma, a phlegmasia alba dolens occurring in the leg or arm will put an end to your doubt and you will be able to assert positively that cancer is present.' This latter occurrence is termed 'Trousseau's phenomenon' or 'Trousseau's syndrome', in which thrombophlebitis (phlegmasia alba dolens) is regarded as an epiphenomenon of hidden gastric or visceral carcinoma. Trousseau himself experienced thrombophlebitis of the leg in January 1867 and recognized the prognosis of the disorder.

After this 'light in the darkness', we have to wait until 1935 for the reported observation by Illtyd James and Matheson[4] that VTE may be a sign of occult malignancy. In 1944, Cooper and Barker re-emphasized the point, reporting that, in the absence of known risk factors, spontaneous peripheral thrombophlebitis, among patients 50 years or older, warrants a careful search for visceral carcinoma.[5] In 1951, a retrospective investigation was published on the prognosis and morbidity of thrombophlebitis.[6]

However, it took another three decades for proper cohort studies to appear in the literature; in 1982, Gore and colleagues observed that in patients with unexplained pulmonary embolism, cancer is often detected within two years of follow-up.[7] Over the last two decades, a number of studies have appeared in the literature, which have clearly demonstrated that the incidence of cancer after confirmation of VTE is higher than that of the general population. Moreover, studies performed over the past two decades have clearly demonstrated that the incidence of newly dis-

Table 7.1 Incidence of occult cancer after VTE diagnosis.

References	Cancer (all VTE)[a]	Cancer (secondary VTE)[a]	Cancer (idiopathic VTE)[a]
Aderka et al[8]	11/83 (13.3)	2/48 (4.2)	9/35 (25.7)
Prandoni et al[9]	13/250 (5.2)	2/105 (1.9)	11/145 (7.6)
Ahmed and Mohyuddin[10]	3/196 (1.5)	0/83 (0.0)	3/113 (2.7)
Monreal et al[11]	8/659 (1.2)	4/563 (0.7)	4/96 (4.2)
Hettiarachchi et al[12]	13/326 (4.0)	3/171 (1.8)	10/155 (6.5)
Rajan et al[13]	21/264 (8.0)	8/112 (7.1)	13/152 (8.6)
Schulman et al[14]	111/854 (13.0)	18/230 (5.6)	93/534 (17.0)

[a]Percentages in parentheses.

covered cancer is much higher in the follow-up of patients with idiopathic VTE than in patients suffering from secondary VTE (Table 7.1).[8–14]

Pathogenesis of VTE in cancer

Active cancer is often associated with a hypercoagulable state, which perturbs the homeostatic balance between anticoagulant and procoagulant forces, creating a prothrombotic state. This involves complex tumor-specific clot-promoting mechansims, which have been clearly demonstrated in tumor models in animals and in cell cultures.[15]

The factors believed to raise the thrombotic potential in cancer patients are complex and reflect the interaction of different mechanisms based on the triad first outlined by Virchow: hypercoagulability, vessel-wall injuries, and venous stasis.[16]

Malignant cells can perturb the clotting system, either directly by synthesizing and releasing clot-promoting molecules or indirectly by cellular interactions. All the mechanisms are not entirely understood; however, intensive research on the topic has greatly improved our understanding of tumor cell prothrombotic properties. In fact, the literature describes many procoagulant molecules associated with tumor cells or tumor-associated macrophages. The interaction between tumor cells and host cells involves direct cell–cell interaction or indirect mechanisms by cytokine release.

Vessel-wall injuries in cancer patients may be due to surgical procedures, chemotherapy, or indwelling central venous lines.[15,17]

Venous stasis, also present in cancer patients, is due to immobilization or derives from vessel compression by a bulky tumor; it increases blood viscosity by preventing activated coagulation factors from being eluted and cleared from the normal blood flow.[1,2]

Multidisciplinary research is underway on this topic, since a clear understanding of the pathogenesis of the hypercoagulable state in cancer patients is crucial to future development of antithrombotic strategies in this setting.

Present knowledge

Thanks to etiopathogenetic knowledge and clinical trials addressing the topic of thrombosis and cancer, there is now conclusive evidence of the close relationship between VTE and cancer. It has been established that the incidence of cancer among patients with suspected VTE is higher in patients with objectively confirmed diagnosis than in those in whom the diagnosis was rejected by objective tests. If the presence of VTE does flag for hidden cancer, it could be expected that the incidence of cancer would be increased in the nearly 1-year period following the thrombotic event, and would subside thereafter. These assertions are in keeping with the data outlined in the 1980s by Aderka et al[8] and Goldberg et al,[18] who found the incidence of cancer in these patients to be as high as, respectively, 13% and 5.7% in the 3-year period after the thrombotic event. Two large population-based registries[19,20] have provided clear evidence that the incidence of cancer is increased in patients with VTE during the first year of follow-up. In fact, they provide a standardized incidence ratio (SIR) of newly diagnosed cancers as compared with the general population in the first year as high as 4.4 and 2.1, respectively.

Moreover, studies performed in the past two decades have demonstrated that patients with idiopathic VTE exhibit a higher risk of harboring a neoplasm, as becomes apparent during the follow-up after the thrombotic event, when compared with secondary VTE. Its incidence in patients in whom a routinary initial screening at the time of observation for VTE is negative is as high as about 10% (Table 7.1). These malignancies are not limited to certain subtypes but involve virtually all body systems.

Clinical spinoff

These challenging data and their reverberations in national and international scientific congresses have led physicians to consider with suspicion otherwise-healthy patients presenting with a first episode of idiopathic VTE. At the same time, they have led to a long-standing and continuing debate on the question of whether or not to screen patients presenting with a first episode of idiopathic VTE, to highlight as soon as possible any hidden neoplasm. In fact, to give a convincing answer to the question, we need to answer other important questions: we need to know what percentage of cancers can be detected by the extensive screening, and at what stage. Moreover, given the fact that patients undergoing extensive screening procedures may suffer discomfort and morbidity from the screening procedures themselves, and that the costs are high, extensive screening may be widely recommended if it demonstrates an impact on cancer-related mortality, thereby modifying the natural history of the pathology.

At present and in the recent past, attending physicians, aware of the possible presence of a hidden cancer among patients presenting with idiopathic VTE and conscious of its importance, have adopted a high index of suspicion of the presence of underlying malignancy in these patients when performing simple, safe, and inexpensive routine tests. Other physicians have ordered some additional tests aimed at detecting treatable cancers, guided by good clinical practice or relying on the very few available data on the topic, given the fact that no guidelines are available.

Concomitant diagnosis of cancer

By routine assessment

In patients presenting with VTE, the prevalence of cancer, not known before the thrombotic event and disclosed by routine assessment at the time of referral, is documented by literature data that vary among the available studies[9-11] (Table 7.2). These variations may derive from different routine schedules (some more extended and others less extended) performed at baseline. Anyway, the average routine screening performed comprised a careful medical history, physical examination, simple hematochemical laboratory tests, urinalysis, and chest radiography. Variations between studies may reflect different patient characteristics in different study cohorts (especially differences in age, since it is well known that the prevalence of cancers varies widely over age-grouped people).

By additional tests

The available literature data seem to support the performance of additional tests after the routine schedule usually performed at the time of referral for index VTE. Four studies have systematically performed additional screening procedures for cancer at the time of thrombosis among patients presenting with VTE. Moreover, the frequency of newly discovered malignancy was impressively high, especially for idiopathic VTE (Table 7.2). Bastounis and colleagues combined physical examinations, and hematochemical analysis with carcinoembryonic antigen (CEA) and CT of abdomen and pelvis in all patients with DVT.[21] A neoplastic disease was found at the time of referral for index DVT in 22/293 patients.

Table 7.2 Cancer identification at the time of VTE.

References	Cancer by routine assessment[a]	Cancer by routine plus extensive screening[a]
Bastounis et al[21]	13/293 (4.4)	22/293 (7.5)
Monreal et al[22]	8/113 (7.1)	12/113 (10.6)
Monreal et al[11]	7/112 (6.3)	22/112 (19.6)
Sanella and O'Connor[23]	4/21 (19.0)	11/21 (52.4)

[a]Percentages in parentheses.

The two studies by Monreal et al,[22] which employed as additional tests abdominal ultrasound and CT, together with esophago-gastro-duodenoscopy (EGDS), had the same results. In a retrospective evaluation of 237 patients with DVT, 21 of whom experienced idiopathic DVT, Sanella and colleagues[23] have found that cancer was present in 4 patients in whom routine tests were abnormal, and in 7/17 patients who were asymptomatic, with the help of a CT scan. The striking fact is that in these studies, when performing additional tests at baseline, more cancers were identified and there was a lower incidence of cancers detected later. In view of these data, it seems worthwhile to perform extensive screening batteries in this setting; it should be noted that these nonrandomized studies could not give any probative information on patient survival, which could be addressed only by prospective, randomized, follow-up studies.

In 1987, Barosi et al published a decision analysis,[24] testing for occult cancer in patients with idiopathic VTE and observing a possible gain in life expectancy thanks to dedicated screening programs in males over 60 for cancer of the prostate, bladder, and colon, and for females over 60 for cancer of the endometrium, breast, and colon.

The SOMIT study

With the aim of contributing to the solution of this important problem, a multicenter, randomized clinical trial[25] bas been undertaken comparing the strategy of an extensive screening (Table 7.3) with no further testing for malignant disease. Patients allocated to the non-extensive group (and their physicians) were not discouraged from searching for malignant disease, and any additional test performed for this purpose among this group was carefully recorded. Hence, 201 patients with idiopathic VTE in whom a routine initial evaluation did not reveal malignancy were randomly allocated to either extensive diagnostic screening ($n = 99$) or no further testing ($n = 102$), and were followed up for 2 years. In the extensive

Table 7.3 Extensive screening battery in the SOMIT study.

Ultrasound of abdomen and pelvis
CT scan of abdomen and pelvis
Gastroscopy or double-contrast barium swallow
Colonoscopy or sigmoidoscopy followed by barium enema
Hemoccult
Sputum cytology and tumor markers (carcinoembryonic antigen, α-fetoprotein, CA125)
Mammography and Pap smear test for women
Transabdominal ultrasound of the prostate and prostate-specific antigen for men

screening group, 13 patients (13.1%) had an early detection of a histolog-ically confirmed malignancy (in 10 cases revealed by CT scan of the abdomen and pelvis), and a further malignancy (1%) became apparent during follow-up. Therefore, 13 of the 14 malignancies, which became apparent in the extensive screening group, were identified at the time of screening, showing a sensitivity of initial screening of 93%. In the control group, a total of 10 (9.8%) malignancies became symptomatic during fol-low-up. Cancer-related mortality occurred in 2 (2%) of the 99 patients of the extensive screening group versus 4 (3.9%) of the 102 control patients, for an absolute difference of 1.9% (95% confidence interval [CI] −5.5 to 10.9%). The cluster of cancer-related mortality, presence of objectively documented residual, or recurrent malignancy occurred in 5 (5.1%) of the 99 patients of the extensive screening group as compared with 8 (7.9%) of the 102 control patients, for an absolute difference of 2.8% (95% CI, ± 6.3–13.4%).

From the results of this prospective study, we can say that the use of extensive screening for malignancy in patients with idiopathic VTE is worthwhile to identify hidden malignancies, since a substantial propor-tion of occult cancer has been discovered, and many of these cases were in a relatively early phase, allowing possible curative treatment. If we stratify patients by group, we can say that the risk of occult cancer was higher in elderly patients and in those without thrombophilic condi-tions. Given the relatively low number of patients included in the study, it is impossible to give firm evidence of an impact on cancer-related mor-tality, but only to present a positive trend toward it.

Future perspectives

Research has provided firm evidence of two important principles:

(1) The risk of cancer in patients with VTE is much higher in idiopathic VTE than secondary.
(2) Extensive screening to detect hidden malignancies is worthwhile in this category of patients.

Further steps are needed to highlight fully the topic and to provide diagnostic measures to improve treatment.

First of all, given that an extensive screening battery, like that presented in the SOMIT study, appears to be recommended for cancer identification, we must consider that it is costly to society and may cause discomfort and inconvenience to the patient, especially in an outpatient setting (problems of waiting lists, minor test-related side effects, and psychological burden). However, there is increasing evidence of home treatment options. Hence, in view of the results of any single test for cancer identification in the SOMIT study, a further step will be to consider less extended screening batteries for the same result to be achieved (for example, using only tests that have had the best results in the latter study).

Prognosis of patients with cancer and VTE

Another important problem is the impact of the screening battery on cancer-related mortality. In fact, it has been asserted by several studies that cancer patients experiencing a VTE event have a 4–8-fold higher risk of dying after the event, regardless of treatment modality, than patients with cancer but without VTE. This observation is supported by two recent population-based evaluations. In fact, in the report by Heit et al,[26] the presence of cancer was an independent predictor of survival in patients with VTE. A study by Sorensen et al[27] compared the survival rate of patients whose cancer was diagnosed in the first year after the thrombotic event in comparison with that of cancer patients without thrombosis, finding an increased mortality rate in the former group. Also, patients in whom cancer was detected at the time of hospital admission for index VTE had a poor prognosis. In view of the evidence that patients with advanced and disseminated cancer have a poor prognosis, it seems that VTE is an independent predictor of worse survival in this setting. Possible explanations of this assertion are that cancer patients experience VTE late in the course of the malignant disease or that thrombotic complications are particularly severe in these patients. The problem of retrospective evaluations, however, is that it is often difficult clearly to distinguish patients in whom cancer was still overt and already symptomatic, and hence immediately detectable by routine simple tests, from patients in whom no advice of malignancy was present at the time of index VTE. In fact, only the latter can be considered to have idiopathic VTE. This distinction is neither formal nor academic, but carries important and substantial implications. In fact, only the early detection of occult cancer, when the disease is still totally asymptomatic, is likely to yield a more favorable clinical outcome.

Anyway, as a consequence of this continuing debate, some physicians question the usefulness of an early detection of cancer after the thrombotic event, since life expectancy seems to be poor. The SOMIT study, which has enrolled patients with idiopathic VTE in whom no sign of malignancy was found in routine tests, has provided clear evidence of the possibility of early cancer identification through extensive screening procedures, and has shown a positive indication of the impact on cancer-related mortality.

Even if these results cannot be considered conclusive, they could have a high impact on patients' prognoses. The early disclosure of cancer seems to be crucial, especially as innovations in therapeutic protocols are increasing the chances of succcess in the eradication of malignant disease.

References

1. Prandoni P, Piccioli A, Girolami A. Cancer and venous thromboembolism: an overview. Haematologica 1999; **84**:437–45.

2. Piccioli A, Baccaglini U, Prandoni P. Cancer and deep vein thrombosis. Scope Phlebol Lymphol 2002; **9**:363–67.

3. Trousseau A. Phlegmasia alba dolens. In: Baillière J, ed. Clinique Medicale de l'Hôtel-Dieu de Paris. (Paris, 1865)654–712.

4. Illtyd James T, Matheson NM. Thrombophlebitis in cancer. Practitioner 1935; **134**:683–84.

5. Cooper T, Barker NW. Recurrent venous thrombosis: an early complication of obscure visceral carcinoma. Minn Med 1944; **27**:31–6.

6. Ackerman RF, Estes JE. Prognosis in idiopathic thrombophlebitis. Ann Intern Med 1951; **34**:902–10.

7. Gore JM, Appelbaum JS, Greene HL et al. Occult cancer in patients with acute pulmonary embolism. Ann Intern Med 1982; **96**:556–60.

8. Aderka D, Brown A, Zelicovski A et al. Idiopathic deep vein thrombosis in an apparently healthy patient as a premonitory sign of occult cancer. Cancer 1986; **57**:1846–9.

9. Prandoni P, Lensing AWA, Buller HR et al. Deep vein thrombosis and the incidence of subsequent symptomatic cancer. N Engl J Med 1992; **327**:1128–33.

10. Ahmed Z, Mohyuddin Z. Deep vein thrombosis as a predictor of cancer. Angiology 1996; **47**:261–5.

11 Monreal M, Fernandez-Liamazares J et al. Occult cancer in patients with venous thromboembolism: which patients, which cancers? Thromb Haemost 1997; **78**:1316–18.

12. Hettiarachchi RJ, Lok J, Prins MH et al. Undiagnosed malignancy in patients with deep vein thrombosis: incidence, risk indicators, and diagnosis. Cancer 1998; **83**:180–5.

13. Rajan R, Levine M, Gene M et al. The occurrence of subsequent malignancy in patients presenting with deep vein thrombosis: result from a historical cohort study. Thromb Haemost 1998; **79**:19–22.

14. Schulman S, Lindmarker P. Incidence of cancer after prophylaxis with warfarin against recurrent

venous thromboembolism. N Engl J Med 2000; **343**:1953–8.

15. Rickles FR, Falanga A. Molecular basis for the relationship between thrombosis and cancer. Thromb Res 2002; **102**(Suppl):V215–24.

16. Donati MB, Falanga A. Pathogenetic mechanisms of thrombosis in malignancy. Acta Haematol 2001; **106**:18–24.

17. Falanga A. Tumor cell prothrombotic properties. Haemostasis 2001; **31**(Suppl):1–4.

18. Goldberg RJ, Seneff M, Gore JM et al. Occult malignant neoplasms in patients with deep vein thrombosis. Arch Intern Med 1987; **147**:251–3.

19. Baron JA, Gridley G, Weiderpass E et al. Venous thromboembolism and cancer. Lancet 1998; **351**: 1077–80.

20. Sorensen HT, Mellem Kjaer L, Steffensen FH et al. The risk of a diagnosis of cancer after primary deep vein thrombosis or pulmonary embolism. N Engl J Med 1998; **338**:1169–73.

21. Bastounis EA, Karayiannakis AJ, Makri GG et al. The incidence of occult cancer in patients with deep venous thrombosis: a prospective study. J Intern Med 1996; **239**: 153–6.

22. Monreal M, Lafoz E, Casals A et al. Occult cancer in patients with deep venous thrombosis. Cancer 1991; **67**:541–5.

23. Sanella NA, O'Connor DJ. Idiopathic deep venous thrombosis: the value of routine abdominal and pelvic computed tomographic scanning. Ann Vasc Surg 1991; **5**:218–22.

24. Barosi G, Marchetti M, Dazzi L et al. Testing for occult cancer in patients with idiopathic deep vein thrombosis—a decision analysis. Thromb Haemost 1997; **78**: 1319–26.

25. Piccioli A, Lensing AWA, Prins MH et al. Extensive screening for occult malignant disease in idiopathic venous thromboembolism. Pathophysiol Haemost Thromb 2002; **32**(Suppl 2):50.

26. Heit JA, Silverstein MD, Mohr DN et al. Predictors of survival after deep vein thrombosis and pulmonary embolism: a population-based cohort study. Arch Intern Med 1999; **159**:445–53.

27. Sorensen HT, Mellemkjaer L, Olsen JH et al. Prognosis of cancer associated with venous thromboembolism. N Engl J Med 2000; **343**:1846–50.

8

Thrombotic complications of overt cancer

Gilles Lugassy and Boris Yoffe

Frequency of thromboembolism in untreated cancer patients

Over 135 years after the original description by Armand Trousseau, who observed that deep-vein thrombosis of the extremities often accompanies visceral cancer, thromboembolism in overt cancer patients is usually underdiagnosed before death. While autopsy results almost uniformly show a 50% frequency of thromboembolism in cancer patients, the reported clinical incidence rises to 15% for untreated patients.[1]

Most clinical studies designed to determine the true incidence of thromboembolism in cancer patients are neither prospective nor selective of untreated patients. Most series include both treated and untreated patients, and patients with occult or overt cancers, indiscriminantly. Moreover, the results of such studies are usually not compared with the frequency of thromboembolism in nonmalignant patients of otherwise similar thrombotic risk. The use of such different diagnostic and methodological criteria for epidemiological estimations, ranging from simple clinical suspicion to more invasive procedures, results in considerable differences in the rate of reported thrombotic complications.

Levitan et al[2] studied the association between venous thromboembolism and the presence of malignant or nonmalignant diseases. The authors used the Medicare Provider Analysis and Review Record database for patients hospitalized during 1988–1990. Among more than 8 000 000 Medicare patients admitted with a diagnosis of nonmalignant disease, some 46 800 suffered also from venous thromboembolism. Among the more than 1 200 000 patients hospitalized with malignancy, 7200 also had venous thromboembolism. The percentage of patients with thromboembolism was higher among those with malignancy than those with nonmalignant diseases: 0.6% versus 0.57% ($p = 0.001$).

The probability of readmission within 6 months with recurrent venous thromboembolism was highest for patients with a prior thrombotic event and malignancy (0.22), followed by those with malignancy alone (0.14), nonmalignant disease (0.08), and isolated thromboembolism (0.06). The probability of death among patients with venous thromboembolism and malignancy was much higher than among those with thrombosis and no malignancy: 0.94 versus 0.29 ($p = 0.001$).

Recently, Sallah et al[3] reported the frequency of venous thromboembolism among 1041 patients with solid tumors hospitalized in three major medical centers. Deep-vein thrombosis, pulmonary embolism, or both were diagnosed on 81 patients (7.8%). These observations need to be compared with the estimated frequency of venous thromboembolism among patients suffering from medical diseases hospitalized in general wards.

In the Medenox study, the incidence of asymptomatic peripheral venous thromboembolism was assessed by bilateral ascending contrast venography in a cohort of acutely ill medical patients with intermediate thrombotic risk. The cohort also included cancer patients.[4] Venous thromboembolism was found in 14.9% of these patients. This incidence is higher than the usually reported frequency of venous thromboembolism among cancer patients, but one should not forget that most studies of cancer patients report symptomatic, overt venous thrombosis, while the Medenox study systematically investigated the asymptomatic presence of venous thrombosis.

Few clinical studies have estimated the occult prevalence of deep-vein thrombosis in the cancer population. Johnson et al[5] screened 298 hospice patients with advanced cancer, using light-reflection rheography. Deep-vein thrombosis was found in 52% of the examined patients, mainly among those with poor mobility, low serum albumin levels, and renal dysfunction.

In a retrospective analysis of three prospective studies, Lee et al[6] assessed the prevalence of deep-vein thrombosis in a population of 1068 outpatients, using D-dimer testing, impedence plethysmography, compression ultrasonography, or contrast venography. Their results confirm, with a rare degree of similarity, the reports by Johnson et al[5] and the Medenox study[4]—deep-vein thrombosis was found in 48.8% of 121 patients with cancer and in 14.6% of 947 patients without cancer. Patients at greatest risk of venous thromboembolism include those with mucin-secreting tumors (pancreas and gastrointestinal tract); cancer of the lung, kidney, brain, prostate, and ovary; acute promyelocytic leukemia; myeloproliferative disorders; and lymphomas.

According to Levitan et al,[2] the malignancies associated with the lowest incidence of thrombosis include cancers of the head and neck, bladder, breast, esophagus, uterus, and cervix.

Paraneoplastic arterial thrombosis is less frequent than venous thrombosis. Among the 41 cancer patients with arterial emboli reported by

Sack et al,[7] 24 had pancreatic, 10 lung, and 4 colon cancer, and 3 had adenocarcinoma of unknown primary site.

Clinical characteristics of thrombosis in cancer patients

The signs and symptoms of the prothrombotic state in cancer patients range from asymptomatic abnormal coagulation tests to massive thromboembolism and disseminated intravascular coagulation (DIC) in critically ill patients. The systemic manifestations of thrombosis are reviewed in Chapter 9, thromboembolism in surgery, is covered in Chapter 13, and chemotherapy-associated thrombosis is covered in Chapter 14.

Venous thromboembolism

Deep venous thrombosis is by far the most frequent thromboembolic complication of cancer. Diagnosis may be difficult in some cases. The presence of tumoral masses, or enlarged abdominal or pelvic lymph nodes may cause extrinsic compression of large veins, mimicking uni- or bilateral deep-vein thrombosis of the legs, with false-positive results on impedence plethysmography and compression ultrasonography.

Recommended procedures for diagnosing venous thrombosis usually include the combination of clinical features at presentation (Wells index), venous ultrasonography, and D-dimer testing.[8] Nevertheless, the cardinal importance attributed to D-dimer testing for diagnosis of venous thrombosis has important drawbacks in cancer patients. D-dimer can be elevated in cancer patients with no suspicion of thrombosis (see Chapter 5). Moreover, the study by Lee et al[6] has shown that a negative D-dimer test in patients with cancer does not reliably exclude venous thrombosis, since the negative predictive value of the test is lower in these patients than in patients without cancer. Therefore, the diagnostic approach in cancer patients should be 'personalized' and should include a clinical assessment, according to the Wells model, together with ultrasonography. In situations where the clinical probability is high (common in cancer patients), but the ultrasonography is negative or inconclusive, venography should be performed to confirm or refute the diagnosis. An intraluminal filling defect surrounded by contrast material is considered to be evidence of recent thombus. Venography has been proven to be a safe procedure in large clinical studies, some of which included cancer patients.[4,9] Injection of contrast material should always be avoided in patients with multiple myeloma and in patients with kidney dysfunction.

Upper extremity venous thrombosis occurs in cancer patients. Differential diagnosis includes external obstruction of the venous outflow by Pancoast tumor or by an axillary mass. Use of indwelling central catheters and intensive cytotoxic therapy are associated with high rates of upper extremity venous thrombosis (see Chapters 12 and 14).

The diagnosis of pulmonary embolism in cancer patients may be complicated by the presence of pulmonary metastasis and underlying lung disease secondary to radio/chemotherapy. Moreover, presenting symptoms and radiological features of pulmonary embolism are usually not specific enough to differentiate between pulmonary embolism and tumor embolism to the lung. The stomach is the most common primary site of cancer causing microembolic carcinoma to the lungs.[10] Less common primary sites include the bronchus, breast, prostate, and pancreas.

The following deep venous thromboses occur less commonly in cancer patients:

- superior vena caval thrombosis, which needs to be distinguished from external compression by lung cancer or lymphoma (T-lymphoblastic type)
- inferior vena caval thrombosis
- hepatic venous thrombosis and portal venous thrombosis seen in patients with hemato-oncological disorders, mostly in myeloproliferative diseases.

Migratory superficial thrombophlebitis is an uncommon, although characteristic, neoplastic thrombotic syndrome involving unusual superficial veins (upper extremities and chest wall) in patients suffering from head and neck, lung, prostatic, pancreatic, or gastrointestinal cancers.[7]

Arterial thrombosis

Arterial thrombosis is much less frequently encountered than venous thrombosis in cancer patients. Patients diagnosed with myeloproliferative disorders do have a tendency to develop arterial thrombosis and therefore will be described in a separate section.

Stroke

A recent study by Chaturvedi et al[11] concluded that cancer patients do not suffer from cerebral strokes more often than nonmalignant patients.

Peripheral and coronary arterial disease

Naschitz et al have extensively studied the epidemiology and clinical features of peripheral and coronary arterial diseases in the cancer population.[12-16] Although most of their studies dealt with the issue of arterial disease preceding the diagnosis of cancer, their comparisons between paraneoplastic (preceding cancer diagnosis) and cancer-associated arterial thromboembolism have improved our knowledge of this rarely reported manifestation. The clinical course of cancer-associated peripheral arterial disease is usually aggressive, often requiring recurrent vascular surgery for limb salvage, with a high incidence of graft occlusion. Effective cytotoxic therapy of the underlying malignancy may improve the evolution of the vascular disorder.[17] An interesting observation is that cancer patients with accelerated arterial disease suffer from a low incidence of venous thrombosis.[12,17]

Coronary disease is a frequently encountered late complication of malignancy, especially in patients with Hodgkin's lymphoma. Its incidence, however, in the early stages of cancer seems to be quite low. Thompson et al[18] found gynecological cancer to be a risk factor for developing coronary disease. Coronary thrombosis has been estimated to occur in 5% of patients with metastatic terminal cancer.[19] Myocardial infarction has been attributed to coronary embolism that originates from a clot that adheres to the valvular endocardium.

Nonbacterial thrombotic endocarditis is mostly observed in patients with mucin-producing adenocarcinoma. Microvascular arterial thrombosis is observed in patients with myeloproliferative disorders (MPD), mostly polycythemia vera and essential thrombocythemia.

Thromboembolism in MPD

Patients with MPD may suffer from both bleeding and thrombotic complications.[20] MPD patients may be either 'bleeders' or thrombosis-prone, or both, or may shift from being a bleeder to being thrombosis-prone.[21] Thrombotic events are most frequently deep venous thrombosis and pulmonary embolism, but cerebrovascular, coronary, and peripheral vascular thromboses also occur in polycythemia vera and essential thrombocythemia.[22] Patients with MPD develop venous thrombosis at unusual sites: hepatic, splenic, portal, and mesenteric. MPD represent the most frequent etiology of Budd–Chiari syndrome (hepatic vein thrombosis).[21]

Since hepatic venous thrombosis has been reported also in association with paroxysmal nocturnal hemoglobinuria, a rare stem-cell disorder with no abdominal organomegaly, it seems that systemic hemostatic disturbances, rather than local factors, play an important role in the development of hepatic venous thrombosis in MPD.

Two clinical syndromes frequently complicate polycythemia vera and essential thrombocythemia, and are specific to thrombocytosis-associated monoclonal disorders. The first one, erythromelalgia, is caused by platelet-mediated arteriolar inflammation and thrombotic occlusion, with no evidence of pre-existing vascular disorder.[23] It is characterized by warm, red, congested limbs and painful burning sensations. Warmth worsens the symptoms while cold provides relief. Erythromelalgia may lead to acrocyanosis and peripheral gangrene. Most of the symptoms of erythromelalgia are relieved by aspirin. The long-acting (up to 3 days) effect of a single dose of aspirin is so specific that it is used as a diagnostic criterion.[24] The second clinical syndrome, transient neurological manifestations, is frequently reported in association with polycythemia vera and essential thrombocythemia.[25] Platelet-mediated arterial thromboses lead to transient ischemic attacks, stroke, headaches, visual disturbances, ataxia, and seizures. There seems to be a correlation between the occurrence of these manifestations and the platelet count, with a higher frequency when the platelets are in excess of 1000×10^9/liter. Response to therapy with aspirin and platelet-reducing medications is favorable, with few long-term recurrences.

In patients with essential thrombocythemia, thromboembolism in normal coronary arteries may cause myocardial infarction. Coronary disease may be seen in essential thrombocythemia patients who suffered previous transient cerebral ischemic attacks or erythromelalgia 1–5 years before.[26]

Finally, the risk of severe thrombotic complications occurring during surgery in MDP patients should be emphasized, since it exceeds that attributed to the postoperative thrombotic state encountered in other conditions.

References

1. Dhami MS, Bona RD. Thrombosis in patients with cancers. Postgrad Med 1999; 93:131–40.

2. Levitan N, Dowlati A, Remick SC et al. Rates of initial and recurrent thromboembolic disease among patients with malignancy versus those without malignancy. Risk analysis using Medicare claims data. Medicine 1999; 78:285–91.

3. Sallah S, Wan JY, Nguyen NP. Venous thrombosis in patients with solid tumors: determination of frequency and characteristics. Thromb Haemost 2002; 87:575–9.

4. Samama MM, Cohen AT, Darmon JY et al. A comparison of enoxaparin with placebo for the prevention of venous thromboembolism in acutely ill medical patients. N Engl J Med 1999; 341:793–800.

5. Johnson MJ, Sproule M, Paul J. The prevalence and associated variables of deep venous thrombosis in patients with advanced cancer. Clin Oncol 1999; 11:105–10.

6. Lee AY, Julian JA, Levine MN et al. Clinical utility of a rapid whole blood D-dimer assay in patients with cancer who present with suspected acute deep venous thrombosis. Ann Intern Med 1999; 131:417–23.

7. Sack GH, Levin J, Bell WB. Trousseau's syndrome and other manifestations of chronic disseminated coagulopathy in patients with neoplasms: clinical, pathophysiologic and therapeutic features. Medicine 1977; 56:1–37.

8. Hirsh J, Lee AYY. How we diagnose and treat deep vein thrombosis. Blood 2002; 99:3102–110.

9. Bergqvist D, Agnelli G, Cohen AT et al. Duration of prophylaxis against

venous thromboembolism with Enoxaparin after surgery for cancer. N Engl J Med 2002; **46**:975–80.

10. Markovitz DH, Mark EJ. A 43 year old man with renal carcinoma and worsening dyspnea. Case Record of the Massachusetts General Hospital. N Engl J Med 2002; **346**:1309–17.

11. Chatuverdi S, Ansell J, Recht L. Should cerebral ischemic events in cancer patients be considered a manifestation of hypercoagulability? Stroke 1994; **25**:1215–18.

12. Naschitz JE, Schechter L, Chang JB. Intermittent claudication associated with cancer. Angiology 1987; **38**:696–704.

13. Naschitz JE, Yeshurun D, Abrahamson MB. Ischemic heart disease precipitated by occult cancer. Cancer 1992; **69**:2712–20.

14. Naschitz JE, Yeshurun D. Arterial occlusive disease in occult cancer. Am Heart J 1992; **124**:738–45.

15. Naschitz JE, Yeshurun D, Lev LM. Thromboembolism in cancer. Changing Trends Cancer 1993; **71**:1384–90.

16. Naschitz JE, Yeshurun D, Eldar S et al. Diagnosis of cancer associated vascular disorders. Cancer 1996; **77**:1759–67.

17. Rickles FR, Edward RL, Barb C et al. Abnormalities of blood coagulation in patients with cancer. Cancer 1983; **51**:301–7.

18. Thompson SG, Greenberg G, Meade TW. Risk factors for stroke and myocardial infarction in women in the United Kingdom as assessed in general practice: a case control study. Br Heart J 1989; **61**:403–9.

19. Kopelson G, Herwig KJ. The etiologies of coronary artery disease in cancer patients. Int J Radiat Oncol Biol Phys 1978; **4**:905–6.

20. Colombi M, Radaelli F, Zocchi L et al. Thrombotic and hemorrhagic complications in essential thrombocythemia. Cancer 1991; **67**:2926–30.

21. Schaefer AI. Bleeding and thrombosis in the myeloproliferative disorders. Blood 1984; **64**:1–12.

22. Lugassy G. Essential thrombocythemia—update on pathogenesis and therapy. Cancer J 1998; **11**:57–9.

23. Michiels JJ, van Joost T. Erythromelalgia and thrombocythemia: a causal relation. J Am Acad Dermatol 1990; **1**:107–11.

24. van Genderen PJJ, Michiels JJ, van Strik R et al. Platelet consumption in thrombocythemia complicated by erythromelalgia: reversal by aspirin. Thromb Haemost 1995; **73**:210–14.

25. Michiels JJ, Kandstaal PJ, Mulder AH et al. Transient neurologic and ocular manifestations in primary thrombocythemia. Neurology 1993; **43**:1107–110.

26. Scheffer MG, Michiels JJ Simons ML et al. Thrombocythemia and coronary artery disease. Am Heart J 1991; **122**:573–6.

9
Systemic microangiopathies in the cancer patient

Marcel Levi

Introduction

The association between cancer and thrombosis has been known for years. Besides the well-recognized connection between venous thromboembolism and malignancies, there are, however, also other manifestations of (micro)vascular dysfunction in combination with an activated coagulation system in cancer patients. In fact, coagulation derangements and vascular disturbances in patients with cancer cover a wide spectrum of diseases and various clinical manifestations. In this review, we will highlight the mechanisms that play a role in the systemic activation of coagulation in cancer patients, in its most severe form manifested as disseminated intravascular coagulation. Furthermore, the role of perturbed endothelium, in particular in the setting of cancer and chemo- or radiotherapy, in the pathogenesis of microvascular dysfunction and microangiopathy will be discussed.

Clinical presentation and incidence

Activation of coagulation in patients with sepsis is very common but may result in widely variable clinical manifestations. Activation of coagulation is mostly subclinical and will not lead to serious complications, although laboratory tests may be seriously abnormal. In more severe forms, clinically significant systemic activation of coagulation or even frank disseminated intravascular coagulation (DIC) may occur.[1] Clinically, DIC in cancer has generally a less fulminant presentation than the types of DIC complicating sepsis and trauma. A more gradual, but also more chronic, systemic activation of coagulation can proceed subclinically. Eventually, this process may lead to exhaustion of platelets and coagulation factors, and bleeding (for example, at the site of the tumor) may be the first clinical symptom indicating the presence of DIC. If the function of the liver is not compromised, then enhanced synthesis of coagulation proteins may mask the ongoing consumption of factors; in that case, thrombocytopenia is the most prominent sign of ongoing DIC. Measurement of fibrin-related markers (such as soluble fibrin or fibrin-degradation products) may be helpful in establishing the diagnosis in a routine setting; however, the specificity of these tests in cancer-related DIC has not been established so far.

Overt venous thromboembolism is common in patients with cancer, with an estimated annual incidence of up to 10%. It is not clear to what extent the manifestation of clinically overt thromboembolism can be ascribed to malignancy-associated DIC. There is ample evidence of a procoagulant state in virtually all patients with advanced malignant disease; however, the incidence of overt DIC appears to be much lower.[2] The incidence of DIC in consecutive patients with solid tumors was found to be 7% in a recent clinical study;[3] in patients presenting with acute leukemia, in particular acute lymphoblastic leukemia, DIC can be diagnosed in 15–20%.[4] Some reports indicate that the incidence of DIC in acute leukemia patients might further increase during remission induction with chemotherapy.[4] In patients with acute promyelocytic leukemia (AML M3), DIC may be diagnosed in more than 90% of patients at the time of diagnosis or after initiation of remission induction.[5]

Pathogenesis of coagulation activation in cancer patients

The coagulopathy that accompanies acute promyelocytic leukemia is often seen as one of the most straightforward forms of DIC complicating malignancy.[6] However, this form of leukemia-associated hemostatic derangement can be considered to be an exceptional type of DIC, characterized by systemic activation of coagulation in combination with marked hyperfibrinolysis. The clinical presentation of severe bleeding associated with laboratory findings of low fibrinogen level, very high levels of fibrin split products and fibrinogen-degradation products, and massive consumption of plasminogen and α_2-antiplasmin (leading to inordinately high levels of plasmin–α_2-antiplasmin complex levels) supports that notion.[5,7] The precise pathogenesis of this hyperfibrinolysis has, however, not been elucidated. Plasma levels of physiological plasminogen activators (such as urokinase-type plasminogen activator [u-PA] and tissue-type plasminogen activator [t-PA]) cannot explain the massive plasminogen activation, nor is a role of leukocytic elastase-mediated hyperfibrinolysis likely.

Hypothetically, a receptor for fibrinolytic proteins, annexin II, which is expressed on the surface of leukemic cells in patients with acute promyelocytic leukemia, may play a role, although the in vivo relevance of these observations is less clear.[8] Annexin II may facilitate plasmin generation at the surface of the cells and may thereby play a pivotal role in the development of the hyperfibrinolytic state. Despite the prominent role of hyperfibrinolysis in patients with acute promyelocytic leukemia, there is mounting evidence that this derangement is superimposed on a more common presentation of DIC, characterized by coagulation activation and fibrin deposition. Indeed, diffuse thrombosis is found in 15–25% of cases at autopsy, and recent studies have demonstrated tissue-factor (TF)-dependent activation of coagulation in this patient category.

Solid-tumor cells can express different procoagulant molecules, including TF, which assembles with factor VII(a) to activate factors IX and X, and cancer procoagulant (CP), a cysteine protease with factor X-activating properties.[9] Recent studies show that TF occurs in vascular endothelial cells as well as tumor cells in breast cancer, while not appearing in material from patients with benign fibrocystic breast disease, while TF was functionally active.[10] It should be noted that the role of TF in pathophysiology is still only partly understood. Independently of its clotting cofactor function, TF appears to be involved in tumor metastasis and angiogenesis,[11,12] processes that may directly influence the course of malignancy and affect the occurrence of thrombosis. CP is an endopeptidase that is found in extracts of neoplastic cells but also in the plasma of patients with solid tumors. The exact role of CP in the pathogenesis of cancer-related coagulation abnormalities is unclear. Another mechanism by which tumor cells may contribute to the pathogenesis of coagulation abnormalities is by expressing fibrinolytic proteins. Despite the ability of many malignant cells to express plasminogen activators, such as u-PA and t-PA, most tumors induce a hypofibrinolytic state. Since DIC is commonly characterized by a shutdown of the fibrinolytic system (mostly due to high levels of the fibrinolytic inhibitor PAI-1), this may represent an alternative mechanism for the development of DIC in cancer.

Cellular factors presumably precipitate coagulation activation in patients with, in most cases, solid tumors. In addition, in a series of patients with malignant neoplasms, high endothelin plasma levels correlated well with progression of coagulation abnormalities, suggesting that this protein may influence the development of coagulation abnormalities in cancer.[13]

Virtually all pathways that contribute to the occurrence of DIC are driven by cytokines. Interleukin-6 (IL-6) has been identified as one of the most important proinflammatory cytokines that is able to induce TF expression on cells. Indeed, inhibition of IL-6 results in an inhibition of endotoxin-stimulated activation of coagulation. In contrast, changes in fibrinolysis and microvascular physiological anticoagulant pathways are mostly dependent on tumor necrosis factor α (TNF-α). Other cytokines that participate in the systemic activation of coagulation are IL-1β and

IL-8, whereas anti-inflammatory cytokines, such as IL-10, are able to inhibit DIC. Since many types of tumors have the ability to synthesize and release cytokines or to stimulate other cells to activate the cytokine network, it is likely that cytokine-dependent modulation of coagulation and fibrinolysis plays a role in cancer-related DIC.

Thrombotic microangiopathy in cancer and chemotherapy

With the use of autologous and allogeneic stem-cell support to overcome the bone-marrow toxicity of (high-dose) chemotherapy, and the adoption of more intensive treatment regimens, other types of chemotherapy-related organ toxicity appear to occur more frequently. Thrombotic microangiopathy is a serious complication of this sort that is occurring in an increasing number of patients after high-dose chemotherapy in combination with autologous or allogeneic stem-cell transplantation.[14,15] In recent years, more than 200 cases have been reported in some 30 publications, and initial prospective (laboratory-based) studies indicate that the incidence of the syndrome ranges from 2% to 8% of patients receiving high-dose chemotherapy.[15–21] Thrombotic microangiopathy encompasses a number of syndromes that closely resemble each other, such as hemolytic uremic syndrome (HUS) and thrombotic thrombocytopenic purpura (TTP). Moreover, some features of veno-occlusive disease (VOD) are similar to those observed in thrombotic microangiopathy. These syndromes are characterized by platelet adhesion to endothelial cells, followed by massive platelet aggregation and activation (resulting in consumptive thrombocytopenia), subsequent activation of the coagulation system leading to fibrin formation and deposition, and inadequate fibrin removal due to impaired function of the fibrinolytic system. The formed thrombi in the (micro)-vasculature cause impaired organ function (leading, for example, to renal or hepatic insufficiency) and red-cell fragmentation due to microangio-pathic hemolysis.[22]

Remarkably, the condition arises, in general, 2–9 months after cessation of chemotherapy, when the cancer itself is also in remission. Historically, the syndrome appeared to be restricted to specific types of antineoplastic chemotherapy, such as mitomycin C, but now a large number of different types of chemotherapy have been associated with the occurrence of thrombotic microangiopathy.[15,16,23] The dose of the chemotherapy appears to be important, a factor which explains the increasing incidence of the syndrome, since the widespread clinical application of stem-cell transplantation (bone-marrow transplantation or peripheral stem-cell transplantation) enables the use of much higher doses of chemotherapy. Furthermore, simultaneous total-body irradiation and the use of cyclosporin A are associated with a higher incidence of postchemotherapy thrombotic microangiopathy.[18,22,24] The prognosis of this particular complication of high-dose chemotherapy is poor: of all affected patients, the mortality rate was 31% and the direct thrombotic microangiopathy-related mortality rate was 23%.[15,20] In addition, survivors may suffer from persistent or even progressive renal insufficiency.

The pathogenesis of thrombotic microangiopathy remains to be elucidated. It may be hypothesized that the endothelial toxicity of the chemotherapy plays a central role in the development of the syndrome. Endothelial damage and subsequent dysfunction have been implicated in various reports dealing with chemotherapy-related thrombotic microangiopathy; however, there is no definitive proof for this hypothesis, nor is it clear how the endothelial dysfunction may result in thrombotic microangiopathy.[15] To achieve rational strategies for treatment or prophylaxis of this complication, detailed insight in the various pathogenetic processes is required.

A pivotal role of endothelium in cancer-related and chemotherapy-induced thrombotic microangiopathy?

Vascular endothelium plays a central role in the processes of hemostasis, coagulation, and fibrinolysis. Endothelial cells are the primary source of von Willebrand factor, which is the adhesive protein responsible for interaction of the vessel wall with the glycoprotein Ib receptor on the platelet surface. In thrombotic microangiopathy, increased plasma levels of von Willebrand factor are found,[24,25] potentially contributing to the initiation of platelet activation. In vitro studies have shown that chemotherapy enhances endothelial cell reactivity to platelets, mediated by cytokine-induced expression of endothelial adhesion molecules.[26] Endothelial cells may also express TF (the main initiator of coagulation) and thrombomodulin (which modulates the activation of protein C, an important physiological inhibitor of the coagulation system) on their surface.[27] Defective regulation of TF and/or thrombomodulin expression on endothelial cells may result in facilitated thrombin generation, leading to fibrinogen-to-fibrin conversion and further enhancement of platelet activation. In addition, endothelial cells synthesize, store and release both t-PA and u-PA and the main inhibitor of fibrinolysis, plasminogen activator inhibitor type 1 (PAI-1).[28] Dysfunction of endothelial cells results in impaired fibrinolysis and may lead to the inadequate removal of fibrin depositions. Finally, a whole series of adhesion molecules expressed by endothelial cells can mediate the binding and activation of white blood cells to the endothelium, resulting in the release of various cytokines that are able to induce activation of blood coagulation and depression of fibrinolytic function.[29]

Among other agents found to be toxic to endothelial cells, cyclosporin A has been extensively studied. The observation that simultaneous treatment with cyclosporin A may aggravate chemotherapy-induced thrombotic microangiopathy further strengthens the hypothesis that damage to the endothelium by chemotherapy is the pivotal process in the pathogenesis of this syndrome.

In conclusion, vascular endothelial cells play a pivotal role in all processes that appear to be important in the pathogenesis of chemotherapy-induced thrombotic microangiopathy, and in vitro observations indicate that chemotherapy induces endothelial damage and subsequent dysfunction. Therefore, endothelial cells appear to be the point of impact of high-dose chemotherapy in the pathogenesis of this syndrome. In the following discussion, the potential effects of damage to the endothelium on primary hemostasis and von Willebrand factor, blood coagulation, and fibrinolysis will be outlined more specifically.

Effects of cancer-related and chemotherapy-induced endothelial damage on primary hemostasis and von Willebrand factor

Endothelial cells synthesize and release von Willebrand factor, which plays an important role in platelet adhesion to the vessel wall. Damage to the endothelium is associated with an increase in circulating von Willebrand factor. Indeed, in a recent study, increased plasma levels of von Willebrand factor were found in cancer patients who developed thrombotic microangiopathy.[24,30] The multimeric pattern of von Willebrand factor determines its biological activity; that is, high-molecular-weight von Willebrand multimers are functionally more potent than other forms of von Willebrand factor. Remarkably, in 'conventional' TTP and HUS, particularly high-molecular-weight multimers of von Willebrand factor are found, which may contribute to the increased platelet reactivity observed.[18] Reports on the multimeric pattern of von Willebrand factor in cancer and after high-dose chemotherapy are controversial.[31,32]

Effects of chemotherapy-induced endothelial damage on coagulation

Endothelial cells are important for the regulation of blood coagulation because of the expression of both procoagulant and anticoagulant mediators.[27] Recently, it has become clear that TF is the principal initiator of coagulation activation. TF is able to bind to and activate factor

VII, and the TF–factor VIIa complex will activate both factors X and IX, leading to direct and indirect prothrombin-to-thrombin conversion and subsequent fibrin formation.[33] TF can be expressed on activated mononuclear cells and—probably even more important—endothelial cells. It has been shown that cytokine-activated endothelial cells in cancer patients show enhanced TF expression and TF-dependent procoagulant activity.[34] Patients with 'conventional' TTP show enhanced levels of TF antigen in blood.[35] There are no published data on the effect of chemotherapy on TF expression on endothelial cells of patients with cancer. In addition, the main regulator of the TF pathway, TF pathway inhibitor (TFPI) is also present on the surface of endothelial cells. Reduction in TFPI activity results in enhanced thrombin generation in vitro and in experimental coagulation activation in vivo. Damage to endothelial cells may result in loss of TFPI on the endothelial cell surface, and it has been shown that plasma levels of TFPI are decreased in patients with TTP.[36] There are no data available on TFPI activity in patients with cancer or chemotherapy-induced thrombotic microangiopathy. In conclusion, there is evidence that the TF pathway and its inhibitor may play an important regulatory role in chemotherapy-induced thrombotic microangiopathy.

Another important role of endothelial cells in the regulation of blood coagulation is by means of thrombomodulin expression on their surface.[37] After (thrombin-mediated) activation of thrombomodulin at the endothelial surface, circulating protein C is converted to activated protein C and may act as an important inhibitor of blood coagulation, due to proteolytic degradation of the cofactors V and VIII. The central role of the protein C system in the regulation of blood coagulation is illustrated by the occurrence of thrombotic disease in patients with a defective protein C system. It has been shown in vitro that endothelial cells may react to certain stimuli, such as toxic substances or cytokines, with downregulation of thrombomodulin expression, thereby reducing the formation of activated protein C and blocking this inhibitory pathway.[38] It is likely that these mechanisms are operative in cancer patients as well. The use of high-dose chemotherapy has been associated with impaired function of the protein C system; however, the mechanism has not been elucidated.[39,40] An important role of the protein C system in the development of thrombotic microangiopathy has also been suggested. Finally, cyclosporin A-induced damage to endothelial cells has been associated with altered function of the protein C system in vivo.[41] From these data taken together, it may be hypothesized that chemotherapy-induced endothelial damage may result in a downregulation of thrombomodulin with subsequent inhibition of the protein C system and facilitation of coagulation activation.

Effects of cancer-related and chemotherapy-induced endothelial damage on fibrinolysis

Endothelial cells are the principal site of production, storage and release of fibrinolytic activators, that is, u-PA and t-PA. Impaired release of plasminogen activators from the endothelium results in a reduction in fibrinolytic activity in vivo and may contribute to the pathogenesis of thrombus formation.[42] In addition, endothelial cells may produce PAI-1, the main inhibitor of plasminogen activation, and it has been shown in vitro that activation of endothelial cells results in enhanced production and release of this inhibitor of fibrinolysis. Elevated levels of PAI-1 are associated with the occurrence of thrombotic disease.[43] Recent reports indicate that endothelial damage may result in endothelial dysfunction, leading to impaired release of plasminogen activators and increased levels of PAI-1, and thus resulting in an overall antifibrinolytic state. For example, it has been shown that cyclosporin A-induced damage to endothelial cells results in a reduction of fibrinolytic activity caused by these mechanisms.[44] In cancer patients with TTP, a similar pattern has been shown regarding the fibrinolytic activation and inhibition: impaired release of plasminogen activators and enhanced levels of PAI-1.[45,46] There are only limited data in the literature on endothelial function as related to fibrinolysis after treatment with high-dose chemotherapy;[47] however, on the basis of the above-mentioned observations, it may be hypothesized that chemotherapy-induced endothelial injury results in an antifibrinolytic condition that may contribute to the pathogenesis of thrombotic microangiopathy.

Conclusion

The presence of cancer may result in activation of coagulation and endothelial cell perturbation, leading to microvascular dysfunction that may present as DIC or microangiopathic disease. The clinical presentation may vary widely among patients. Pathogenetic pathways that seem to play a central role in the development of microangiopathy in cancer patients include TF-mediated thrombin generation, downregulation of endothelial cell-associated physiological anticoagulant pathways, deranged fibrinolysis, and dysfunctional endothelial cells.

References

1. Levi M, ten Cate H. Disseminated intravascular coagulation. N Engl J Med 1999; **341**:586–92.

2. Colman RW, Rubin RN. Disseminated intravascular coagulation due to malignancy. Semin Oncol 1990; **17**:172–86.

3. Sallah S, Wan JY, Nguyen NP et al. Disseminated intravascular coagulation in solid tumors: clinical and pathological study. Thromb Haemost 2001; **86**:828–33.

4. Sarris AH, Kempin S, Berman E et al. High incidence of disseminated intravascular coagulation during remission induction of adult patients with acute lymphoblastic leukemia. Blood 1992; **79**: 1305–10.

5. Avvisati G, ten Cate JW, Sturk A et al. Acquired alpha-2-antiplasmin deficiency in acute promyelocytic leukaemia. Br J Haematol 1988; **70**:43–8.

6. Tallman MS. The thrombophilic state in acute promyelocytic leukemia. Semin Thromb Hemost 1999; **25**:209–15.

7. Rodeghiero F, Castaman G. The pathophysiology and treatment of hemorrhagic syndrome of acute promyelocytic leukemia. Leukemia 1994; **8**(Suppl 2):S20–6

8. Menell JS, Cesarman GM, Jacovina AT et al. Annexin II and bleeding in acute promyelocytic leukemia. N Engl J Med 1999; **340**:994–1004

9. Donati MB. Cancer and thrombosis: from phlegmasia alba dolens to transgenic mice. Thromb Haemost 1995; **74**:278–81.

10. Contrino J, Hair G, Kreutzer DL et al. In situ detection of tissue factor in vascular endothelial cells: correlation with the malignant phenotype of human breast disease. Nat Med 1996; **2**:209–15.

11. Bromberg ME, Konigsberg WH, Madison JF et al. Tissue factor promotes melanoma metastasis by a pathway independent of blood coagulation. Proc Natl Acad Sci USA 1995; **92**:8205–9.

12. Zhang Y, Deng Y, Luther T et al. Tissue factor controls the balance of angiogenic and antiangiogenic properties of tumor cells in mice. J Clin Invest 1994; **94**:1320–7.

13. Ishibashi M, Ito N, Fujita M et al. Endothelin-1 as an aggravating factor of disseminated intravascular coagulation associated with malignant neoplasms. Cancer 1994; **73**:191–5.

14. Doll DC, Yabro JW. Vascular toxicity associated with antineoplastic agents. Semin Oncol 1992; **19**: 580–96.

15. Pettitt AR, Clarck RE. Thrombotic microangiopathy following bone marrow transplantation. Bone Marrow Transplant 1994; **14**: 495–504.

16. Snyder HW, Mittelman A, Oral A et al. Treatment of cancer chemotherapy-associated thrombotic thrombocytopenic purpura/hemolytic uremic syndrome by protein A immunoadsorption of plasma. Cancer 1993; **71**:1882–92.

17. Guinan EC, Tarbell NJ, Niemeyer CM et al. Intravascular hemolysis and renal insufficiency after bone marrow transplantation. Blood 1988; **72**:451–5.

18. Chappel ME, Keeling MD, Prentice HG et al. Haemolytic uraemic syndrome after bone marrow transplantation: an adverse effect of total body irradiation? Bone Marrow Transplant 1988; **3**: 339–47.

19. Antignac C, Gubler MC, Leverger G et al. Delayed renal failure with extensive mesangiolysis following

bone marrow tranplantation. Kidney Int 1989; **35**:1336–44.

20. Rabinowe SN, Soiffer RJ, Tarbel NJ et al. Hemolytic uremic syndrome following bone marrow transplantation in adults for hematological malignancies. Blood 1991; **77**: 1837–44.

21. Jucket M, Perry EH, Daniels BS et al. Hemolytic uremic syndrome following bone marrow transplantation. Bone Marrow Transplant 1991; **7**:405–9.

22. Neild G. The hemolytic uremic syndrome; a review. Q J Med1987; **63**:367–76.

23. Jackson AM, Rose BD, Graff LG et al. Thrombotic microangiopathy and renal failure associated with antineoplastic chemotherapy. Ann Intern Med 1984; **101**:803–7.

24. Holler E, Kolb HJ, Hiller E. Microangiopathy in patients on cyclosporin prophylaxis who developed acute graft-versus-host disease after HLA-identical bone marrow transplantation. Blood 1989; **73**:2018–24.

25. Collins PW, Gutteridge CN, O'Driscoll A. Von Willebrand factor as a marker of endothelial cell activation following BMT. Bone Marrow Transplant 1992; **10**:499–506.

26. Bertomeu MC, Gallo S, Lauri D et al. Chemotherapy enhances endothelial cell reactivity to platelets. Clin Exp Metastasis 1990; **8**:511–18.

27. Jaffe EA. Biochemistry, immunology and cell biology of the endothelium. In: Colman RW, Hirsh J, eds. Hemostasis and Thrombosis: Basic Principles and Clinical Practice, 3rd edn. (JB Lippincott: Philadelphia, 1994)718-44.

28. Levi M, ten Cate JW, Dooijewaard G et al. DDAVP induces systemic release of urokinase-type plasminogen activator. Thromb Haemost 1989; **62**:686–9.

29. Carlos TM, Harlan JM. Leucocyte-endothelial adhesion molecules. Blood 1994; **84**:2068–101.

30. Seeber CH, Hiller E, Holler E, Kolb HJ. Increased levels of tissue plasminogen activator (t-PA) and tissue plasminogen activator inhibitor (PAI) correlate with tumor necrosis factor alpha (TNFα)-release in patients suffering from microangiopathy following allogeneic bone marrow transplantation (BMT). Thromb Res 1992; **66**:373–83.

31. Cohen H, Bull HA, Seddon A. Vascular endothelial cell function and ultrastructure in thrombotic microangiopathy following allogeneic bone marrow transplantation. Eur J Haematol 1989; **43**: 207–14.

32. Charba D, Moake JL, Harris MA et al. Abnormalities of von Willebrand factor multimers in drug-associated thrombotic microangiopathies. Am J Hematol 1993; **42**:268–77.

33. ten Cate H, Bauer KA, Levi M et al. The activation of factors IX and X by recombinant factor VIIa is mediated by tissue factor. J Clin Invest 1993; **92**:1207–12.

34. Gregory SA, Morrissey JH, Edgington TS. Regulation of tissue factor gene expression in the monocyte procoagulant response to endotoxin. Mol Cell Biol 1989; **9**:2752–5.

35. Koyama T, Nishida K, Ohdama S et al. Determination of plasma tissue factor antigen and its clinical significance. Br J Haematol 1994; **87**: 343–7.

36. Kobayashi M, Wada H, Wakita Y et al. Decreased plasma tissue factor pathway inhibitor levels in patients with thrombotic thrombocytopenic purpura. Thromb Haemost 1995; **73**:10–4.

37. Esmon CT, Owen WG. Identification of an endothelial cell cofactor for the thrombin-catalyzed activation of protein C. Proc Natl Acad Sci USA 1981; **78**:2249–56.

38. Conway EM, Rosenberg RD. Tumor necrosis factor suppresses transcription of the thrombomodulin gene in endothelial cells. Mol Cell Biol 1988; **8**:5588–92.

39. Kaufman PA, Jones RB, Greenberg CS et al. Autologous bone marrow transplantation and factor XII, factor VII and protein C defieciencies. Report of a new association and its possible relationship to endothelial cell injury. Cancer 1990; **66**: 515–21.

40. Bazarbachi A, Scrobohaci ML, Gisselbreacht C et al. Changes in protein C, factor VII and endothelial markers after autologous bone marrow transplantation: possible implications in the pathogenesis of veno-occlusive disease. Nouv Rev Fr Hematol 1993; **35**:135–40.

41. Vanrenterghem Y, Roels L, Lerut T et al. Thromboembolic complications and haemostatic changes in cyclosporin-treated cadaveric kidney allograft recipients. Lancet 1985; **i**:999–1003.

42. Levi M, Lensing AWA, Büller HR et al. Deep vein thrombosis and fibrinolysis. Defective urokinase-type plasminogen activator release. Thromb Haemost 1991; **66**:426–9.

43. Juhan Vague I, Alessi MC. Plasminogen activator inhibitor 1 and atherothrombosis. Thromb Haemost 1993; **70**:138–143.

44. Levi M, Wilmink JM, Büller HR et al. Impaired fibrinolysis in cyclosporin-treated renal transplant patients: analysis of the defect and beneficial effect of fish-oil. Transplantation 1992; **54**:978–83.

45. Menzel D, Levi M, Peters M et al. Impaired fibrinolysis in haemolytic uremic syndrome of childhood. Ann Haematol 1994; **68**:43–8.

46. van de Kar NC, van Hinsbergh VW, Brommer EJ et al. The fibrinolytic system in the hemolytic uremic syndrome: in vivo and in vitro studies. Pediatr Res 1994; **36**:257–64.

47. Wada H, Kaneko T, Ohiwa M et al. Increased levels of vascular endothelial cell markers in thrombotic thrombocytopenic purpura. Am J Hematol 1993; **44**:101–5.

10

Thrombophilia and the risk of venous thromboembolism in cancer

Ron Hoffman and Benjamin Brenner

Introduction

The term 'thrombophilia' is designated to describe situations where there is a tendency to thrombosis. In the past, this term was reserved for thromboembolic episodes of unknown etiology (idiopathic), thrombosis in the young, or a major thrombotic event. Only recently, with significant progress having been made in understanding the biochemical and molecular mechanisms of the pathogenesis of thrombosis, have we been able to identify a great proportion of causes and defects that lead to thrombotic events. While the term 'thrombophilia' is usually reserved for inherited thrombophilic risk factors (Table 10.1), acquired hypercoagulable states (Table 10.2) are more commonly associated with thromboembolic episodes.

Inherited and acquired defects frequently act in synergy in the formation of thrombus, as a temporary, acquired hypercoagulable state exposes the patient with inherited thrombophilia to the development of an overt clinical thrombotic event. The prevalence of inherited thrombophilia in healthy subjects and patients with thrombosis is depicted in

Table 10.1 Causes of inherited thrombophilia.

Protein C deficiency
Protein S deficiency
Antithrombin deficiency
Factor V Leiden (R506Q
Prothrombin gene polymorphism G20210A
Hyperhomocysteinemia due to genetic enzymatic defects
Homocysteinuria
Elevated factor VIII
Dysfibrinogenemia

Table 10.2 Acquired thrombophilic states.

Surgery
Oral contraceptives and hormone-replacement treatment
Cancer and its treatment (chemo- or hormonal therapy)
Myeloproliferative disorders
Trauma
Immobility
Antiphospholipid syndrome
Pregnancy and puerperium
Long travel
Heart failure
Stroke
Nephrotic syndrome
Inflammatory bowel disease
Behçet's disease

Table 10.3. The risk of thromboembolism varies according to the type of thrombophilia, as shown in Table 10.4.

The relationship between cancer and thrombosis has been known since 1865, when Trousseau first described 'a particular condition of the blood which predisposed it to spontaneous coagulation'.[1] Multiple prothrombotic pathogenic processes are involved in malignancy, including activation of the coagulation cascade and fibrinolytic system, procoagulant activation of tumor cells, and tumor-cell interaction with blood cells and endothelium, as well as clinical situations with increased risk of thrombosis (for example, chemotherapy, immobilization, surgery, and infection).[2] While the role of acquired thrombophilia as one of the possible pathogenic mechanisms in venous thromboembolism (VTE) in cancer, has been thoroughly explored (see Chapter 2), the issue of thrombophilia as a cause or additional contributor to the hypercoagulable state in cancer patients has not been fully investigated. This chapter

Table 10.3 Prevalence of inherited thrombophilia among healthy subjects and unselected patients with venous thrombosis.

Type of thrombophilia	Healthy subjects (%)	Unselected patients (%)
Antithrombin deficiency	0.02	1–2
Protein C deficiency	0.2–0.4	3–4
Protein S deficiency	?	2
Factor V Leiden	5	20
Prothrombin G20210A	2–3	7
Elevated factor VIII levels	11	25
Hyperhomocysteinemia	5	10

Data based on[32–34]

Table 10.4 The risk of venous thrombosis in hereditary thrombophilia.

Type of thrombophilia	Odds ratio	95% confidence interval
Antithrombin deficiency	2.2	1–4.7
Protein C deficiency	3.1	1.4–7
Protein S deficiency	1.6	0.6–4
Factor V Leiden: heterozygous	6.6	3.6–12
Factor V Leiden: homozygous	80	22.0–289
Prothrombin G20210A	2.8	1.4–5.6
Hyperhomocysteinemia	2.5	1.2–5.2

Data based[35]

focuses on the association of inherited thrombophilia and VTE in patients with cancer and briefly mentions other acquired thrombophilic states that may influence the hypercoagulable state associated with cancer.

APC resistance and factor V Leiden (FVL)

Dahlback was the first to notice the phenomenon of activated protein C resistance (APC-R), which is the most common cause of inherited thrombophilia.[3,4] Later, Bertina et al[5] found the molecular basis of APC-R, namely, the factor V Leiden (FVL) mutation, R506Q, in which arginine (R) is replaced by glutamine (Q) at position 506 in the factor V gene. The mutant FVL is more slowly inactivated by protein C than wild-type factor V.[6] APC-R, which is not related to this mutation (acquired APC-R), has also been found to be an independent risk factor for VTE.[7,8] Acquired APC-R is associated with a number of clinical conditions, including pregnancy,[9] oral contraceptive use,[10] and antiphospholipid syndrome.[11]

Only a few studies have investigated whether the prevalence of APC-R is different in cancer patients than in patients without cancer. Otterson et al[12] reported a 5% prevalence of the FVL mutation in oncology patients, similar to the 8% rate observed among cancer patients with VTE, and concluded that this mutation was not associated with thrombosis in cancer patients. Two other small studies[13,14] suggested that APC-R is relatively common in cancer patients without a history of VTE. In these studies, acquired APC-R was detected in 10% of patients with various types of advanced cancer and in 50% of patients with advanced gastrointestinal cancer. Weitz et al[15] reported three patients with breast cancer who developed thromboembolic complications while receiving tamoxifen. All patients carried the FVL mutation.

Our group performed a prospective study designed to evaluate the prevalence of inherited and acquired APC-R in cancer patients with previous episodes of VTE as well as in cancer patients without VTE and in controls.[16] Fifty-five consecutive cancer patients with deep-vein thrombosis (DVT), 58 cancer patients with no history of DVT, 54 patients with DVT without cancer, and 56 healthy controls were included in the study. The prevalence of the FVL mutation in cancer patients with VTE (2%) did not differ significantly from cancer patients without VTE (7%) or normal subjects (4%), but it was significantly lower than in patients with VTE without cancer (33%, $p < 0.001$). The prevalence of acquired APC-R was significantly greater in cancer patients with VTE (54%, $p = 0.001$) than in the other groups.

The conclusion is that while FVL is not a major risk factor for VTE in cancer patients, acquired APC-R is a common risk factor potentially contributing to the thrombotic tendency in these patients. We further tried to explain the mechanisms for acquired APC-R in cancer patients. It was found that elevated levels (>150 u/dl) of coagulation factor V and factor VIII were significantly more common in cancer patients than controls (21% vs 3% and 40% vs 0%, $p = 0.03$ and $p = 0.02$ respectively).[17]

Recently, a prospective randomized trial was conducted to examine the incidence of APC-R in multiple myeloma (MM) patients and its relation to VTE.[18] Sixty-two newly diagnosed MM patients were tested at baseline for hypercoagulability, including activated protein C sensitivity ratio (APC-SR) and the FVL mutation. The patients underwent an intensive chemotherapy regimen with or without thalidomide in a randomized fashion. During the induction phase, 12 patients (19%) developed DVT, which was significantly more common in the thalidomide arm (36%) than in the control group (3%, $p = 0.001$). Fourteen patients (23%) were found to have reduced APC-SR at baseline in the absence of the FVL mutation. A significantly higher proportion of patients with APC-R developed DVT (5/14 vs 7/38, $p = 0.04$) irrespective of thalidomide administration. The risk of DVT (50%) was highest in patients with APC-R on thalidomide. Thus, acquired APC-R was present in almost a quarter of newly diagnosed MM patients, and thalidomide significantly increased the risk of DVT, highlighting the question of prophylaxis with anticoagulants in this setting.

To elucidate the interaction of cancer with the FVL mutation and its effect on the occurrence of thrombosis, Blom et al[19] conducted a retrospective study among 1267 patients with a first event of DVT/pulmonary embolism from five anticoagulation clinics. Their partners served as controls. Eleven percent of patients died because of cancer. It was found that the FVL mutation increased the risk of VTE by 2.9-fold (95% confidence interval [CI] 1.9–4.4) and cancer by 2.7-fold (95% CI: 1.9–4), and the combination of FVL and cancer increased the risk by the sum of the separate effects. The conclusion is that, regarding VTE, the combination of cancer and FVL is additive but not multiplicative.

Thrombophilia polymorphisms

The impact of FVL, prothrombin mutation (PTM), and methylenetetrahy-drofolate reductase (MTHFR) polymorphism on thrombosis risk was determined in another study, which included a cohort of 175 patients with gastrointestinal adenocarcinoma.[20] An increased prevalence of PTM was found in patients compared with the normal population (5.7% vs 0.8%, $p = 0.028$). One hundred and forty-seven patients did not have VTE (group A), whereas 28 of patients had VTE during the period follow-ing tumor diagnosis (group B). Only 6.8% of group A patients, but 21.4% of the patients in group B, had thrombosis before the diagnosis of cancer (OR = 3.7, $p = 0.025$). Heterozygosity for the FVL mutation was present in 4.8% of the patients in group A and in 17.9% of group B (OR = 4.4, $p = 0.026$). This study demonstrated a significant effect of FVL on thrombosis in patients with malignancy and also suggested that PTM may be a risk factor in cancer thrombosis.

A study from Italy[21] performed thrombophilia work-up and a search for occult cancer in 360 consecutive patients with VTE. Twenty-three occult cancers were discovered (7%). No increased rate of congenital thrombophilia in the cancer patients was found, suggesting that the cancer itself was responsible for the hypercoagulable state.

The natural anticoagulants

In one study, 50 consecutive cancer patients with gastrointestinal or pelvic malignancy and 50 healthy controls were enrolled.[22] In the cancer group, the frequency of inherited coagulation defects, including protein C (PC), protein S (PS), antithrombin (AT), the FVL mutation, MTHFR C677T polymorphisms, and the prothrombin G20210A mutation, did not differ from the control group.

Several studies demonstrated reduced levels of the natural anticoagu-lants, namely, PC, PS, and AT, in cancer patients.[23] This may stem from decreased hepatic production or increased consumption, it may be sec-ondary to chemotherapy (L-asparaginase) and hormonal treatment (tamoxifen), or it may be due to low-grade disseminated intravascular coagulation (DIC). No specific association between hereditary deficiency of PC, PS, and AT and thrombosis in cancer patients has been found.[24,25]

Antiphospholipid antibodies (APA)

There is a clear association between thrombotic events in cancer patients and antiphospholipid antibodies (APA), which encompass lupus anticoagulant (LA), anticardiolipin antibodies (ACA), and other antiphospholipids detected by ELISA. A large prospective study from France[26] has provided important data on the occurrence of malignancy in APA-positive patients. Among 1014 patients admitted to a department of internal medicine, 72 patients (7.1%) were found to be APA-positive, as expected. The most frequently associated disease in these patients was cancer (19%).

Zuckerman et al,[27] estimated the prevalence of ACA in 216 patients with solid and nonsolid tumors and 88 healthy controls. ACA levels were measured and related to thromboembolic phenomena that occurred within 1 year of the diagnosis of cancer. Forty-seven patients with cancer had elevated ACA levels (22%), as compared with 3% in the control group ($p \leq 0.0001$). The ACA-positive cancer patients had a significantly higher rate of thromboembolic events than the ACA-negative cancer patients (28% vs 14%, $p < 0.05$), and the risk of VTE correlated positively with high titers of ACA.

In conclusion, regarding the association between APA and cancer, patients with APA should undergo a search for underlying malignancy.[28]

Hyperhomocysteinemia (HHC) and cancer

Hyperhomocysteinemia (HHC) is a risk factor for VTE and arterial thrombosis.[29,30] Inherited enzyme defects in homocysteine metabolism and several acquired conditions may cause HHC. Cancers of the breast, ovary, and pancreas, as well as acute lymphoblastic leukemia, result in marked elevation of homocysteine levels.[31] No studies have been conducted in this regard, but it is possible that, as cancer and HHC are independent risk factors for VTE, the combination of the two may further increase the thromboembolic risk. However, a direct relation between HHC, cancer, and the risk of VTE has not been established.

Summary

There is no evidence yet of a higher frequency of thrombophilia in cancer patients. Recent studies suggest that the prevalence of acquired APC-R is higher in cancer patients than in patients without cancer. It is possible that thrombophilia coexists with cancer, and this situation may lead to an increased risk of thrombosis. More studies are needed to determine a possible relation between cancer, thrombophilia, and VTE.

References

1. Trousseau A. Phlegmasia alba dolens. In: Lectures on Clinical Medicine, Delivered at the Hôtel-Dieu, Paris. (New Sydenham Society: London, 1872) 281–95.

2. Falanga A, Rickles F. Pathophysiology of the thrombophilic state in the cancer patient. Semin Thromb Haemost 1999; **25**:173–82.

3. Dahlback B, Carlsson M. Svensson PJ. Familial thrombophilia due to a previously unrecognized mechanism characterized by poor anticoagulant response to activated protein C: prediction of a cofactor to activated protein C. Proc Natl Acad Sci USA 1993; **90**:1004–8.

4. Koster T, Rosendaal FR, de Ronde H et al. Venous thrombosis due to poor anticoagulant response to activated protein C: Leiden Thrombophilia Study. Lancet 1993; **342**:1503–6.

5. Bertina RM, Koeleman BP, Koster T et al. Mutation in blood coagulation factor V associated with resistance to activated protein C. Nature 1994; **369**:64–7.

6. Tosetto A, Misssiaglia E, Gatto E et al. The VITA project: phenotypic resistance to activated protein C and factor V Leiden mutation in the general population. Vicenza Thrombophilia and Atherosclerosis. Thromb Haemost 1997; **78**: 859–63.

7. Rodeghiero F, Tosetto A. Activated protein C resistance and factor V Leiden mutation are independent risk factors for venous thromboembolism. Ann Intern Med 1991; **130**:643–50.

8. de Visser MCH, Rosendaal FR, Bertina RM. A Reduced sensitivity for activated protein C in the absence of factor V Leiden increases the risk of venous thrombosis. Blood 1999; **93**:1271–76.

9. Cumming AM, Tait RC, Fildes S et al. Development of resistance to activated protein C during pregnancy. Br J Haematol 1995; **90**: 725–27.

10. Rosing J, Tans G, Nicolaes GA et al. Oral contraceptives and venous thrombosis: different sensitivities to activated protein C in women using second- and third-generation oral contraceptives. Br J Haematol 1997; **97**:233–8.

11. Rand JH. Antiphospholipid antibody syndrome: new insights on thrombogenic mechanisms. Am J Med Sci 1998; **316**:142–51.

12. Otterson GA, Monahan BP, Harold N et al. Clinical significance of the FV: Q506 mutation in unselected oncology patients. Am J Med 1996; **101**:406–12.

13. Green D, Maliekel K, Sushko E et al. Activated protein C resistance in cancer patients. Hemostasis 1997; **27**:112–18.

14. De Lucia D, De Vita F, Orditura M et al. Hypercoagulable state in patients with advanced gastrointestinal cancer: evidence for an acquired resistance to activated protein C. Tumori 1997; **83**: 948–52.

15. Weitz IC, Israel VK, Libman HA. Tamoxifen-associated venous thrombosis and activated protein C resistance due to factor V Leiden. Cancer 1997; **79**:2024–27.

16. Haim N, Lanir N, Hoffman R et al. Acquired activated protein C resistance is common in cancer patients and is associated with venous thromboembolism. Am J Med 2001; **10**:91–6.

17. Michaeli Y, Lanir N, Sarig G et al. Mechanisms for acquired activated

protein C resistance in cancer patients. Haemostasis 2001; **31** (Suppl 1):91 (abst).

18. Zangari M, Saghafifar F, Anaissie E et al. Activated protein C resistance in the absence of factor V Leiden mutation is a common finding in multiple myeloma and is associated with an increased risk of thrombotic complications. Blood Coagul Fibrinolysis 2002; **13**:187–92.

19. Blom JW, Doggen CJM, Rosendaal FR. The risk of venous thrombosis in cancer patients with or without the factor V Leiden mutation. Haemostasis 2001; **31**(Suppl 1):73 (abst).

20. Pihusch R, Danzl G, Scholz M et al. Impact of thrombophilic gene mutations on thrombosis risk in patients with gastrointestinal carcinoma. Cancer 2002; **94**:3120–6.

21. Thibault-Gouin I, Achkar A, Samama MM. The thrombophilic state in cancer patients. Acta Haematol 2001; **106**:33–42.

22. Battistelli S, Ranalli M, Battistini S et al. The prevalence of inherited thrombophilia in patients with cancer: Preliminary findings. Haemostasis 2001; **31** (Suppl 1):91 (abst).

23. Rickles FR, Levine M, Edwards RL. Hemostatic alterations in cancer patients. Cancer Metastasis Rev 1992; **11**:237–48.

24. Schmitt M, Kuhn W, Harbeck N et al. Thrombophilic state in breast cancer. Semin Thromb Hemost 1999; **25**:157–72.

25. Lee AYY, Levine MN. The thrombophilic state induced by therapeutic agents in the cancer patient. Semin Thromb Hemost 1999; **25**:137–46.

26. Schved JF, Dupuy-Fons C, Biron C et al. Prospective epidemiological study of the occurrence of antiphospholipid antibody; the Montpellier Antiphopholipid (MAP) study. Haemostasis 1994; **24**: 175–82.

27. Zuckerman E, Toubi E, Golan TD et al. Increased thromboembolic incidence in anti-cardiolipin positive patients with malignancy. Br J Cancer 1995; **72**:447–51.

28. Asherson RA. Antiphospholipid antibodies, malignancies and paraproteinemias. J Autoimmun 2000; **15**:117–22.

29. den Heijer M, Koster T, Blom HJ et al. Hyperhomocyteinemia as a risk factor for deep vein thrombosis. N Engl J Med 1996; **334**:759–62.

30. Welch GN, Loscalzo J. Homocysteine and artherothrombosis. N Engl J Med 1998; **338**:1042–50.

31. Wu LL, Wu JT. Hyperhomocysteinemia is a risk factor for cancer and a new potential tumour marker. Clin Chim Acta 2000; **322**:21–8.

32. Lane DA, Mannucci PM, Bauer KA et al. Inherited thrombophilia: Part 1. Thromb Haemost 1996; **76**: 651–2.

33. Seligsohn U, Lubetsky A. Genetic susceptibility to venous thrombosis. N Engl J Med 2001; **344**: 1222–31.

34. Rosendaal FR. Risk factors for enous thrombotic disease. Thromb Haemost 1999; **82**:610–19.

35. Koster T, Rosendaal FR, Briet E et al. Protein C deficiency in a controlled series of unselected outpatients: an infrequent but clear risk factor for venous thrombosis (Leiden Thrombophilia Study). Blood 1995; **85**:2756–61.

11

Long-term thrombotic complications in cancer-treated patients: The problem of recurrent venous thromboembolism

Graham F Pineo and Russell D Hull

Introduction

Numerous studies have identified cancer as a significant risk factor for the development of venous thromboembolism (VTE), deep venous thrombosis (DVT), and pulmonary embolism (PE). Furthermore, a small percentage of patients presenting with idiopathic DVT or PE go on to develop clinical evidence of cancer in the subsequent 1–2 years. In patients entered into recent treatment trials for DVT or PE, the incidence of cancer is in the range of 10–25%. Short-term or long-term follow-up of patients in these trials and in cohort studies continues to demonstrate that recurrent VTE remains a problem even with the best current management. Therefore, one of the unmet needs with respect to the treatment of VTE is to find better ways to prevent recurrent VTE, and this is of particular relevance to patients with cancer.

Risk factors predisposing to recurrent VTE

The various risk factors that predispose to VTE have been well documented (Table 11.1).[1] To this list, we now add various forms of thrombophilia.[2] In many cases, patients presenting with VTE have multiple risk factors, and all epidemiological studies include cancer as one of those risk factors.

Many of the risk factors that predispose to the initial development of VTE also predispose to recurrent events.[3,4] In all studies, cancer is identified as a risk factor for recurrent VTE. In a follow-up study of 738 consecutive patients with documented DVT, the overall recurrence rate over 5 years was 21.5%. In a multivariate analysis, proximal DVT,

Table 11.1 Prevalence of risk factors for venous thromboembolism among hospitalized patients. (Reproduced from Archives of Internal Medicine with permission.[1])

Risk factor	Percentage	No. of risk factors (mean + SD)
Age > 40 years	59.1	2.1 + 1.0
Obesity	27.6	2.4 + 1.0
Major surgery	22.8	2.3 + 1.1
Prolonged immobilization	14.2	3.0 + 1.1
Cancer	9.3	2.8 + 1.0
Congestive heart failure	7.8	2.8 + 0.9
Myocardial infarction	2.9	3.3 + 0.9
Fracture (hip or leg)	2.2	3.7 + 1.3
History of venous thromboembolism	1.8	3.0 + 1.0
Trauma	1.6	2.1 + 1.5
Stroke	1.5	3.3 + 1.3
Estrogen-replacement therapy	0.4	2.0 + 0.8

cancer, and a history of thromboembolism independently predicted an increased risk of recurrent events, with the relative risks being 2.40, 1.97, and 1.71, respectively.[4] As in other studies, DVT secondary to surgery had a lower relative risk of recurrence than the three previous risk factors.[4] In the database described by White et al using linked California state hospital discharge records, the 6-month cumulative incidence of hospitalization for recurrent VTE was around 5.5%, depending on the length of initial hospitalization.[5] Multivariate modeling revealed that recurrent VTE was associated with the length of hospitalization, presence of cancer, older age, dementia, and hospitalization for multiple injuries within 3 months and surgery within 3 months. The odds ratio for readmission for recurrent VTE and the presence of cancer was 1.58 (95% confidence interval [CI] 1.46–1.68), the highest of any of the risk categories. In a prospective study of 296 consecutive patients with PE, logistic regression was used to predict death, recurrent thromboembolic events, or major bleeding over the initial 3-month period. Factors associated with an adverse outcome in order of magnitude were systolic blood pressure less than 100 mm mercury, cancer, presence of DVT, and ultrasound showing previous DVT and heart failure.[6]

The location of the initial DVT has an impact on the incidence of recurrence. Thus, the presence of iliofemoral vein thrombosis has a rate of recurrent VTE of 11.8%, compared with 5.1% for popliteal vein thrombosis.[7] In the report by Breddin et al,[8] there was a high correlation between venographic results as measured by the Marder[9] score and recurrence of the DVT. Of the 490 patients classified as having no response on venography, 34% had recurrent VTE, whereas only 5 (1.05%) of 476 patients classified as having a response had such a recurrent event.

There are a number of reasons why patients with cancer are prone to develop recurrent VTE.[10–12] The same risk factors predisposing to the initial episode in most cases persist and are often aggravated by administration of chemotherapy, insertion of central lines, repeat surgery, and compression of pelvic veins by malignant tumors, as well as the worsening condition of the patient. The impact of either hereditary or acquired thrombophilic states is yet to be assessed. Although early reports suggest that thrombophilia in addition to cancer may be associated with an increased thrombotic risk,[13–15] further studies are required to clarify the role of these and other risk factors in the initial and recurrent development of VTE in cancer patients.

Diagnosis of recurrent VTE

The diagnosis of recurrent DVT or PE is problematic because of abnormalities persisting from the initial diagnosis.[16] This problem is taken into account in diagnostic algorithms for DVT and PE. Thus, for the diagnosis of recurrent DVT, if a new segment is identified on ultrasound or venography, if there is extension of a previous clot, or if the defect is in the opposite leg, a firm diagnosis of a new DVT can be made. The diameter of the involved vein on compression ultrasonography has recently been shown to be a useful finding.[17,18] In a follow-up study of 205 consecutive patients presenting with suspected recurrent DVT in the same leg, the ultrasound was positive for recurrent DVT if a previously normalized vein had become noncompressible or if the residual vein diameter in the venous segment had enlarged 2 mm or more compared with the previous assessment. All three patients with this abnormality had recurrent VTE confirmed by venography.[18]

For patients with previous PE, diagnosis can be established if there is a new perfusion defect indicating high probability of PE or if the leg ultrasound is positive for DVT. New techniques identifying the thrombus directly, such as spiral CT or MRI, may identify a new PE. Finally, blood tests, such as D-dimer and cardiac troponin-1 levels, may be useful in establishing a diagnosis.[19–21] Furthermore, a recent study has shown that D-dimer could be used in conjunction with ultrasonography in patients who had cancer to rule out DVT.[22] The presence of active cancer (treatment ongoing or within the previous 6 months, or patients on palliative care) is one of the scoring points for the pretest probability assessment of both DVT and PE.[23,24]

Treatment of VTE

The initial treatment of DVT and PE is the same: either unfractionated heparin or low-molecular-weight heparin.[25] The suggestive evidence that the prognosis for long-term survival and recurrent VTE is worse with patients presenting with PE than DVT may be a reason to treat patients presenting with PE more aggressively in the future, but, at present, the anticoagulant management is identical.[26,27] A selected group of patients with acute massive or submassive PE may be candidates for thrombolysis. A recent study has shown that heparin plus alteplase was significantly better than heparin plus placebo in increasing the probability of event-free survival (with 'event' being defined as in-hospital death or clinical deterioration requiring an escalation of treatment after termination of the infusion of the study drug).[28] However, as with previous trials of thrombolysis in acute PE, there was no significant decrease in mortality with the use of thrombolysis. Except for patients who present with an acute episode of isolated femoral or ileofemoral DVT, there are no indications for thrombolysis in the treatment of DVT.[29]

Low-molecular-weight heparin or unfractionated heparin

In a number of large, multicenter, randomized clinical trials, low-molecular-weight heparin in fixed doses given by subcutaneous injection once or twice daily without laboratory monitoring (apart from platelet counts) has been compared with unfractionated heparin given by continuous intravenous infusion, in most cases with a prescriptive heparin nomogram.[30,31] There has been only one large, randomized clinical trial comparing fixed-dose low-molecular-weight heparin given by subcutaneous injection once daily with unfractionated heparin for the initial treatment of acute PE.[32] These studies have been reviewed in a number of meta-analyses.[33–36] The conclusions from these systematic reviews is that low-molecular-weight heparin is at least as effective and safe as unfractionated heparin in terms of recurrent VTE and major bleeding. They demonstrate that there is a small but significant mortality advantage for patients receiving low-molecular-weight heparin when compared with unfractionated heparin. The studies also indicate that once-daily is as safe and effective as twice-daily administration of low-molecular-weight heparin.[35] Randomized clinical trials and cohort studies indicate that many patients presenting with DVT or PE can be safely managed out of hospital.[34–36] The incidence of heparin-induced thrombocytopenia is lower in patients receiving low-molecular-weight heparin than unfractionated heparin, although heparin-induced thrombocytopenia may still occur with the various low-molecular-weight heparins.[37,38] There is evidence from laboratory experiments[39,40] and clinical trials[41–43] that low-molecular-weight heparin has less tendency to cause osteoporosis than unfractionated heparin. Unfractionated heparin has the advantage that the anticoagulant effect can be more readily blocked by protamine sulfate than can that of low-molecular-weight heparin,[44–46] and the infusion can be discontinued should bleeding occur, but it has the disadvantage of requiring careful monitoring.

Warfarin treatment

Warfarin with a targeted international normalized ratio (INR) of 2.0–3.0 is the agent most commonly used for long-term anticoagulation in patients with VTE.[25] This agent is often difficult to manage because of the narrow therapeutic window, and long-term treatment studies demonstrate a close correlation with thrombosis when the INR is less than 2 and increased major bleeding complications when the INR is elevated, particularly when it is above 4.5.[47,48] Furthermore, compliance is an issue, as many clinical trials indicate that patients are within the predicted therapeutic range only around 40% of the time.

A number of studies have addressed the issue of safety of oral anticoagulant therapy in patients with cancer.[49–54] In a prospective cohort study, Bona et al observed that the rates of major bleeding, minor bleeding, and recurrent thrombosis were not significantly different in patients treated with long-term oral anticoagulation either with or without cancer.[51] However, therapeutic INRs were more difficult to sustain in cancer patients. In their review of data from the ISCOAT study, Palareti et al showed that the rate of major and minor bleeding was significantly greater in patients with cancer than in those without cancer.[53] Bleeding was more frequently a cause of anticoagulation withdrawal in cancer patients as well (4.2% versus 0.7%). In addition, Hutten et al, from a review of two randomized clinical trials, indicated that the incidence of major bleeding was 13.3 per 100 patient-years compared with 2.1 per 100 patient-years in the cancer patients versus those without cancer ($p = 0.002$).[54] Not all studies demonstrated a close correlation of bleeding with over-anticoagulation. For example, Hutten et al demonstrated a higher incidence of bleeding complications with an INR greater than 3 in patients without cancer, but this pattern was not demonstrated in patients with cancer.[54]

In patients with idiopathic DVT, the duration of initial anticoagulation has a significant impact on the development of recurrent DVT. Thus, in trials comparing 4 weeks with 12 weeks, 6 weeks with 6 months, or 3 months with 12 months or indefinite anticoagulation, the longer oral anticoagulants are used, the lower the incidence of recurrent VTE.[55–60] In the study by Agnelli et al, comparing 3 months with 12 months of oral anticoagulation following an initial episode of idiopathic DVT, patients treated for 3 months had an increased rate of recurrent DVT over the subsequent 9 months, but those patients treated for 12 months had recurrences when their oral anticoagulants were stopped, and by 36 months the recurrent VTE rates were the same.[60] Thus, it would appear that there are a significant number of patients with DVT who have a tendency to have recurrent VTE. This is particularly true in patients who have VTE related to cancer. Indeed, in the Sixth American College of Chest Physicians Consensus Conference on Antithrombotic Therapy, the recommendation was, for patients with an initial episode of VTE with a continuing risk factor such as cancer, that anticoagulant treatment should be continued for 12 months or longer.[25] In most cases, these patients are continued on oral anticoagulants indefinitely or until it becomes unsafe to continue this kind of treatment.

Patients with brain metastases who require oral anticoagulation are always a concern, and many of these patients have inferior vena cava filters inserted.[61-64] In one report of an experience from a single institution, 51 patients experienced VTE. Of the 42 patients who received oral anticoagulation, 2 had devastating intracranial hemorrhage and another had minor deterioration.[63] Other bleeding complications were infrequent. The authors concluded that oral anticoagulation was acceptably safe when patients were maintained within the therapeutic range in the presence of brain metastases and VTE.

Recurrent VTE in patients with cancer

A number of studies have confirmed that the incidence of recurrent VTE is higher in patients with cancer than in those without cancer.[61-65] In one of the early clinical trials comparing low-molecular-weight heparin with unfractionated heparin, there was a significant decrease in the incidence of recurrent DVT and death in those patients receiving low-molecular-weight heparin.[30] Data from two large, randomized clinical trials comparing the efficacy and safety of low-molecular-heparin with unfractionated heparin in the treatment of proximal DVT were reviewed by Hutten et al.[54] Their aim was to assess the incidence of recurrent VTE and major bleeding among patients with VTE, with particular reference to cancer and the achieved INR. There were 264 patients with malignancy among the 1303 eligible patients. The incidence of recurrent VTE was 27.1% versus 9.0% in the cancer versus noncancer patients (95% CI 1.5–5.9, $p = 0.003$). The relation of INR to recurrent VTE was also assessed. In both treatment groups, there was a higher incidence of VTE when the INR was in the lowest range. The excess risk of recurrent VTE for patients with malignancy was 35.1 per 100 patient-years compared with 8.7 per 100 patient-years for patients without malignancy during those periods when the INR was less than 2.0. The effect of malignancy on the risk of recurrent VTE was not influenced by the percentage of time spent within the target range.[54]

Palareti and colleagues reviewed data from the ISCOAT Study Group in Italy.[53] This study compared outcomes of anticoagulation initially with heparin or low-molecular-weight heparin and then long-term oral anticoagulation in 95 patients with cancer and 733 patients without cancer, all of whom had documented acute VTE. Patients were within the targeted INR range 70% of the time, but cancer patients were above the therapeutic range more of the time than were those without cancer (8.8% versus 4.5%, respectively). More patients without cancer completed the prescribed anticoagulation course than those with cancer (61.9% versus 39.0%). The two main reasons for early withdrawal of anticoagulation therapy in the cancer group versus the noncancer group were death (32.6% versus 2.5%) and the significantly higher bleeding rate (4.2% versus 0.7%). The incidence of recurrent thromboembolism was 6.8% in the cancer group versus 2.5% in the noncancer group (95% CI 0.9–6.5). The incidence of thrombosis was higher in both groups when the INR was less than 2.0. However, in the cancer group, the relative risk of recurrent VTE with an INR of less than 2.0, compared with an INR of greater than 2.0, was 5.2, whereas in the patients without cancer the relative risk was 3.0, both of which were statistically significant. In this review, cancer was the most common cause of death, but only 6.5% of deaths were attributed to PE.

Long-term low-molecular-weight heparin treatment

An alternative to the use of warfarin for long-term treatment of patients with VTE is daily subcutaneous low-molecular-weight heparin.[66] Data comparing the efficacy and safety of warfarin with low-molecular-weight heparin for the long-term treatment of symptomatic VTE were reviewed by van den Heijden et al for the Cochrane Database.[66] The doses of low-molecular-weight heparin were not therapeutic doses; rather they were doses used for prevention of VTE in moderate- to high-risk surgical patients. It was concluded that low-molecular-weight heparin, as used in these studies, had an improved safety profile possibly related to the somewhat low dosage used. However, the studies did not provide conclusive evidence on whether treatment with low-molecular-weight heparin was as effective as warfarin treatment, again because of the low doses used.

Recently reported in abstract form were a number of studies comparing low-molecular-weight heparin with warfarin for 3–6 months in patients with VTE with or without cancer. One clinical trial compared low-molecular-weight heparin (tinzaparin 175 Xa units/kg, once daily by subcutaneous injection) with long-term warfarin in patients with proximal

DVT.[67] All patients received tinzaparin initially for 5–6 days. It was concluded that long-term therapeutic low-molecular-weight heparin was as effective and safe as warfarin, but quality of life was improved.

In the long-term treatment study, low-molecular-weight heparin (tinzaparin 175 Xa units/kg per day by subcutaneous injection) was compared with initial intravenous heparin followed by warfarin, with both treatment arms continuing for 3 months in patients with proximal DVT.[68] Randomization was stratified for cancer and by treatment site. This study indicated that low-molecular-weight heparin treatment resulted in a significant reduction in the rates of recurrent VTE in cancer patients, when compared with warfarin therapy, without any increase in the rates of bleeding.

In a randomized clinical trial in patients with cancer and VTE, low-molecular-weight heparin (dalteparin, 200 units/kg once daily for 5–7 days) with overlapping warfarin continued for 6 months, with a target INR of 2.5, was compared with dalteparin alone for 6 months (200 IU/kg per day for the first month followed by 150 IU kg/per day for the remaining 5 months).[69] This study indicated that low-molecular-weight heparin treatment resulted in a significant reduction in the rate of recurrent VTE, when compared with warfarin therapy, without any increase in the rate of bleeding.

Inferior vena cava filters in patients with recurrent VTE

In the past, there was widespread use of inferior vena cava filters in patients who experienced bleeding or recurrent VTE while within the therapeutic range on warfarin.[70–72] This was particularly common in patients with VTE and cancer where it was expected that there would be a greater tendency to recurrent VTE and fatal PE. In the only randomized clinical trial to date, patients with proximal DVT were randomized to insertion of an inferior vena cava filter or no filter, and all patients were treated with initial low-molecular-weight heparin and warfarin long-term.[72] The rates of recurrent VTE, death, and major bleeding were analyzed at 12 days and at 2 years. At 12 days, symptomatic or asymptomatic PE was confirmed in two patients who had received a filter (1.1%) versus nine patients who did not receive a filter (4.8%)—OR 0.22 (95% CI 0.05–0.90). However, at 2 years, 37 patients assigned to the filter group (20.8%), versus 21 patients without a filter (11.6%), had recurrent DVT—OR 1.87 (95% CI 1.10–3.20). There was no difference in mortality or major bleeding. Currently, the main indications for inferior vena cava filters are contraindication to anticoagulants, recurrent PE despite adequate anticoagulation, and prophylactic placement in high-risk patients, such as those with multiple traumas.[25] In the higher-risk category are patients with cor pulmonale or previous history of PE who are placed in high-risk situations, such as acetabular fracture, or patients who have active cancer.

Conclusions

VTE is a common problem in patients with cancer, particularly those with active and ongoing disease. The use of standard heparin or low-molecular-weight heparin followed by warfarin is effective in most of these patients, but the incidence of both major and minor bleeding and of recurrent VTE is higher when VTE occurs in cancer patients than in those without cancer. At present, warfarin is the only agent used widely for the secondary prevention of VTE, but there is current interest in the use of once-daily low-molecular-weight heparin, particularly in those patients who have recurrent VTE while within the therapeutic INR range on warfarin. Recent reports support the use of low-molecular-weight heparin in place of warfarin in cancer patients with VTE. A number of new antithrombotic agents are under active investigation, and many of these are oral agents not requiring laboratory monitoring or dose adjustments. It remains to be seen whether they will be able to replace warfarin for the long-term treatment of VTE. In the meantime, further effort is required to maximize both the efficacy and safety of the current agents used for the management of VTE in cancer to decrease the considerable morbidity and mortality suffered by these patients.

References

1. Anderson FA Jr, Wheeler HB, Goldberg RJ et al. Prevalence of risk factors for venous thromboembolism among hospital patients. Arch Intern Med 1992; **152**: 1660–4.

2. Bauer KA. The thrombophilias: well-defined risk factors with uncertain therapeutic implications. Ann Intern Med 2001; **135**:367–73.

3. Prandoni P, Lensing AWA, Cogo A. The long-term clinical course of acute deep venous thrombosis. Ann Intern Med 1996; **125**:1–7.

4. Hansson PO, Sorbo J, Eriksson H. Recurrent venous thromboembolism after deep vein thrombosis. Arch Intern Med 2000; **160**: 769–74.

5. White RH, Zhou H, Romano PS. Length of hospital stay for treatment of deep venous thrombosis and the incidence of recurrent thromboembolism. Arch Intern Med 1998; **158**:1005–10.

6. Wicki J, Perrier A, Perneger TV et al. Predicting adverse outcome in patients with acute pulmonary embolism: a risk score. Thromb Haemost 2000; **84**:548–52.

7. Douketis JD, Crowther MA, Foster GA et al. Does the location of thrombosis determine the risk of disease recurrence in patients with proximal deep vein thrombosis? Am J Med 2000; **110**:515–19.

8. Breddin HK, Hach-Wunderle V, Nakov R et al. Effects of a low-

molecular weight heparin on thrombus regression and recurrent thromboembolism in patients with deep-vein thrombosis. N Engl J Med 2001; **344**:626–31.

9. Marder VJ, Soulen RL, Atchartakarn V et al. Quantitative venographic assessment of deep vein thrombosis in the evaluation of streptokinase and heparin therapy. J Lab Clin Med 1977; **89**:1018–29.

10. Prandoni P, Lensing AWA, Piccioli A et al. Recurrent venous thromboembolism and bleeding complications during anticoagulant treatment in patients with cancer and venous thrombosis. Blood 2002; **100**:3484–8.

11. Rickles FR, Levine MN. Epidemiology of thrombosis in cancer. Acta Haematol 2001; **106**: 6–12.

12. Prandoni P, Lensing AWA, Prins MH et al. Residual venous thrombosis as a predictive factor of recurrent venous thromboembolism. Ann Intern Med 2002; **137**:955–60.

13. Gouin-Thibeult I, Achkar A, Samama MM. The thrombophilic state in cancer patients. Acta Haematol 2001; **106**:33–42.

14. Haim N, Lanir N, Hoffman R et al. Acquired activated protein C resistance is common in cancer patients and is associated with venous thromboembolism. Am J Med 2001; **110**:91–6.

15. Zangari M, Saghafifar F, Anaissie E et al. Activated protein C resistance in the absence of factor V Leiden mutation is a common finding in multiple myeloma and is associated with an increased risk of thrombotic complications. Blood Coagul Fibrinolysis 2002; **13**:187–92.

16. Huisman MV. Recurrent venous thromboembolism: diagnosis and management. Pulm Med 2000; **6**:330–4.

17. Prandoni P, Cogo A, Bernardi E et al. A simple ultrasound approach for detection of recurrent proximal-vein thrombosis. Circulation 1993; **88**:1730–5.

18. Prandoni P, Lensing AWA, Bernardi E et al. The diagnostic value of compression ultrasonography in patients with suspected recurrent deep vein thrombosis. Thromb Haemost 2002; **88**:402–6.

19. Wells PS, Anderson DR, Rodger M et al. Excluding pulmonary embolism at the bedside without diagnostic imaging: management of patients with suspected pulmonary embolism presenting to the emergency department by using a simple clinical model and D-dimer. Ann Intern Med. 2001; **135**: 98–107.

20. Dieter RS, Ernst E, Ende DJ et al. Diagnostic utility of cardiac troponin-1 levels in patients with suspected pulmonary embolism. Angiology 2002; **53**:583–5.

21. Meyer T, Binder L, Hruska N et al. Cardiac troponin 1 elevation in acute pulmonary embolism is associated with right ventricular dysfunction. J Am Coll Cardiol 2000; **36**:1632–6.

22. ten Wolde M, Kraaijenhagen A, Prins MH et al. The clinical usefulness of D-dimer testing in cancer patients with suspected deep venous thrombosis. Arch Intern Med 2002; **162**:1880–4.

23. Wells PS, Anderson DR, Bormanis J et al. Application of a diagnostic clinical model for the management of hospitalized patients with suspected deep-vein thrombosis. Thromb Haemost 1999; **81**:493–7.

24. Wells PS, Anderson DR, Rodger M et al. Derivation of a simple clinical model to categorize patients' probability of pulmonary embolism: increasing the model's utility with the SimpliRED D-dimer. Thromb Haemost 2000; **83**:416–20.

25. Hyers T, Agnelli G, Hull R et al. Antithrombotic therapy for venous thromboembolic disease. Chest 2001; **119**:S176–93.

26. Douketis DID, Foster GA, Crowther MA et al. Clinical risk factors and timing of recurrent venous thromboembolism during the initial 3 months of anticoagulant therapy. Arch Intern Med 2000; **160**:3431–6.

27. Douketis DID, Kearon C, Bates S et al. Risk of fatal pulmonary embolism in patients with treated venous thromboembolism. JAMA 1998; **279**: 458–62.

28. Konstantinides S, Geibel A, Heusel G et al. Heparin plus alteplase compared with heparin alone in patients with submassive pulmonary embolism. N Engl J Med 2002; **347**:1143–50.

29. Wells PS, Forster AJ. Thrombolysis in deep vein thrombosis: is there still an indication? Thromb Haemost 2001; **86**:499–508.

30. Hull RD, Raskob GE, Pineo GF et al. Subcutaneous low-molecular-weight heparin compared with continuous intravenous heparin in the treatment of proximal-vein thrombosis. N Engl J Med 1992; **326**:975–83.

31. Prandoni P, Lensing AW, Buller HR et al. Comparison of subcutaneous low-molecular-weight heparin with intravenous standard heparin in proximal deep-vein thrombosis. Lancet 1992; **339**:411–15.

32. Simonneau G, Sors H, Charbonnier B, et al. A comparison of low-molecular-weight heparin with unfractionated heparin for acute pulmonary embolism. The THESEE Study Group. N Engl J Med 1997; **337**:663–9.

33. Hettiarachchi RJ, Prins MH, Lensing AW et al. Low molecular weight heparin versus unfractionated heparin in the initial treatment of venous thromboembolism. Curr Opin Pulm Med 1998; **4**:220–5.

34. Gould MK, Dembitzer AD, Doyle RL et al. Low-molecular-weight heparins compared with unfractionated heparin for treatment of acute deep venous thrombosis. A meta-analysis of randomized, controlled trials. Ann Intern Med 1999; **130**:800–9.

35. Dolovich LR, Ginsberg JS, Douketis JD et al. A meta-analysis comparing low-molecular-weight heparins with unfractionated heparin in the treatment of venous thromboembolism: examining some unanswered questions regarding location of treatment, product type, and dosing frequency. Arch Intern Med 2000; **160**:181–8.

36. van den Belt AG, Prins MH, Lensing AW et al. Fixed dose subcutaneous low-molecular weight heparin versus adjusted dose unfractionated heparin for venous thromboembolism. Cochrane Database Syst Rev 2000; CD001100.

37. Warkentin TE, Levine MN, Hirsh J et al. Heparin-induced thrombocytopenia in patients treated with low-molecular-weight heparin or unfractionated heparin. N Engl J Med 1995; **332**:1330–76.

38. Lindhoff-Last E, Nakov R, Misselwitz F et al. Incidence and clinical relevance of heparin-induced antibodies in patients with deep vein thrombosis treated with unfractionated or low-molecular-weight heparin. Br J Haematol 2002; **118**:1137–42.

39. Shaughnessy SG, Young E, Deschamps P et al. The effects of low molecular weight and standard heparin on calcium loss from fetal rat calvaria. Blood 1995; **86**:1368.

40. Bhandari M, Hirsh J, Weitz JI et al. The effects of standard and low molecular weight heparin on bone nodule formation in vitro. Thromb Haemost 1998; **80**:413–17.

41. Monreal M, Lafox E, Salvador R et al. Adverse effects of three different

forms of heparin therapy: thrombocytopenia, increased transaminases, and hyperkalaemia. Eur J Clin Pharmacol 1989; **37**:415–18.

42. Pettila V, Kaaja R, Leinonen P, et al. Thromboprophylaxis with low molecular weight heparin (dalteparin) in pregnancy. Thromb Res 1999; **96**:275–82.

43. Pettila V, Leinonen P, Markkola A et al. Postpartum bone mineral density in women treated for thromboprophylaxis with unfractionated heparin or LMW heparin. Thromb Haemost 2002; **87**:182–6.

44. Hirsh J, Warkentin TE, Shaughnessy SG et al. Heparin and low-molecular-weight heparin: mechanisms of action, pharmacokinetics, dosing, monitoring, efficacy and safety. Chest 2001; **119**(Suppl 1):65S–94S.

45. Massonnet-Castel S, Pelissier E, Bara L et al. Partial reversal of low molecular weight heparin (PK 10169) anti-Xa activity by protamine sulfate: in vitro and in vivo study during cardiac surgery with extracorporeal circulation. Haemostasis 1986;**16**:139–46.

46. Crowther MA, Berry LR, Monagle PT et al. Mechanisms responsible for the failure of protamine to inactivate low-molecular-weight heparin. Br J Haematol 2002; **116**:178–86.

47. Hylek EM, Heiman H, Skates SJ et al. Acetaminophen and other risk factors for excessive warfarin anticoagulation. JAMA 1998; **279**: 657–62.

48. Beyth RJ, Cohen AM, Landefeld CS. Long-term outcomes of deep vein thrombosis. Arch Intern Med 1995; **155**:1031–37.

49. Jarrett BP, Dougherty MJ, Calligaro KD. Inferior vena cava filters in malignant disease. J Vasc Surg 2002; **36**:704–7.

50. Clarke-Pearson DL, Synan IS, Creasman WT. Anticoagulation therapy for venous thromboembolism in patients with gynecologic malignancy. Am J Obstet Gynecol 1983; **147**:369–75.

51. Bona RD, Sivjee KY, Hickey AD et al. The efficacy and safety of oral anticoagulation in patients with cancer. Thromb Haemost 1995; **74**:1055-8.

52. Chan A, Woodruff RK. Complications and failure of anticoagulation therapy in the treatment of venous thromboembolism in patients with disseminated malignancy. Aust NZ J Med 1992; **22**:119–22.

53. Palareti G, Legnani C, Lee A et al. A comparison of the safety and efficacy of oral anticoagulation for the treatment of venous thromboembolic disease in patients with or without malignancy. Thromb Haemost 2000; **84**:805–10.

54. Hutten BA, Prins MH, Gent M et al. Incidence of recurrent thromboembolic and bleeding complications among patients with venous thromboembolism in relation to both malignancy and achieved international normalized ratio: a retrospective analysis. J Clin Oncol 2000; **18**:3078–83.

55. Fennerty AG, Dolben J, Thomas P et al. A comparison of 3 and 6 weeks anticoagulation in the treatment of venous thromboembolism. Clin Lab Haematol 1987; **9**:17–21.

56. Research Committee of the British Thoracic Society: optimum duration of anticoagulation for deep-vein thrombosis and pulmonary embolism. Lancet 1992; **340**: 873–6.

57. Levine MN, Hirsh J, Gent M et al. Optimal duration of oral anticoagulation therapy: a randomized trial comparing four weeks with three months of warfarin in patients with proximal deep vein thrombosis. Thromb Haemost 1995; **74**:606–11.

58. Schulman S, Rhedin AS, Lindmarker P et al. A comparison

of six weeks with six months of oral anticoagulation therapy after a first episode of venous thromboembolism. N Engl J Med 1995; **332**:1661–5.

59. Kearon C, Gent M, Hirsh J et al. Extended anticoagulation prevented recurrence after a first episode of idiopathic venous thromboembolism. N Engl J Med 1999; **34**: 901–7.

60. Agnelli G, Prandoni P, Gabriella M et al. Three months versus one year of oral anticoagulant therapy for idiopathic deep venous thrombosis. N Engl J Med 2001; **345**: 165–9.

61. Schiff D, DeAngelis LM. Therapy of venous thromboembolism in patients with brain metastases. Cancer 1994; **73**:493–8.

62. Altschuler E, Moose H, Seiker RG et al. The risk of efficacy of anticoagulant therapy in the treatment of thromboembolic complications in patients with primary malignant brain tumors. Neurosurgery 1990; **27**:74–6.

63. Levin JM, Schiff D, Loeffler JS et al. Complications of therapy for venous thromboembolic disease in patients with brain tumors. Neurology 1993; **43**:1111–14.

64. Norris LK, Grossman SA. Treatment of thromboembolic complications in patients with brain tumors. J Neuro oncol 1994; **22**:127–37.

65. Levine M, Rickles FR. Treatment of venous thromboembolism in cancer patients. Haemostasis 1998; **28**:66–70.

66. van der Heijden JF, Hutten BA, Buller HR et al. Vitamin K antago-

nists or low-molecular-weight heparin for the long-term treatment of symptomatic venous thromboembolism. Cochrane Database Syst Rev 2002; 1.

67. Hull R, Pineo G, Mah A et al. The LITE Investigators. Long-term low-molecular-weight heparin treatment with oral anticoagulant therapy for proximal deep vein thrombosis. Blood 2000; **96**:449a.

68. Hull RD, Pineo GF, Mah AF et al. The LITE Investigators. A randomized trial evaluating long-term low-molecular-weight heparin therapy for three months versus intravenous heparin followed by warfarin. Blood 2002; **100**:556a.

69. Levine MN, Lee AY, Baker R et al. The CLOT Investigators. A randomized trial of long-term dalteparin low-molecular-weight heparin (LMWH) versus oral anticoagulant (OA) therapy in cancer patients with venous thromboembolism (VTE). Blood 2002; **100**: 298a.

70. Greenfield LJ, Proctor MC, Saluja A. Clinical results of Greenfield filter use in patients with cancer. Cardiovasc Surg 1997; **5**:145–9.

71. Ihnat DM, Mills JL, Hughes JD et al. Treatment of patients with venous thromboembolism and malignant disease: should vena cava filter placement be routine? J Vasc Surg 1998; **28**:800–7.

72. Decousus H, Leizorovicz A, Parent F et al. A clinical trial of vena caval filters in the prevention of pulmonary embolism in patients with proximal deep-vein thrombosis. N Engl J Med 1998; **338**:409–15.

12

Prevention of cancer-associated thrombosis: An overview

Mark Levine

Patients with cancer who undergo surgery are at increased risk of venous thromboembolism (VTE). In addition, 'medical' cancer patients who receive chemotherapy, hormonal therapy, and/or radiation therapy are also prone to develop VTE. Finally, cancer patients with central venous catheters (CVC) can develop CVC-associated thrombosis. Prophylaxis with antithrombotic agents can be problematic in cancer patients because they are also at increased risk of anticoagulant-induced bleeding. In this chapter, we discuss the evidence and provide recommendations for the prevention of VTE in these three clinical settings.

Surgical patients

Among patients with active malignancy, those undergoing surgery have a particularly high risk of thromboembolic disease. In general, prophylaxis with anticoagulant therapy in patients undergoing surgery for malignancy is strongly recommended. However, most of these patients also have a high risk of bleeding. Because malignancy (odds ratio 1.69) and complex surgery (odds ratio 1.62) are risk factors for perioperative bleeding in patients receiving heparin prophylaxis,[1] it is important that anticoagulant therapy be individualized to balance the competing risks of thrombosis and bleeding.

General surgery

Patients who are undergoing major abdominal or pelvic surgery for malignancy are at high risk of postoperative thrombosis.[1] The reason for the high incidence is multifactorial.[2] In addition to their malignancy, these patients often have concurrent risk factors that increase their risk of thrombosis, including advanced age, debility, long and complicated surgery, and often a prolonged postoperative course.

Kakkar and colleagues[3] evaluated the risk of thrombosis following major abdominal surgery, using ^{125}I-fibrinogen leg scanning. This technique is no longer used because of concern over viral transmission and accuracy.[4–6] In addition, many of the thrombi detected with leg scanning were asymptomatic. Kakkar et al showed that the postoperative rate of deep-vein thrombosis (DVT) was higher in patients with malignancy (41%) than in patients undergoing surgery for benign disease (26%).

A significantly higher rate of fatal pulmonary embolism (PE) following surgery has also been reported in cancer patients than noncancer patients.[1] A subgroup analysis of a large multicenter study with more than 4000 patients showed that the rate of fatal PE was 1.6% in patients with cancer and only 0.5% in those without cancer ($p = 0.05$).[7,8]

Pharmacological prophylaxis

The agents used most widely for prophylaxis in surgical patients are unfractionated heparin (UFH) and low-molecular-weight heparin (LMWH). Many clinical trials have compared the efficacy and safety of these agents, and several large meta-analyses of these trials have not detected any significant differences between these agents in reducing postoperative thrombosis and in anticoagulant-related bleeding following major abdominal surgery.[9–12] Although many of these trials included cancer patients, they were usually a small subset, and the results for the two patient groups were not analyzed or reported separately in many of the studies. In the trials of low-dose UFH versus LMWH that did comment on the differences between cancer and noncancer patients, a trend toward more thrombotic complications in cancer patients was consistently reported, independently of the prophylactic agent used.[13–17] In a recent meta-analysis that combined the results for cancer patients from these various trials, Mismetti et al found no significant difference between LMWH and UFH, in cancer patients undergoing surgery, for a number of clinically relevant outcomes, including symptomatic thromboembolism, major bleeding, transfusions, and death.[18]

Several trials have evaluated prophylaxis specifically in cancer patients undergoing general surgery. The largest study was performed by the ENOXACAN Study Group in Sweden.[19] These investigators compared a LMWH (enoxaparin 40 mg once daily) with UFH (5000 U three times a day) in 1115 patients having elective curative surgery for cancer of the abdomen or pelvis. According to mandatory bilateral venography used for outcome assessment, the rates of thrombosis were 14.7% in the enoxaparin group and 18.2% in the UFH group. These results were not statistically different. There were also no differences in the rates of major bleeding and the 30-day or 3-month mortality.

Taken together, the evidence suggests that once-daily LMWH is as safe and effective as multiple daily injections of UFH for the prevention of postoperative DVT in cancer patients. However, the residual risk of thrombosis with prophylaxis for 5–7 days remains considerable at 10–15%.

To examine whether extended prophylaxis could further reduce the risk of thrombosis, the ENOXACAN II study was conducted. Patients undergoing surgery for abdominal malignancy received 1 week of enoxaparin and then were randomized to enoxaparin or placebo for another 21 days.[20] Bilateral venography was performed at the end of treatment. Extended prophylaxis statistically significantly reduced the rate of DVT from 12% to 4.8%. However, most of these thrombi were asymptomatic, and the 1-year follow-up showed no difference in overall survival.[21] Therefore, although extended prophylaxis is efficacious in reducing postoperative DVT in cancer patients, additional clinical trials are required before extended prophylaxis can be recommended after cancer surgery.

Mechanical methods

Devices such as external pneumatic compression and graduated compression stockings are effective in reducing thrombosis after general surgery.[22–26] In a meta-analysis of 11 randomized clinical trials in abdominal and gynecological surgery and neurosurgery, graduated compression stockings were found to have a risk reduction of 68%.[22] Although it is effective, the major limitation of external pneumatic compression is its inconvenience and interference with early mobilization. Therefore, clinicians usually reserve it for patients with active hemorrhage or a high risk of bleeding after surgery. Mechanical devices can also be used in combination with UFH or LMWH in patients with a particularly high risk of thrombosis, such as those with a history of VTE, but evidence showing additive or synergistic effects is lacking.

In summary, pharmacological and mechanical methods of prophylaxis are effective and are recommended in cancer patients undergoing general surgery. Thromboprophylaxis should be initiated before surgery and continued throughout the acute, and possibly the extended, postoperative period. UFH and LMWHs appear to be equally safe and effective, but LMWHs have the major advantage of once-daily administration. Graduated compression stockings are effective and may improve the efficacy of pharmacological prophylaxis alone. External pneumatic compression is an acceptable alternative in patients in whom anticoagulant use is contraindicated. In the cancer patient undergoing general surgery, once-daily LMWH plus graduated compression stockings is recommended.

Neurosurgery

There is a general reluctance in neurosurgery to use anticoagulant prophylaxis because of the risk of intracranial or intraspinal bleeding. As a result, mechanical methods—such as external pneumatic compression, with or without graduated compression stockings—have typically been the preferred prophylactic measures in these patients.[27,28] However, the rate of postoperative thrombosis with compression stockings alone is approximately 30% on the basis of mandatory bilateral venography.[29,30]

Two randomized, placebo-controlled trials have compared the combined use of LMWH and graduated compression stockings with stockings alone in patients undergoing elective neurosurgery.[29,30] More than 80% of the patients in each study were having surgery for a brain or spinal-cord tumor. In both studies, the added administration of LMWH, starting within 24 hours after surgery, significantly improved the efficacy of stockings alone without a concomitant increase in the rate of major bleeding. However, despite a relative risk reduction of 30–40% with LMWH, about 18% of the patients who received LMWH and stockings still had evidence of thrombosis on mandatory bilateral venography approximately 1 week after surgery. This high residual risk may be due to the potent thrombogenic stimulus generated from large amounts of tissue factor released during neurosurgery, the delay in starting anticoagulant prophylaxis until after surgery, and the protracted immobilization after surgery.

In contrast, preoperative administration of LMWH may be associated with an increased risk of intracranial hemorrhage.[31] In an open-label study, patients with an intracranial neoplasm undergoing a neurosurgical procedure were randomized to receive enoxaparin, a sequential compression device, or both. After 66 patients were enrolled, the study was terminated prematurely when 3 patients in the combined therapy group and 1 in the enoxaparin group experienced clinically significant intracerebral bleeding, and 1 patient in the enoxaparin group suffered an epidural hematoma. There were no bleeding episodes in the mechanical prophylaxis group.

Based on the results of the two randomized trials, the most recent American College of Chest Physicians (ACCP) consensus guidelines, published in 2001, concluded that the combination of LMWH and a mechanical method may be more effective than either a pharmacological or mechanical method alone.[32] Nonetheless, there is a widespread reluctance to use LMWH within the perioperative period in these patients because of the risk of bleeding. It remains paramount that all cases be assessed individually, and those patients with an increased risk of bleeding should be treated with mechanical prophylaxis alone. Thus, to summarize, for cancer patients undergoing neurosurgery, LMWH commencing no sooner than 24 hours postoperatively, as well as mechanical prophylaxis (graduated compression stockings or intermittent pneumatic compression) or mechanical prophylaxis alone is recommended.

Gynecological surgery

The early studies in this patient group were a series of small, open-label, controlled trials in which women with gynecological cancers were randomized to receive prophylaxis versus no treatment.[33-36] Using ^{125}I-fibrinogen leg scanning or impedance plethysmography for screening, these studies found that the incidence of postoperative venous thrombosis after surgery for gynecological malignancy without prophylaxis ranged from 12% to 35%. Various prophylactic regimens, including low-dose UFH commencing 2 hours preoperatively, UFH commencing 16 hours preoperatively, and external pneumatic compression, were found to be effectively in reducing this risk by 20–60%.

Other investigators have compared LMWH with UFH in patients undergoing surgery for gynecological malignancy.[37,38] In these trials, no difference was detected between LMWH and UFH. The major shortcomings of most of these studies were the insufficient statistical power as a result of small sample sizes and the use of noninvasive leg testing for screening DVT. Nonetheless, the limited evidence demonstrates that the risk of thrombosis following gynecological surgery for cancer is substantial and that prophylaxis with anticoagulant therapy is indicated. The available data are also consistent with the observations in general surgery and suggest that once-daily LMWH administration is likely to be as efficacious and safe as UFH given in multiple injections. For patients undergoing extensive surgery for malignancy, the ACCP guidelines of 2001 recommend either low-dose heparin three times a day, with or without compression stockings or intermittent pneumatic compression, or LMWH.[32] For cancer patients undergoing gynecological surgery, LMWH as well as compression stockings is recommended for most patients and it is suggested that LMWH in addition to pneumatic compression be reserved for patients at especially high risk of thrombosis (such as with a past history of VTE.)

Medical patients

When considering the prevention of VTE in the medical cancer patient, the physician should be prepared to deal with two main clinical situations: the ambulatory patient who is receiving chemotherapy or radiation therapy and the patient who is bedridden for prolonged periods of time.

Much fewer data are available on the primary prevention of thrombosis in ambulatory cancer patients than on prevention after cancer surgery. Levine and colleagues[39] showed that low-dose warfarin is effective in reducing the rate of thrombosis during chemotherapy. In a double-blind, randomized trial, 311 patients with stage IV breast cancer were given either very low-dose warfarin or placebo while they were receiving chemotherapy. The warfarin dose was 1 mg daily for 6 weeks and was then adjusted to have the international normalized ratio (INR) maintained at 1.3–1.9. The average duration of therapy was 6 months. Seven patients in the placebo group and one in the warfarin group experienced a thrombotic event during follow-up. This relative risk reduction of 85% was statistically significant (p = 0.031) and was not associated with an increase in bleeding.

Despite this study, oncologists do not commonly practice prophylaxis with oral anticoagulants during chemotherapy. The most likely reasons are the risk of bleeding and the logistics of laboratory monitoring and dose adjustments, which are frequently required to compensate for changes in the platelet count and interaction with concomitant medications. An alternative is to reserve prophylaxis for high-risk situations (such as previous history of VTE or a pelvic mass causing poor venous drainage from the lower limbs). Although there are a number of trials that have evaluated long-term LMWH as secondary prophylaxis in patients with established venous thrombosis, there have been no trials reported that evaluated it for long-term primary prevention of VTE.

Similarly, no studies have evaluated long-term prophylaxis in bedridden cancer patients. Low-dose UFH and LMWH have been found to be effective in patients hospitalized with acute medical illnesses (such as myocardial infarction and ischemic stroke).[32] Samama and colleagues[40] demonstrated that short-term prophylaxis with LMWH in hospitalized medical patients significantly reduced the rate of DVT detected by screening venography. There was a trend, however, for an increase in overall bleeding. Thus, based on these considerations, it would seem reasonable that patients with advanced malignancy who are bedridden would benefit from prophylaxis with low-dose UFH or LMWH. The feasibility and cost-effectiveness of long-term subcutaneous administration, however, remain uncertain.

Catheter-related thrombosis

Long-term indwelling central venous catheters (CVCs) are commonly used in cancer patients for the administration of chemotherapy, parenteral nutrition, and blood products, and for facilitating the drawing of blood. One of the complications of CVCs is venous thrombosis related to the catheter. The extent of thrombosis associated with a CVC can involve the catheter tip (ball-valve clot), the length of the catheter (fibrin sheath), the catheterized vessel in the upper limb, the central vasculature of the neck or mediastinum, or a combination of these sites.

Although a number of studies have reported on the incidence of CVC-related thrombosis, the rates have varied between studies, and hence the true incidence in cancer patients is uncertain.[41] The discrepancy is due to a number of factors, including the retrospective nature and small size of most of the studies, differences in the populations studied, and variation in the diagnostic tests used to detect CVC-related thrombosis.

Four randomized studies have been performed to evaluate the safety and efficacy of prophylactic anticoagulation in patients with CVCs; two investigated low-dose warfarin and two examined LMWH. The first open-label study using low-dose warfarin was reported in 1990 by Bern et al,[42] who randomized 84 cancer patients to receive 1 mg warfarin daily or no treatment. Mandatory contrast venography was performed at 90 days or sooner if patients had symptoms suggestive of thrombosis. The rate of thrombosis was 37% in the control group and 10% in the warfarin group ($p < 0.001$). The majority of the patients with thrombosis were symptomatic by 30 days. There was no difference in the bleeding rates between the two groups, but four patients (10%) in the warfarin group required vitamin K to reverse a prolonged prothrombin time. In contrast, Couban et al demonstrated no difference between 1 mg of warfarin and placebo in a more recent and larger study with 255 patients.[43] The risk of symptomatic CVC-related thrombosis was approximately 4% in both groups.

Conflicting evidence has also been reported for LMWH. Monreal et al[44] performed an open-label randomized study that evaluated low-dose LMWH in patients with CVCs. Patients requiring a port device for chemotherapy infusion were treated with dalteparin 2500 IU subcutaneously once daily or received no prophylaxis. Based on blinded venographic assessment at day 90, patients who received the LMWH had a much lower incidence of catheter-related thrombosis. The study was terminated early by the safety committee because of a large difference in the thrombotic rates between the groups. Of the 16 patients randomized to LMWH, 1 (6%) developed thrombosis, compared with 8 of 13 patients (62%) in the control group ($p = 0.002$). This is contrary to more recent evidence suggesting that low-dose LMWH does not reduce the risk of CVC-related thrombosis. Reichart et al studied 425 cancer patients with CVCs who were randomized to 16 weeks of dalteparin or placebo.[45] Venography or ultrasound was performed at 16 weeks. The rate of catheter-associated thrombosis was very low in both groups: 3.7% and 3.4%, respectively. The reasons for the much lower rates of CVC-related thrombosis reported in recent trials are uncertain, but improved catheter material and advances in insertion techniques may be contributory.

Most clinicians do not routinely prescribe thromboprophylaxis in cancer patients with CVCs. In addition to the conflicting data from the above trials, there is concern about bleeding related to the anticoagulant. It also remains uncertain where asymptomatic catheter-related thrombi may be clinically relevant in terms of catheter function and lifespan, PE, and long-term complications such as postphlebitic syndrome.

Finally, there is the inconvenience and cost of long-term antithrombotic prophylaxis. Low-dose warfarin therapy requires INR monitoring, and LMWH requires daily subcutaneous injections. For patients with cancer who may need an indwelling CVC for months, these latter limitations are significant quality-of-life issues. On the other hand, CVC-related thrombosis can complicate the clinical management of cancer patients because of the need for anticoagulant therapy. It therefore follows that prevention of CVC-associated thrombosis is prudent. The ACCP guidelines of 2001 recommend low-dose warfarin or LMWH for preventing CVC-related thrombosis; however, in view of the evidence from the recent randomized trials, this recommendation is likely to be challenged. Additional randomized trials are required to clarify the many unanswered questions in this clinical setting.

Summary

Cancer patients undergoing surgery are at high risk of postoperative VTE. Effective methods of prophylaxis, including low-dose UFH, LMWH, and mechanical methods, are available. The prophylactic method used should be tailored to the patient's underlying risk of both thrombosis and bleeding. There is much less information available on long-term primary prophylaxis in ambulatory cancer patients. One study demonstrated that low-dose warfarin is effective and safe in women with advanced breast cancer. Further research is required to evaluate prolonged antithrombotic prophylaxis in the medical cancer population and in patients with central venous catheters.

References

1. Kakkar AK, Williamson RC. Prevention of venous thromboembolism in cancer patients. Semin Thromb Haemost 1999; 25: 239–43.

2. Gallus AS. Prevention of post-operative deep leg vein thrombosis in patients with cancer. Thromb Haemost 1997; 78:126–32.

3. Kakkar VV, Howe CT, Nicolaides AN et al. Deep vein thrombosis of the leg: is there a 'high risk' group? Am J Surg 1970; 120:527–30.

4. Agnelli G, Radicchia S, Nenci GG. Diagnosis of deep vein thrombosis in asymptomatic high-risk patients. Haemostasis 1995; 25:40–8.

5. Cruickshank MK, Levine MN, Hirsh J et al. An evaluation of impedance plethysmography and ^{125}I-fibrinogen leg scanning in patients following hip surgery. Thromb Haemost 1989; 62:830–4.

6. Lensing AW, Hirsh J. ^{125}I-fibrinogen leg scanning: reassessment of its role for the diagnosis of venous thrombosis in post-operative patients. Thromb Haemost 1993; 69:2–7.

7. Prevention of fatal postoperative pulmonary embolism by low doses of heparin: an international multicentre trial. Lancet 1975; ii:45–51.

8. Rahr HB, Sorensen JV. Venous thromboembolism and cancer. Blood Coagul Fibrinolysis 1992; **3**:451–60.

9. Palmer AJ, Schramm W, Kirchhof B et al. Low molecular weight heparin and unfractionated heparin for prevention of thromboembolism in general surgery: a meta-analysis of randomised clinical trials. Haemostasis 1997; **27**:65–74.

10. Koch A, Bouges S, Ziegler S et al. Low molecular weight heparin and unfractionated heparin in thrombosis prophylaxis after major surgical intervention: update of previous meta-analyses. Br J Surg 1997;**84**: 750–9.

11. Nurmohamed MT, Rosendaal FR, Buller HR et al. Low-molecular-weight heparin versus standard heparin in general and orthopaedic surgery: a meta-analysis. Lancet 1992; **340**:1526.

12. Leizorovicz A, Haugh MC, Chapuis FR et al. Low molecular weight heparin in prevention of perioperative thrombosis. BMJ 1992; **305**: 913–20.

13. Bergqvist D, Burmark US, Flordal PA et al. Low molecular weight heparin started before surgery as prophylaxis against deep vein thrombosis: 2500 versus 5000 XaI units in 2070 patients. Br J Surg 1995; **82**:496–501.

14. Koppenhagen K, Adolf J, Matthes M et al. Low molecular weight heparin and prevention of postoperative thrombosis in abdominal surgery. Thromb Haemost 1992; **67**:627–30.

15. The European Fraxiparin Study (EFS) Group. Comparison of a low molecular weight heparin and unfractionated heparin for the prevention of deep vein thrombosis in patients undergoing abdominal surgery. Br J Surg 1988; **75**:1058–63.

16. Kakkar VV, Cohen AT, Edmonson RA et al. Low molecular weight versus standard heparin for prevention of venous thromboembolism after major abdominal surgery. The Thromboprophylaxis Collaborative Group. Lancet 1993; **341**:259–65.

17. Nurmohamed MT, Verhaeghe R, Haas S et al. A comparative trial of a low molecular weight heparin (enoxaparin) versus standard heparin for the prophylaxis of postoperative deep vein thrombosis in general surgery. Am J Surg 1995; **169**:567–71.

18. Mismetti P, Laporte S, Darmon JY et al. Meta-analysis of low molecular weight heparin in the prevention of venous thromboembolism in general surgery. Br J Surg 2001; **88**:913–30.

19. ENOXACAN Study Group. Efficacy and safety of enoxaparin versus unfractionated heparin for prevention of deep vein thrombosis in elective cancer surgery: a double blind randomized multicentre trial with venographic assessment. Br J Surg 1997; **84**:1099–103.

20. Eldor A, Bergqvist D, Agnelli G et al. Prolonged thromboprophylaxis in patients undergoing abdominal cancer surgery with enoxaparin: the Enoxacan II Study. Blood 2000; **98**:706a.

21. Bergqvist D, Agnelli G, Cohen AT et al. Duration of prophylaxis against venous thromboembolism with enoxaparin after surgery for cancer. N Engl J Med 2002; **346**:975–980.

22. Wells PS, Lensing AW, Hirsh J. Graduated compression stockings in the prevention of postoperative venous thromboembolism: a meta-analysis. Arch Intern Med 1994; **154**:67-72.

23. Roberts VC, Cotton LT. Prevention of postoperative deep vein thrombosis in patients with malignant disease. BMJ 1974; **i**:358–60.

24. Allan A, Williams JT, Bolton JP et al. The use of graduated compression stockings in the prevention of

postoperative deep vein thrombosis. Br J Surg 1983; **70**:172–4.

25. Clagett GP, Reisch JS. Prevention of venous thromboembolism in general surgical patients: results of meta-analysis. Ann Surg 1988; **208**:227–40.

26. Cisek LJ, Walsh PC. Thromboembolic complications following radical retropubic prostatectomy: influence of external sequential pneumatic compression devices. Urology 1993; **42**:406–8.

27. Hamilton MG, Hull RD, Pineo GF. Venous thromboembolism in neurosurgery and neurology patients: a review. Neurosurgery 1994; **34**:280–96.

28. Clagett GP, Anderson FA, Jr, Geerts W et al. Prevention of venous thromboembolism. Chest 1998; **114**:531S-60S.

29. Nurmohamed MT, van Riel AM, Henkens CM et al. Low molecular weight heparin and compression stockings in the prevention of venous thromboembolism in neurosurgery. Thromb Haemost 1996; **75**:233–8.

30. Agnelli G, Piovella F, Buoncristiani P et al. Enoxaparin plus compression stockings compared with compression stockings alone in the prevention of venous thromboembolism after elective neurosurgery. N Engl J Med 1998; **339**:80–5.

31. Dickinson LD, Miller LD, Patel CP et al. Enoxaparin increases the incidence of postoperative intracranial hemorrhage when initiated preoperatively for deep venous thrombosis prophylaxis in patients with brain tumors. Neurosurgery 1998; **43**:1074–81.

32. Geerts WH, Heit JA, Clagett GP, et al. Prevention of venous thromboembolism. Chest 2001; **119**: 132S–75S.

33. Clarke-Pearson DL, Creasman WT, Coleman RE et al. Perioperative external pneumatic calf compression as thromboembolism prophylaxis in gynecologic oncology: report of a randomized controlled trial. Gynecol Oncol 1984; **18**: 226–32.

34. Clarke-Pearson DL, Synan IS, Hinshaw WM et al. Prevention of postoperative venous thromboembolism by external pneumatic calf compression in patients with gynecologic malignancy. Obstet Gynecol 1984; **63**:92–8.

35. Clarke-Pearson DL, Synan IS, Creasman WT. Anticoagulation therapy for venous thromboembolism in patients with gynecologic malignancy. Am J Obstet Gynecol 1983; **147**:369–75.

36. Clarke-Pearson DL, DeLong E, Synan IS, Soper JT, Creasman WT, Coleman RE. A controlled trial of two low-dose heparin regimens for the prevention of postoperative deep vein thrombosis. Obstet Gynecol 1990; **75**:684–9.

37. Fricker JP, Vergnes Y, Schach R et al. Low dose heparin versus low molecular weight heparin (Kabi 2165, Fragmin) in the prophylaxis of thromboembolic complications of abdominal oncological surgery. Eur J Clin Invest 1988; **18**:561–7.

38. Heilmann L, von Tempelhoff GF, Kirkpatrick C et al. Comparison of unfractionated versus low molecular weight heparin for deep vein thrombosis prophylaxis during breast and pelvic cancer surgery: efficacy, safety, and follow-up. Clin Appl Thromb Hemost 1998; **4**: 268–73.

39. Levine M, Hirsh J, Gent M et al. Double blind randomised trial of a very-low-dose warfarin for prevention of thromboembolism in stage IV breast cancer. Lancet 1994; **343**:886–9.

40. Samama MM, Cohen AT, Darmon JY et al. A comparison of enoxaparin with placebo for the prevention of venous thromboembolism in acutely ill medical

patients. Prophylaxis in Medical Patients with Enoxaparin Study Group. N Engl J Med 1999; **341**: 793–800.

41. Bona RD. Thrombotic complications of central venous catheters in cancer patients. Semin Thromb Haemost 1999; **25**:147–55.

42. Bern MM, Lokich JJ, Wallach SR, et al. Very low doses of warfarin can prevent thrombosis in central venous catheters: a randomized prospective trial. Ann Intern Med 1990; **112**:423–8.

43. Couban S, Goodyear M, Burnell M et al. A randomized double-blind placebo-controlled study of low dose warfarin for the prevention of symptomatic central venous catheter-associated thrombosis in patients with cancer. Blood 2002; **100**:2769 (abst).

44. Monreal M, Alastrue A, Rull M et al. Upper extremity deep venous thrombosis in cancer patients with venous access devices—prophylaxis with a low molecular weight heparin (Fragmin). Thromb Haemost 1996; **75**:251–3.

45. Reichart P, Kretzschmar A, Biakhov M et al. A phase III double blind, placebo-controlled study evaluating the efficacy and safety of daily low-molecular-weight heparin (dalteparin sodium, Fragmin) in preventing catheter-related complications in cancer patients with central venous catheters. Proc Am Soc Clin Oncol 2002; **21**:1474.

13

Thromboprophylaxis in cancer surgery

Ajay K Kakkar and Gloria A Petralia

Introduction

Survival and quality of life have considerably improved among the cancer population during the last decades, while more effective adjuvant and neoadjuvant therapies have shifted the balance towards intervention. The number of cancer patients falling under the surgeon's hand is therefore increasing further and further, and their management is becoming more demanding. In patients with shorter life expectancy, treatment will have to prioritize quality of life, whereas where there is a reasonable chance of longer-term survival, prevention of life-threatening conditions needs to be addressed. Therapeutic choices have to take into account that cancer patients may be immobile for significantly longer periods than the non-cancer surgical population, either whilst undergoing interventions requiring the patient to be immobilized or just out of sheer debilitation. In this picture, a pivotal role is played by venous thromboembolism (VTE), whose manifestations may range from asymptomatic calf vein thrombosis to acute, life-threatening, massive pulmonary embolism (PE). Its association with malignant disease was first described by Armand Trousseau in 1865[1] and has been validated many times since.

The pathogenesis of thrombosis

During the same period, Virchow[2] described three key factors in the formation of thrombus: venous stasis, vascular trauma, and blood hypercoagulability, and the same mechanisms are recognizable in the cancer population.

Tumor-associated hypercoagulability

The hypercoagulable state identified in malignancy is multifactorial; for instance, tumors have the ability to express procoagulant molecules.

Some tumor cells produce molecules such as cysteine and serine proteases that promote coagulation directly by activating factor X.[3] Other tumors secrete physiological tissue factor (TF), which is responsible for the activation of the extrinsic coagulation pathway; this, in turn, can lead to subclinical or overt thrombosis in some cases or disseminated intravascular coagulation (DIC) in others.[4-6]

Tumor cells can also promote coagulation indirectly by secreting tumor necrosis factor or interleukin-like proteins[7] that act on endothelial and mononuclear cells, stimulating the secretion of procoagulant molecules that may have a role in platelet activation.[3]

Vascular trauma and venous stasis

It is easy to understand how, by its mere presence, a mass could cause venous stasis by external compression. Both stasis and vascular trauma may result from direct invasion of a blood vessel by tumor cells; a well-known example of this is a renal cell carcinoma causing thrombosis of the inferior vena cava;[3] this produces a prothrombotic state that may be aggravated by local secretion of vascular permeability factors.[8] The ever more common use of a central line is a direct cause of mechanical insult and slowing of blood flow. The prothrombotic effect that certain chemotherapeutic agents exert may be in part mediated by damage to the endothelial cells.[9]

Furthermore, the network of aberrant vessels associated with some tumors able to induce angiogenesis creates a maze where flow is slowed and disordered, clearance of activated coagulation factors is impaired, and hypoxia is present, all of which can be responsible for a procoagulant state.[7]

Epidemiology

Whether symptomatic or not, VTE is much more likely in the cancer patient; in fact, about 15% of cancer patients experience a symptomatic thromboembolic event[3,10,11] in the course of their illness. To treat those episodes, we end up using 6% of inpatient day usage on medical oncology wards[10] alone. Furthermore, 6-month death probability rises from 15% in patients diagnosed with cancer alone to 80% when VTE is associated.[12]

In patients with malignant disease, VTE is estimated to be the second most common cause of death,[3,11] with up to 60% of thromboembolic deaths occurring at an otherwise-favorable time in the history of the cancer. It has been calculated that one in seven patients dies of avoidable PE, rather than because of the cancer itself.[13] The risk of PE seems also to be dependent on tumor histology;[14] in addition, the incidence of

DIC requiring intervention in cancer patients has been estimated to be 9–15%[10] (Chapter 9). Radiotherapy,[15,16] chemotherapy[17–20] (Table 13.1) (Chapter 12), and the use of central lines[9,21–23] (Chapter 14) further contribute to the thromboembolic risk.

A number of studies have shown that cancer patients undergoing surgery have a substantially higher risk of postoperative deep-vein thrombosis (DVT) (Table 13.2) and PE (fatal PE after major surgery, 1.6% vs 0.4%; $p < 0.05$)[24] than noncancer patients. The risk of bleeding is also higher in patients receiving anticoagulant therapy than in noncancer patients (16.1% vs 7.4%).[25]

Table 13.1 VTE rates in patients undergoing chemotherapy for breast cancer.

Reference	Stage	Number	%	Type
Weiss et al, 1981[79]	II	433	5.0	Venous
Goodnough et al, 1984[80]	IV	159	17.6	Venous and arterial
Levine et al, 1988[17]	II	205	6.8	Venous and arterial
Wall et al, 1989[81]	II, III	1014	1.3	Arterial
Fisher et al, 1990[82]	II	383	3.1	Venous
Saphner et al, 1991[19]	I, II	2352	5.4	Venous and arterial
Clahsen et al, 1994[18]	I, II	1292	2.1	Venous
Rifkin et al, 1994[83]	II	603	2.5	Venous and arterial
Levine et al, 1994[84]	IV	159	4.4	Venous and arterial
Pritchard et al, 1996[20]	II	353	9.6	Venous and arterial
Tempelhoff et al, 1996[85]	II	50	10.0	Venous
Orlando et al, 2000[86]	Various	182	7.7	Venous

Table 13.2 Incidence of postoperative VTE: comparison of cancer and noncancer patients.

Reference	Cancer[a]		Noncancer[a]	
Kakkar et al, 1970[71]	24/59	(41.0)	38/144	(26.0)
Hills et al, 1972[72]	8/16	(50.0)	7/34	(21.0)
Walsh et al, 1974[73]	16/45	(35.0)	22/217	(10.0)
Rosemberg et al, 1975[45]	28/66	(42.0)	29/128	(23.0)
Rem et al,1975[74]	16/30	(53.0)	16/65	(28.0)
Gallus et al, 1976[75]	17/76	(22.0)	49/36	(16.0)
Allan et al, 1983[47]	41/100	(31.0)	21/100	(21.0)
Sasahara, 1984[76]	62/304	(20.0)	113/707	(16.0)
Kakkar and Murray 1985[77]	21/310	(6.7)	10/597	(1.6)
Sue-Ling et al, 1986[78]	12/23	(52.0)	16/62	(26.0)
Kakkar et al, 1993[25]	25/1407	(1.8)	16/2402	(0.7)
Total	270/2436	(11.0)	337/3898	(8.6)

[a]Percentages in parantheses.

The American College of Chest Physicians[26] collected evidence on surgical cancer patients over the last four decades and found high rates of proximal vein thrombosis and clinical PE, with alarming rates of fatal PE (1–5%) in the absence of any form of thromboprophylaxis, rendering this mandatory in that setting.

Available drugs

Aspirin

Mechanism of action
Aspirin inactivates platelet cyclooxygenase. It is cheap, easy to administer, and has few side effects; but it is generally ineffective in preventing VTE in surgical patients.

Dextran

Mechanism of action
Dextran is adsorbed onto the platelet surface, increasing its negative charge. This leads to the formation of a blood clot more susceptible to lysis by plasmin. It is used in cases of hypovolemic shock to expand blood volume, but it is expensive and requires intravenous administration.

Dermatan sulfate

Mechanism of action
Dermatan sulfate is a glycosaminoglycan that selectively inhibits thrombin through heparin cofactor II. It is effective on both fibrin-bound and free thrombin.

Oral onticoagulants (warfarin)

Mechanism of action
Vitamin K antagonists prevent the post-translational carboxylation of factors II, VII, IX, and X in the liver. In clinical practice, their use is bound to dose adjustments according to the international normalized ratio (INR). Elevated loading doses may produce excessive anticoagulation and therefore risk of bleeding, without achieving corresponding levels of thromboprophylaxis.[27] In the cancer population, a risk of bleeding could be unacceptable, especially as prophylactic INR levels are more difficult to obtain (56.9% of the time vs 43.3%; $p < 0.0001$).[28]

Unfractionated heparin (UFH)

Mechanism of action

The pentasaccharide sequence binds to the endogenous anticoagulant protein antithrombin (AT), greatly increasing the ability of AT to inhibit thrombin and factor Xa. However, AT is unable to inhibit thrombin that is bound to fibrin and platelet-bound factor X. It can increase circulating levels of tissue plasminogen activator and TF pathway inhibitor (TFPI) by releasing them from their binding sites on the surface of endothelial cells. TFPI is a tridomain protein that binds to the TF–FVIIa–FX complex that suppresses the generation of factor Xa by TF.[29] As TF plays a major role in the coagulation process in cancer patients, this may account for the activity of UFH in these patients. Used intravenously, UFH has the advantage of being easily and rapidly reversed by stopping the infusion and using protamine sulfate if necessary.[30] But it does require intra-venous administration and costly laboratory monitoring of activated partial thromboplastin time (APTT) to site-specific controls; moreover, it may give rise to heparin resistance and can be complicated by heparin-induced thrombocytopenia with thrombosis (HITT).[31–33]

Low-molecular-weight heparin (LMWH)

Mechanism of action

LMWH is similar in action to UFH, but with diminished inhibition of thrombin. Prepared by chemical or enzymatic degradation of UFH, LMWH has an average molecular mass of 5000 Da that allows it to be effectively absorbed from the subcutaneous tissue. Its affinity for plasma proteins, platelets, macrophages, and endothelium is reduced, render-ing it more predictable thanks to a longer plasma half-life (3.5–4.5 hours) and increased bioavailability (>85%). APTT is not affected, rendering any requirement for dose monitoring superfluous, increasing cost-effective-ness, and allowing simple subcutaneous administration, which is ideal even in outpatient settings. In addition, LMWH has a reduced incidence of HITT,[31,34] and a lower risk of bleeding,[35–39] and has not been associ-ated with osteoporosis.[40–43]

VTE prevention

Thromboprophylaxis is essential as a means of achieving reduced rates of mortality and morbidity and to maintain the quality of life in those patients whose life expectancy may be short. An effective prevention program needs to target underlying factors predisposing to VTE, mini-mize any secondary effects, be well tolerated by the patient, and be feasible from both a logistical and an economical point of view.[44]

In addition to the usual strategies that can be adopted to reduce the risk of thromboembolism in the surgical patient (elevation of the lower extremities, leg exercise, early ambulation, and pressure prevention), mechanical and pharmacological measures are recommended, especially in the oncological subpopulation.

Mechanical modes of prevention

Electrical stimulation of the calf muscles during surgery has been shown to be beneficial in reducing stasis-related problems, but not in patients with malignancy.[45] Intermittent pneumatic compression (IPN) has proved beneficial in a small study of cancer patients: 9% (2/23) versus 40% (8/20) in the control group, where the confidence intervals were extremely wide.[46] The graduated static compression stocking significantly reduces the incidence of postoperative VTE[47] but is less effective in cancer patients. Inferior vena cava filters should not be considered as an alternative method, as patients are more prone to recurrent DVT,[48] which can occur after thrombosis of the filter itself. Furthermore, fatal PE has been reported to occur in cancer patients with filters in place.[49,50]

Pharmacological modes of prevention

Low-dose heparin is usually administered subcutaneously (5000 U) 2 hours before surgery and every 8–12 hours thereafter. It has proven beneficial in cancer patients (Table 13.3); in a meta-analysis, it showed significant reduction in VTE rates when compared to placebo (13.6% vs 30.6%, $p < 0.001$);[51] and in an international randomized trial it reduced mortality due to PE (1.6% vs 0.4%).[52]

LMWH is recommended for patients with cancer undergoing minor operations or, for whatever reason, confined to bed.[26] It proved more effective than and as safe as UFH in many studies containing a high percentage of cancer patients (Table 13.4). Higher doses (5000 U vs 2500 U) are more effective in thromboprophylaxis (8.5% vs 14.9%, $p = 0.001$) without increasing the bleeding risk.[53] Prophylaxis should continue for at least 4 weeks after abdominal or pelvic surgical procedures for cancer,

Table 13.3 VTE incidence in patients receiving UFH thromboprophylaxis.

Reference	Group	UFT[a]	Control[a]	RR
Rem et al,1975[74]	Benign	4/59 (7)	18/65 (28)	25
	Malignant	7/24 (30)	16/30 (53)	55
Gallus et al,1976[75]	Benign	8/304 (3)	49/36 (16)	18
	Malignant	5/58 (9)	17/76 (22)	39

[a]Percentages in parantheses.

Table 13.4 DVT rates in cancer surgical patients: comparison of prophylaxis with LMWH and UFH. (Modified from *Thrombosis and Haemostasis*.[87])

Reference	LMWH	Cancer (%)	LMWH (%)	UFH (%)
Bergqvist et al, 1986[88]	Dalteparin	45	6.4	4.3
EFS Group 1988[89]	Nadroparin	100	4.2	5.4
Bergqvist et al, 1988[90]	Dalteparin	63.3	5.5	8.3
Samama et al, 1988[91]	Enoxaparin	30	3.2	5.0
Liezorovicz et al, 1991[92]	Tinzaparin	38.5	5.8	4.2
Kakkar et al, 1993[25]	Dalteparin	37.6	1.26	1.30
Boneu et al, 1993[93]	Reviparin	52.3	4.6	4.2
Gallus et al, 1993[94]	Danaparoid	100	10.4	14.9
Nurmohamed et al, 1995[95]	Enoxaparin	100	13.6	8.7
Bergqvist et al, 1995[53]	Enoxaparin	100	14.7	18.2

as it will decrease VTE rates at both 4 weeks (4.8% vs 12.0%, $p = 0.02$) and 3 months (5.5% vs 13.8%, $p = 0.01$) when comparedwith 1-week regimens.[54] Even in neurosurgery, where intracranial bleeding is particularly feared, LMWH proved safe and effective in the oncological population, reducing the risk of VTE by 0.51 ($p = 0.004$) without increasing bleeding rates; this has been confirmed in a large meta-analysis showing a 48% VTE risk reduction.[55]

Dermatan sulfate: showed a lower VTE incidence when compared with UFH in 842 patients with cancer (15.0% vs 22.0%).[55]

Prevention of secondary recurrence

Following initial treatment with heparin (either UFH or LMWH), prevention of recurrence can be achieved by pharmacological means. Warfarin is traditionally used for long-term treatment; for this purpose, one aims to maintain an INR of 2.0–3.0.[31] Unfortunately, due to the already mentioned unpredictable pharmacokinetics of coumarin derivatives, this treatment is not compatible with invasive procedures and surgical interventions.

Because LMWH offers better pharmacokinetics, and is not influenced by diet and concomitant therapies, it has been proposed as a valuable alternative to oral anticoagulants after proving effective in patients with warfarin failure. LMWH's flexibility, due to predictable clearance times and rapid onset of action, makes it a valuable tool in the armament of the surgeon for the perioperative period.[31] In the few randomized studies that have compared LMWH with warfarin in long-term usage, recurrence and bleeding appeared to be comparable in the two groups,[57–59] but further evidence is needed.

Table 13.5 Incidence of recurrent VTE in cancer and noncancer patients.

Reference	Cancer patients[a]		Noncancer patients[a]	
Bona et al, 1995[28]	4/44	(9.1)	3/64	(4.6)
Columbus Investigators, 1997[96]	20/232	(8.6)	32/789	(4.1)
Hutten et al, 2000[97]	14/264	(5.0)	21/1039	(2.0)

[a]Percentages in parentheses.

At present, there are no evidence-based guidelines with regard to the duration of anticoagulant therapy in the cancer population. The traditional 3-month course following VTE may be acceptable only when the risk factors behind the thrombotic event are transient, as in trauma or general surgical patients. In patients with idiopathic DVT or PE, treatment shorter then 6 months has been associated with an increased risk of recurrence, and it must be taken into account that idiopathic VTE can be the first manifestation of occult malignancy.[7,56,60] In fact, two large studies found the incidence of cancer in patients with idiopathic VTE to be 1.3 times and 3.2 times higher among the Danish and Swedish populations respectively.[61,62]

Current recommendations are that oral anticoagulant therapy should continue as long as there is active cancer therapy or active cancer and for 6 months thereafter. Thrombotic prophylaxis must be tailored to the actual risk of VTE recurrence (Table 13.5) and balanced against the risk of bleeding or any other contraindications to thromboprophylaxis; for surgical patients, LMWH may be more suitable than coumarin derivatives.

Antithrombotic therapy and cancer survival

Anticoagulant therapy improves quality of life and survival rates by preventing DVT and the fatal PE that would otherwise decimate the cancer population; but is this all that there is to it? An interesting question that has been raised in the literature is whether antithrombotic treatment might in itself possess antineoplastic features; and there is, indeed, evidence that, at least in vitro, warfarin, heparin, and fibrinolytic and antiplatelet agents can inhibit tumor growth and metastasis formation.[63] It is known that fibrin and thrombin play a role in the adhesion and implantation of tumor cells, while fibrin deposit around tumor masses can protect against immune surveillance; this can explain why anticoagulants may interfere with tumor progression.[3] It is also known that TF, vascular endothelial growth factor, and platelet-activating factor play a role in the neoangiogenesis process that occurs in some malignant growths, and the ability of heparin to inhibit all of those may again explain its effectiveness.[3] But how does this translate into clinical practice?

In a prospective, randomized trial, patients with small-cell lung cancer, receiving radiotherapy and chemotherapy, were randomized to warfarin or no antithrombotic therapy. There was a statistically significant benefit in survival (mean 49.5 weeks vs 23.0 weeks).[64] When patients with malignancies nonresponding to chemotherapy, such as prostate, colorectal, head, neck, and non-small-cell lung cancer, were followed up, warfarin failed to show any improvement in life expectancy.[65] Another study focusing on patients with small-cell lung carcinoma analyzed the use of subcutaneous UFH in addition to chemotherapy and found a statistically significant improvement in response (37% vs 23%, $p = 0.004$) and median survival (317 days vs 261 days, $p = 0.01$).[66]

In a meta-analysis[67] of nine randomized clinical trials including data from 629 cancer patients enrolled in these studies, the effects of UFH and LMWH treatments demonstrated a statistically significant difference in 3-month mortality rate of approximately 40% in favor of LMWH (odds ratio 0.39; 95% confidence interval, 0.15–1.02). Retrospective analyses of studies undertaken to compare the safety and efficacy of UFH and LMWH in the treatment of DVT have looked at 3–6-month survival in cancer patients with DVT randomized in these trials. These analyses have demonstrated a trend toward a mortality benefit in those cancer patients receiving LMWH.[68,69] These findings are difficult to explain, given that cancer patients with DVT received only a short course (7–10 days) of LMWH for initial treatment of their DVT, and most were interpreted with caution because the original studies were not designed to evaluate long-term cancer mortality. A recent prospective study evaluating perioperative LMWH prophylaxis in surgery for breast or gynecological malignancy[70] demonstrated a late survival benefit for patients with pelvic malignancy who received thromboprophylaxis with LMWH for up to 2 years after surgery. It appears that LMWH, either by effectively preventing VTE or by directly influencing tumor biology, can improve outcome in cancer patients, and if the results of prospective studies currently assessing the value of prolonged LMWH in cancer patients without thrombosis confirm the previous retrospective analyses, its use may become routine.

Conclusions

Malignancy per se increases the risk of thrombosis, whose burden has often led many cancer patients to an even earlier grave. When one intends to intervene aggressively on those patients, whose risk of bleeding is also increased, appropriate thromboprophylaxis requires careful planning. As standard, it should include the use of graduated compression stockings combined with either UFH or LMWH. If VTE occurs as a first manifestation, or notwithstanding prophylaxis, primary treatment follows the recommendations for noncancer patients in the form of LMWH or UFH for 5 days in noncomplicated cases and 7–10 days in more extensive or complicated ones.

After the first line of treatment, long-term prophylaxis for the prevention of recurrent VTE needs to be continued until active cancer or cancer treatment is present. Unfortunately, for this purpose, warfarin, which is the traditional first-line approach, is unsuitable for patients due to undergo surgery or recovering from a surgical intervention. LMWH is more often employed to prevent symptomatic recurrences in these circumstances, having proven effective in cases of warfarin failure.

Finally, the improvement in survival rates in the oncological population receiving anticoagulant therapy may not only be due to mere prevention of fatal PE, but may also be mediated by direct antineoplastic activity (see Chapter 16). This hypothesis, if proven, would make the anticoagulants effective chemotherapeutic agents that do not increase chemotoxicity.

References

1. Trousseau A. Phlegmasia alba dolens. In: Lectures on Clinical Medicine, Delivered at the Hôtel-Dieu, Paris (New Syndeham Society: London, 1872)282–332.

2. Virchow R. Gesammelte Abhandlungen Zurwissenschaftlichen Medizin [Collected Articles on Scientific Medicine] (Medinger Sohn: Frankfurt, 1856)219–732.

3. Letai A, Kuter DJ. Cancer, coagulation, and anticoagulation. Oncologist 1999; 4:443–9.

4. Kakkar AK, DeRuvo N, Chinswangwatanakul V et al, Extrinsic-pathway activation in cancer with high factor VIIa and tissue factor. Lancet 1995; 346:1004–5.

5. Kakkar AK, Lemoine NR, Scully MF et al. Tissue factor expression correlates with histological grade in human pancreatic carcinoma. Br J Surg 1995; 82:1101–4.

6. Gordon SG, Cancer cell procoagulants and their implications. Hematol Oncol Clin North Am 1992; 6:1359–74.

7. Prandoni P, Piccioli A. Venous thromboembolism and cancer: a two-way clinical association. Front Biosci 1997; 2:e12–20.

8. Edwards RL, Rickles FR, Thrombosis and cancer. In: Hull R, Pineo GF, eds. Disorders of Thrombosis. (WB Saunders: Philadelphia, 1996)374–82.

9. Boraks P, Seale J, Price J et al. Prevention of central venous catheter associated thrombosis using minidose warfarin in patients with hematological malignancies. Br J Haematol 1998; 101:483–6.

10. Harrington KJ, Bateman AR, Syrigos KN et al. Cancer-related thromboembolic disease in patients with solid tumours: a retrospective analysis. Ann Oncol 1997; 8:669–73.

11. Rickles FR, Edwards RL. Activation of blood coagulation in cancer:

Trousseau's syndrome revisited. Blood 1983; **62**:14–31.

12. Sack GH, Levin J, Bell W. Trousseau's syndrome and other manifestations of chronic disseminated coagulopathy in patients with neoplasms: clinical, pathologic, and therapeutic features. Medicine (Baltimore) 1977; **56**:1–37.

13. Shen VS, Pollak EW. Fatal pulmonary embolism in cancer patients: is heparin prophylaxis justified? South Med J 1980; **73**: 841–3.

14. Svendsen E, Karwinski B. Prevalence of pulmonary embolism at necroscopy in patients with cancer. J Clin Pathol 1989; **42**: 805–9.

15. Goldberg PA, Nicholls FJ, Porter NH et al. Long-term results of a randomised trial of short-course low-dose adjuvant pre-operative radiotherapy for rectal cancer: reduction in local treatment failure. Eur J Cancer 1994; **11**:1602–6.

16. Holm T, Singnomklao T, Rutqvist LE et al. Adjuvant preoperative radiotherapy in patients with rectal carcinoma. Adverse effects during long term follow-up of two randomized trials. Cancer 1996; **78**: 968–76.

17. Levine M, Gent M, Hirsh J et al. The thrombogenic effect of anticancer drug therapy in women stage II breast cancer. N Engl J Med 1988; **318**:404–7.

18. Clahsen PC, Van de Velde CJH, Julien JP et al. Thromboembolic complications after perioperative chemotherapy in women with early Breast Cancer: a European Organization for Research and Treatment of breast cancer cooperative group study. J Clin Oncol 1994; **12**:1266–71.

19. Saphner T, Tormey DC, Gray R. Venous and arterial thrombosis in patients who received adjuvant therapy for breast cancer. J Clin Oncol 1991; **9**:286–94.

20. Pritchard KI, Paterson AH, Paul NA et al. Increases thromboembolic complications with current tamoxifen and chemotherapy in a randomized trial of adjuvant therapy for women with breast cancer. National Cancer Institute of Canada Clinical Trials Group Breast Cancer Site Group. J Clin Oncol 1996; **14**:2731–7.

21. Bern MM, Lokich JJ, Wallach SR et al. Very low doses of warfarin can prevent thrombosis in central venous catheters. Ann Intern Med 1990; **112**:423–8.

22. Monreal M, Alastrue A, Rull M et al. Upper extremity deep venous thrombosis in cancer patients with venous access devices—prophylaxis with a low molecular weight heparin (Fragmin). Thromb Haemost 1996; **75**:251–3.

23. Graf AH, Graf B, Brandis MG et al. Oral anticoagulation in patients with gynecological cancer and radiotherapy: a retrospective analysis of 132 patients. Anticancer Res 1998; **18**:2047–51.

24. Rahr HB, Sorensen JV. Venous thromboembolism and cancer. Blood Coagul Fibrinolysis 1992; **3**:451–60.

25. Kakkar VV, Cohen AT, Edmonson RA et al. Low molecular weight versus standard heparin for prevention of venous thromboembolism after major abdominal surgery. Lancet 1993; **341**:259–65.

26. Proceedings of the American College of Chest Physicians 5th Consensus on Antithrombotic Therapy. Chest 1998; **114**:439S–769S.

27. Harrison L, Johnson M, Massicotte MP et al. Comparison of 5-mg and 10-mg loading doses in initiation of warfarin therapy. Ann Intern Med 1997; **126**:133–6.

28. Bona RD, Sivjee KY, Hickey AD et al. The efficacy and safety of oral

anticoagulation in patients with cancer. Thromb Haemost 1995; **74**:1055–8.

29. Baugh RJ, Broze GJ, Krishnaswamy S. Regulation of extrinsic pathway factor Xa formation by TFPI. J Biol Chem 1998; **273**: 4378–86.

30. Lee AY. Treatment of venous thromboembolism in cancer patients. Thromb Res 2001; **101**: V195–V208.

31. Hirsh J, Warkentin TW, Raschke R et al. Heparin and low-molecular-weight heparin: mechanisms of action, pharmacokinetics, dosing considerations, monitoring, efficacy, and safety. Chest 1998; **114**: 489S–510S.

32. Brill-Edwards P, Ginsberg JS, Johnston M et al Establishing a therapeutic range for heparin therapy, Ann Intern Med 1993; **119**: 104–9.

33. Hull RD, Raskob GE, Brant RF et al. Relation between the time to achieve the lower limit of the APTT therapeutical range and recurrent venous thromboembolism during heparin treatment for deep vein thrombosis. Arch Intern Med 1997; **157**:2562–8.

34. Warkentin TE, Levine MN, Hirsh J et al. Heparin-induced thrombocytopenia in patients treated with low-molecular-weight heparin or unfractionated heparin. N Engl J Med 1995; **332**:1330–5.

35. Siragusa S, Cosmi B, Piovella F et al. Low molecular weight heparins and unfractionated heparin in the treatment of patients with acute venous thromboembolism: results of a meta-analysis. Am J Med 1996; **100**:269–77.

36. Lensing AW, Prins MH, Davidson BL et al. Treatment of deep vein thrombosis with low molecular weight heparins. A meta-analysis. Arch Intern Med 1995; **155**: 601–7.

37. Leirozovicz A, Simonneau G, Decousus H et al. Comparison of efficacy and safety of low-molecular-weight heparins and unfractionated heparin in initial treatment of deep vein thrombosis: a meta-analysis. BMJ 1994; **309**: 299–304.

38. Gould MK, Dembitzer AD, Doyle RL et al. Low-molecular-weight heparins compared with unfractionated heparin for treatment of acute deep vein thrombosis: a meta-analysis of randomised, controlled trials. Ann Intern Med 1999; **130**: 800–9.

39. Dolovich LR, Ginsberg JS, Douketis JD et al. A meta-analysis comparing low-molecular-weight heparins with unfractionated heparin in the treatment of venous thromboembolism: examining some unanswered questions regarding location of treatment, product type, and dosing frequency. Arch Intern Med 2000; **160**: 181–8.

40. Kakkar AK, Williamson RC. Prevention of venous thromboembolism in cancer using low-molecular-weight heparins. Haemostasis 1997; **27**:32–7.

41. Muir JM, Hirsh J, Weitz JI et al. A histomorphometric comparison of the effects of heparin and low molecular weight heparin on a cancellous bone in rats. Blood 1997; **89**:3236–42.

42. Shaughnessy SG, Young E, Deschamps P et al. The effects of low molecular weight heparin on calcium loss from fetal rate calvaria. Blood 1995; **86**:1368–73.

43. Monreal M, Lazof E, Olive A et al. Comparison of subcutaneous unfractionated heparin with a low molecular weight heparin (Fragmin) in patients with venous thromboembolism and contraindications to coumarins. Thromb Haemost 1994; **71**:7–11.

44. Kakkar VV. Prevention of venous thromboembolism. In: Bloom AL, ed. Haemostasis and Thrombosis. (Churchill Livingstone: Edinburgh, 1994)1361–79.

45. Rosemberg IL, Evans M, Pollock AV. Prophylaxis of postoperative leg vein thrombosis by low dose subcutaneous heparin or peroperative calf muscles stimulation: a controlled clinical trial. BMJ 1975; i:649–51.

46. Roberts VS, Cotton LT. Prevention of postoperative deep vein thrombosis in patients with malignant disease. BMJ 1974; i:435–48.

47. Allan A, Williams JT, Bolton JP et al. The use of graduated compression stockings in the prevention of postoperative deep vein thrombosis. Br J Surg 1983; 70:172–4.

48. Decousus H, Leizorovicz A, Parent F et al. A clinical trial of vena cava filters in the prevention of pulmonary embolism in patients with proximal deep-vein thrombosis. N Engl J Med 1998; 338:409–15.

49. Athanasoulis CA, Kaufman JA, Halpern EF et al. Inferior vena cava filters: a review of a 26-year single-centre clinical experience. Radiology 2000; 21:54–66.

50. Millward SF, Peterson RA, Moher D et al. LGM (Vena Tech) vena caval filter: experience at a single institution. J Vasc Interv Radiol 1994; 5: 351–6.

51. Clagett PG, Reisch JS. Prevention of venous thromboembolism in general surgical patients. Result of a meta-analysis. Ann Surg 1988; 208:227–40.

52. International Multicentre Trial. Prevention of fatal postoperative pulmonary embolism by low doses of heparin. Lancet 1975; ii:45–51.

53. Bergqvist D, Burmark US, Flordal PA et al. Low molecular weight heparin started before surgery as prophylaxis against deep vein thrombosis: 2500 versus 5000 Xal units in 2070 patients. Br J Surg 1995; 82:496–501.

54. Bergqvist D, Agnelli G, Cohen AT et al, for the ENOXACAN Investigators, Duration of prophylaxis against venous thromboembolism with enoxaparin after surgery for cancer. N Engl J Med 2002; 346: 975–80.

55. Iorio A, Agnelli G. Low molecular weight and unfractionated heparin for prevention of venous thromboembolism in neurosurgery: a meta-analysis. Arch Intern Med 2000; 160:2327–32.

56. Di Carlo V, Agnelli G, Prandoni P, et al. Dermatan sulphate for the prevention of postoperative venous thromboembolism in patients with cancer. DOS (Dermatan sulphate in Oncologic Surgery) Study Group. Thromb Haemost 1999; 82:30–4.

57. Pini M, Aiello S, Manotti C et al. Low molecular weight heparin versus warfarin in the prevention of recurrences after deep vein thrombosis. Thromb Haemost 1994; 72: 191–7.

58. Das SK, Cohen AT, Edmondson RA et al. Low-molecular-weight heparin versus warfarin for prevention of recurrent venous thromboembolism: a randomized trial. World J Surg 1996; 20:521–7.

59. Lopaciuk S, Bielska-Falda H, Noszczyk W et al. Low molecular weight heparin versus acenocoumarol in the secondary prophylaxis of deep vein thrombosis. Thromb Haemost 1999; 81: 26–31.

60. Kakkar AK, Williamson RCN. Antithrombotic therapy in cancer: low molecular weight heparins may have a direct effect on tumours. BMJ 1999; 318:1571–2.

61. Sorensen HT, Mellemkjaer L, Steffensen FH et al. The risk of a diagnosis of cancer after primary deep venous thrombosis or pul-

monary embolism. N Engl J Med 1998; **338**:1169.

62. Baron JA, Gridley G, Weiderpass E et al. Venous thromboembolism and cancer. Lancet 1998; **351**: 1077–80.

63. Hejna M, Radere M, Zielinski CC. Inhibition of metastases by antico-agulants. J Natl Cancer Inst 1999; **91**:22–36.

64. Zacharski LP, Henderson WG, Rickles FR et al. Effect of warfarin on survival in small cell carcinoma of the lung. JAMA 1981; **245**: 831–5.

65. Zacharski LP, Henderson WG, Rickles FR et al. Effect of warfarin anticoagulation on survival in carci-noma of the lung, colon, head and neck, and prostate, Cancer 1984; **53**:2046–52.

66. Lebeau B, Chastang C, Brechot JM et al. Subcutaneous heparin treatment increases survival in small cell lung cancer. Cancer 1994; **74**:38–45.

67. Buller HR, Hettiarachchi RJK, Smoremburg SM, et al, Do heparins do more then just treat thrombosis? The influence of heparins on cancer spread. In: Abstract Book 'Simposio Eparina 2000' (Itlalfarmaco: Bologna, 2000) 11.

68. Walsh-McMonagle D, Green D. Low-molecular-weight heparin in the management of Trousseau's Syndrome. Cancer 1997; **80**: 649–55.

69. Green D, Hull RD, Brant R et al. Lower mortality in cancer patients treated with low-molecular weight versus standard heparin. Lancet 1992; **339**:1476.

70. Von Tempelhoff GF, Harenberg J, Niemann F et al. Effect of low molecular weight heparin (Certoparin) versus unfractionated heparin on cancer survival following breast or pelvic cancer surgery: a prospective randomised double-

blind trial. Int J Oncol 2000; **16**: 815–24.

71. Kakkar VV, Howe CT, Nicolaides AN et al. Deep vein thrombosis of the leg. Is there a 'high risk' group? Am J Surg 1970; **120**:527–30.

72. Hills NH, Pflug JJ, Jeyasingh K et al. Prevention of deep vein throm-bosis by intermittent pneumatic compression of calf. BMJ 1972; i:131–5.

73. Walsh JJ, Bonnar J, Wright FW. A study of pulmonary embolism and deep vein thrombosis after major gynaecological surgery using labelled fibrinogen–phlebography and lung scanning. J Obstet Gynaecol Br Commonw 1974; **81**: 311–6.

74. Rem J, Duckert F, Friedrich R et al. Subkutane kleine Heparindosen zur Thromboseprophylaxe in der allge-meinen Chirurgie and Urologie. Schweiz Med Wochenschr Suppl (1975) **105**:827–35.

75. Gallus AS, Hirsh J, O'Brien SE et al. Prevention of venous thrombo-sis with small subcutaneous does heparin. JAMA 1976; **235**:1980–2.

76. The Multicentre Trial Committee. Dihydroergotamine–heparin pro-phylaxis of postoperative deep vein thrombosis: a multicentre trial, JAMA 1984; **251**:2960–6.

77. Kakkar VV, Murray WJG. Efficacy and safety of low molecular weight heparin (CY216) in preventing post-operative venous thrombo-embolism: a cooperative study. Br J Surg 1985; **82**:724–5.

78. Sue-Ling HM, Johnston D, McMahon MU et al. Preoperative identification of patients at high risk of deep venous thrombosis after elective major abdominal surgery. Lancet 1986; i:1173–6.

79. Weiss RB, Tormey DC, Holland JF et al. Venous thrombosis during multinodal treatment of primary breast carcinoma. Cancer Treat Res 1981; **65**:677–9.

80. Goodnough LT, Saito H, Manni A et al. Increased incidence of thromboembolism in stage IV breast cancer patients treated with a five-drug chemotherapy regimen. Cancer 1984; **54**:1264–8.

81. Wall JC, Weiss RB, Norton L et al. Arterial thrombosis associated with adjuvant chemotherapy for breast cancer: a Cancer and Leukemia Group B study. Am J Med 1989; **87**:501–4.

82. Fisher B, Redmond C, Legault-Poisson R. Postoperative chemotherapy and tamoxifene compared with tamoxifen alone in treatment of positive node breast cancer patients aged 50 years and older with tumors responsive to tamoxifene: results from national adjuvant breast and bowel project B. J Clin Oncol 1990; **8**:1005–18.

83. Rifkin SE, Green S, Metch B et al. Adjuvant CMFVP versus tamoxifen versus concurrent CMFVP and tamoxifen for postmenopausal node positive and estrogen receptor positive breast cancer patients: a Southwest Oncology Group study. J Clin Oncol 1994; **12**: 2078–85.

84. Levine M, Hirsh J, Gent M et al. Double-blind randomised trial of a very-low-dose warfarin for prevention of thromboembolism in stage IV breast cancer, Lancet 1994; **343**:886–9.

85. von Tempelhoff GF, Dietrich M, Hommel G et al. Blood coagulation during adjuvant epirubicin/cyclophosphamide chemotherapy in patients with primary operable breast cancer. J Clin Oncol 1996; **14**:2560–8.

86. Orlando L, Colleoni M, Nole F et al. Incidence of venous thromboembolism in breast cancer patients during chemotherapy with vinorelbine, cisplatin, 5-fluorouracil as continuous infusion (ViFuP regimen): is prophylaxis required? Ann Oncol 2000; **11**:117–8.

87. Gallus AS. Prevention of post-operative deep leg vein thrombosis in patients with cancer. Thromb Haemost 1997; **78**:126–32.

88. Bergqvist D, Burmark US, Frisell J et al. Low molecular weight heparin once daily compared with conventional low-dose heparin twice daily. A prospective double-blind multicentre trial on prevention of postoperative thrombosis. Br J Surg 1986; **73**:204–8.

89. European Fraxiparin Study (EFS) Group. Comparison of a low molecular weight heparin and unfractioned heparin for the prevention of deep vein thrombosis in patients undergoing abdominal surgery. Br J Surg 1988; **75**: 1058–63.

90. Bergqvist D, Matzsch T, Burmark US et al. Low molecular weight heparin given the evening before surgery compared with conventional low dose heparin in the prevention of thrombosis. Br J Surg 1988; **75**:888–91.

91. Samama M, Bernard P, Bonnardot JP et al. Low molecular weight heparin compared with unfractionated heparin in prevention of postoperative thrombosis. Br J Surg 1988; **75**:128–31.

92. Leirozovicz A, Picolet H, Peyrieux JC et al. HBPM Research Group, Prevention of perioperative deep vein thrombosis in general surgery: a multicentre double blind study comparing two doses of logiparin and standard heparin. Br J Surg 1991; **78**:412–6.

93. Boneu B. An international multicentre study: clivarin in the prevention of thromboembolism in patients undergoing general surgery. Blood Coagul Fibrinolysis 1993; **4**:S21–S22.

94. Gallus A, Cade J, Ockelford P et al. Orgaran (Org 10172) or heparin for preventing venous thrombosis after elective surgery for malignant dis-

ease? A double-blind, randomised, multicentre comparison. ANZ– Orgaran Investigators' Group. Thromb Haemost 1993; **70**:562–7.

95. Nurmohamed MT, Verhaege R, Haas S et al. A comparative trial of a low molecular weight heparin (enoxaparin) versus standard heparin for the prophylaxis of post-operative deep vein thrombosis in general surgery. Am J Surg 1995; **169**:567–71.

96. The Columbus Investigators. Low-molecular-weight heparin in the treatment of patients with venous thromboembolism. N Engl J Med 1997; **337**:657–62.

97. Hutten BA, Prins MH, Gent M et al. Incidence of recurrent thromboembolic and bleeding complications among patients with venous thromboembolism in relation to both malignancy and achieved international normalized ratio: a retrospective study analysis. J Clin Oncol 2000; **18**:3078–383.

14

Catheter-related arm-vein thrombosis in patients with cancer

Manuel Monreal

Introduction

Deep venous thrombosis (DVT) of the arm was long believed to be an uncommon disorder caused by malrotation of the upper extremity, especially when associated with strenuous exercise. However, with the increasingly common use of subclavian venous access, arm DVT has been recognized to be more common than previously reported. It has been estimated that 13–35% of patients with subclavian catheters develop arm DVT, with catheterization estimated to account for about 40% of all subclavian vein thromboses.[1]

Clinical presentation

Because central venous catheters are located deep in the mediastinum, thrombosis may be clinically silent until late in its course, and may then be potentially lethal. Sleeve thrombi starting at the point of entry of the catheter into the vein and extending toward the catheter tip are quite common. Although sleeve thrombosis seldom gives rise to any signs or symptoms, its importance should not be underestimated. A fibrin sleeve may occlude the catheter tip and cause catheter malfunction (inability to infuse or withdraw blood). Furthermore, parts of the thrombus may detach and cause pulmonary embolism when the catheter is removed.

Axillosubclavian DVT, which can partially block or occlude the vessel lumen, may lead to more severe clinical problems. These patients may also be asymptomatic, may present with inability to draw blood from the catheter as the only symptom, or may present with a constellation of nonspecific symptoms, including arm swelling with erythema or warmth, pain or fullness in the axilla, jaw pain, neck swelling, headache, collateral vessels on the chest wall, or arm paresthesia.

Incidence and risk factors

Long-term central venous catheterization is often required in cancer patients (frequently with poor peripheral access) for delivery of chemotherapy, blood and blood products, parenteral nutrition, fluids, and other medications. It has led to increased patient comfort as well as enhanced therapeutic options. However, despite many efforts to improve catheter biocompatibility, arm DVT remains a side-effect to be considered.

The true incidence of arm DVT in patients with indwelling central venous catheters is difficult to estimate since there are few studies in which the diagnosis of DVT was based on anything but clinical symptoms. In the literature, its incidence varies widely according to the sensitivity of the examination procedures (when surveillance objective tests were used, the DVT rate was higher than when they were performed only for evaluation of symptoms suggestive of DVT), the diverse types of catheters, the various underlying diseases, and the mean duration of catheterization. Table 14.1 summarizes the results of five prospective studies aiming to evaluate the incidence of complications relating to upper-extremity venous access devices placed in oncology patients primarily for chemotherapy.[2-6]

Numerous risk factors have been established for catheter-related arm DVT. The texture and coating of the catheter is an important factor, since polyurethane and silicone catheters are associated with lower rates of both arm DVT and pulmonary embolism than polyethylene, polyvinylchloride, or Teflon-coated catheters.[7,8] Lower rates of arm DVT are also found in patients with smaller catheter diameters[9,10] or a correct placement of the tip in the superior vena cava DVT.[11] Finally, there

Table 14.1 Prospective studies evaluating the incidence of catheter-related complications placed in cancer patients primarily for chemotherapy.

	Povoski et al[2]	Burbridge et al[3]	Biffi et al[4]	Luciani et al[5]	Harter et al[6]
Patients (n)	82	125	302	145	233
Cancers	Solid	All	Solid	Head and neck	All
Catheters	All	Ports	All	CVC	CVC
Duration	7 months	9 months	8 months	3 months	13 days
Endpoints	Symptoms	Symptoms	CUS	CUS	Symptoms
Malfunction	NA	NA	8%	NA	0.4%
DVT	4%	4%	6%	12%	1.5%
Infection	8%	3.2%	1%	NA	21%

CUS = compression ultrasonography; NA = not available; DVT = deep venous thrombosis; CVC = central venous catheters.

seems to be less risk of arm DVT with implantable ports than with external catheters.[12]

More recently, attention has focused on risk factors that are independent of the catheter. Cancer patients with central venous catheters are more prone to develop catheter-related arm DVT. Additive risk factors include the hypercoagulable state caused by the presence of malignancy, irritation of vessel walls by chemotherapeutic drugs and hormonal therapies, and disease-related complications, including infection and pathological bone fractures. In rare cases, endothelial lesions can be produced by tumor compression or infiltration. Finally, fibrosis of upper-extremity deep veins can be a long-term consequence of the radiotherapy of thoracic cancers, causing stasis and decreased flow. Some of these factors are clearly difficult to control in the cancer patient. In fact, considering the number and frequency of all these contributing factors, the question why arm DVT occurs is less puzzling than why it does not occur more often.

Complications of arm DVT

The significance of arm DVT has received less attention than femoral vein thrombosis, probably due to the erroneous belief that subsequent pulmonary embolism is rare. Accordingly, some authors have questioned the need for anticoagulant therapy in such patients. However, a number of prospective studies have demonstrated that the prevalence of both symptomatic and asymptomatic pulmonary embolism in patients with arm DVT is high, and it is close to that observed in cohorts of patients with lower-extremity DVT.[8,13,14]

Another complication is catheter malfunction. It significantly affects quality of life and exposes patients to multiple venipunctures and peripheral intravenous catheters. This condition has been descibed as a progressive inability to aspirate blood for laboratory tests, and is ascribed to adherence of a fibrin sleeve to the tip of the catheter, thus creating a one-way valve mechanism. Sometimes the catheter needs to be removed, but, since these catheters are often integral to patient care, reinsertion is often required.

The post-thrombotic syndrome in patients with arm DVT is characterized by pain, swelling, and limitation of activity in the affected arm secondary to residual venous obstruction by thrombus or stenosis of the vein. The reported incidence in the literature varies widely and may be as high as 36–50%.[15]

Infection of a thrombus surrounding a catheter may cause septic thrombophlebitis, which can evolve into systemic sepsis. Timsit et al identified catheter-associated sepsis in 19% of patients with catheter-related arm DVT, and in 7.2% of patients with catheters in place but without DVT.[16] Finally, superior vena cava syndrome may also occur in patients with arm DVT: in a series of 59 patients with superior vena cava syndrome, Kee et al found 20% of them to be associated with central venous catheters and pacemakers.[17]

Prophylaxis

Warfarin therapy, with a target international normalized ratio (INR) of 2–3, is commonly used for long-term treatment of DVT. To achieve this, a mean dose of approximately 4.5 mg is required. In 1990, Bern et al reported the results of a clinical trial in which 121 patients with solid tumors and indwelling central venous ports (Port-a-Cath) were randomized to receive or not receive minidose warfarin, beginning 3 days before catheter insertion and continuing for 90 days.[18] Final analysis was available for 82 patients (68%): 4 patients taking warfarin had venogram-proven DVT versus 15 patients in the control group (10 with symptoms). There were no bleeding complications, but warfarin had to be discontinued in 4 patients in whom the prothrombin time became longer than 15.0 seconds. The paper resulted in recommendations for the use of daily minidose warfarin in patients having central venous catheters.[19]

Since then, a number of studies[20-24] have evaluated the same endpoint, with conflicting results (Table 14.2). When considered overall, there were 30 of 357 patients (8.4%) who developed arm DVT despite minidose warfarin prophylaxis, as compared with 84 of 809 patients (10.4%) without warfarin (odds ratio 0.79; 95% confidence interval:

Table 14.2 Clinical studies evaluating the influence of prophylaxis with minidose warfarin in cancer patients with indwelling central venous lines.

	Bern et al[18]	Boraks et al[20]	Ratcliffe et al[21]	Minassian et al[22]	Heaton et al[23]	Kuriakose et al[24]
Design	Prosp.	Retrosp.	Retrosp.	Retrosp.	Prosp.	Retrosp.
Patients (n)	82	223	84	305	88	384
Cancers	Solid	Hematol.	All	Gynecol.	Hematol.	Solid
Catheters	Ports	CVC	CVC	All	CVC	Ports
Duration	3 months	NA	4 months	11 months	3 months	13 months
Endpoints	Venogram	Symptoms	Symptoms	Symptoms	Symptoms	Symptoms
DVT rate:						
Warfarin	4 (10%)	5 (5%)	7 (13%)	4 (4%)	8 (18%)	2 (18%)
Controls	15 (37%)	15 (13%)	3 (10%)	24 (11%)	5 (12%)	22 (6%)
p-value	0.003	0.03	NS	0.04	NS	NS
Bleeding	0	0	3 (5%)	NA	1 (2%)	NA

NA = not available; DVT = deep venous thrombosis; CVC = central venous catheters.

0.50–1.25). By contrast, in some cases, warfarin prophylaxis was asso-ciated with either abnormal INR results[23] or increased bleeding in patients taking warfarin.[21,23]

In fact, routine prophylaxis is not used in many medical centers. Carr and Rabinowitz retrospectively reviewed the practice of prescribing minidose warfarin in cancer patients with central venous catheters at their institution.[25] In the initial review, 39 charts were reviewed, and it was found that only 4 of the patients (10%) had been placed on prophy-lactic minidose warfarin. Then, after notification of the physicians about the policy and benefits of such prophylaxis, only 7 of 35 patients (20%) reviewed were found to have been placed on prophylactic warfarin. Thus, although most physicians universally agree to use prophylactic anticoagulation, their compliance remains poor.

In a study by our group, the effectiveness of a low-molecular-weight heparin in this setting was investigated. In an open, prospective study, patients with cancer who underwent insertion of a Port-a-Cath subcla-vian venous catheter were randomized to receive or not receive 2500 IU of dalteparin once daily for 90 days.[26] Initially, 100 consecutive patients were to be included, but, on the recommendation of the ethics commit-tee, patient recruitment was terminated earlier than planned after inclusion of 32 patients, because of an excess of thrombotic events in patients without prophylaxis. Eight of 13 patients (62%) without prophy-laxis developed DVT, as compared with only 1 of 16 patients (6%) taking dalteparin. Indeed, once-daily administration of LMWH may also have an antitumor effect, though this remains to be proven.[27] However, prophy-laxis with LMWH needs to be further investigated on a large scale. Two large, prospective, randomized clinical trials have been recently con-ducted to test the efficacy of LMWHs in this setting. The results of these studies will greatly improve our knowledge in this field.

Treatment

In patients with catheter dysfunction, one needs to know whether it is due to a thrombus at the tip of the catheter or occlusive thrombosis of a venous segment. Although there are other causes of catheter dysfunc-tion, such as malposition, catheter tip thrombus usually presents with an inability to draw adequately from or infuse into the catheter. This has tra-ditionally been treated with low doses of urokinase instilled into the catheter. If treatment is unsuccesful, diagnostic testing for DVT (ultra-sonography or venography) should be performed. If occlusive DVT is detected, anticoagulant therapy must be considered, with or without catheter removal.[28–30]

Systemic anticoagulation is associated with an increased risk of bleeding, particularly in patients who develop thrombocytopenia as a result of their disease or its treatment. A second approach is to remove the catheter, but cancer patients frequently require central venous access, and removal of the catheter may necessitate replacement with a second catheter. Frank et al have reported the results of a retrospective study in 112 patients with cancer and catheter-related arm DVT.[31] Regardless of therapeutic intervention, including anticoagulation, catheter removal or replacement, or a combination of them, no patients had a major adverse outcome. However, in four patients treated with replacement of the catheter, upper-extremity edema persisted without change. A prospective, randomized trial to evaluate these approaches seems to be warranted.

References

1. Reed JD, Harman JT, Harris V. Regional fibrinolytic therapy for iatrogenic subclavian vein thrombosis. Semin Interv Radiol 1992; 9:183–9.

2. Povoski SP. A prospective analysis of the cephalic vein cutdown approach for chronic indwelling central venous access in 100 consecutive cancer patients. Ann Surg Oncol 2000; 7:496–502.

3. Burbridge B, Krieger E, Stoneham G. Arm placement of the Cook titanium Petite Vital-Port: results of radiologic placement in 125 patients with cancer. Can Assoc Radiol J 2000; 51:163–9.

4. Biffi R, De Braud F, Orsi F et al. A randomized, prospective trial of central venous ports connected to standard open-ended or Groshong catheters in adult oncology patients. Cancer 2001; 92: 1204–12.

5. Luciani A, Clement O, Halimi P et al. Catheter-related upper extremity deep venous thrombosis in cancer patients: a prospective study based on Doppler US. Radiology 2001; 220:655–60.

6. Harter C, Salwender HJ, Bach A et al. Catheter-related infection and thrombosis of the jugular vein in hematologic–oncologic patients undergoing chemotherapy. A prospective comparison of silver-coated and uncoated catheters. Cancer 2002; 94:245–51.

7. Welch GW, McKeel DW, Silverstein P et al. The role of catheter composition in the development of thrombophlebitis. Surg Gynecol Obstet 1974; 138:421–4.

8. Monreal M, Raventós A, Lerma R et al. Pulmonary embolism in patients with upper extremity DVT associated to venous central lines. A prospective study. Thromb Haemost 1994; 72:548–50.

9. Lokich JJ, Becker B. Subclavian vein thrombosis in patients treated with infusion chemotherapy for advanced malignancy. Cancer 1983; 52:1586–9.

10. Grove JR, Pevec WC. Venous thrombosis related to peripherally inserted central catheters. J Vasc Interv Radiol 2000; 11:837–40.

11. James L, Bledsoe L, Hadaway LC. A retrospective look at tip location and complications of peripherally inserted central catheter lines. J Intravenous Nurs 1993; 16:104–9.

12. Hayward SR, Ledgerwood AM, Lucas CE. The fate of 100 prolonged venous access devices. Am Surg 1990; 56:515–19.

13. Monreal M, Lafoz E, Ruiz J et al. Upper-extremity deep venous thrombosis and pulmonary embolism. A prospective study. Chest 1991; **9**:280–3.

14. Prandoni P, Polistena P, Bernardi E et al. Upper-extremity deep vein thrombosis. Risk factors, diagnosis and complications. Arch Intern Med 1997; **157**:57–62.

15. Kommareddy A, Zaroukian MH, Hassouna HI. Upper extremity deep vein thrombosis. Semin Thromb Hemost 2002; **28**:89–99.

16. Timsit JF, Farkas JC, Boyer JM et al. Central vein catheter related thrombosis in intensive care patients. Incidence, risk factors, and relationship with catheter related sepsis. Chest 1998; **114**: 207–13.

17. Kee ST, Kinoshita L, Razavi MK et al. Superior vena cava syndrome: treatment with catheter-directed thrombolysis and endovascular stent placement. Radiology 1998; **40**:370–7.

18. Bern MM, Lokich JJ, Wallach SR et al. Very low doses of warfarin can prevent thrombosis in central venous catheters. A randomized prospective trial. Ann Intern Med 1990; **112**:423–8.

19. Geerts WH, Heit JA, Clagett GP et al. Prevention of venous thromboembolism. Chest 2001; **119**: 132S–75S.

20. Boraks P, Seale J, Price J et al. Prevention of central venous catheter associated thrombosis using minidose warfarin in patients with haematological malignancies. Br J Haematol 1998; **101**:483–6.

21. Ratcliffe M, Broadfoot C, Davidson M et al. Thrombosis, markers of thrombotic risk, indwelling central venous catheters and antithrombotic prophylaxis using low-dose warfarin in subjects with malignant disease. Clin Lab Haematol 1999; **21**:353–7.

22. Minassian VA, Sood AK, Lowe P, Sorosky JI, Al-Jurf AS, Buller RE. Longterm central venous access in gynecologic cancer patients. J Am Coll Surg 2000; **191**:403–9.

23. Heaton DC, Han DY, Inder A. Minidose (1 mg) warfarin as prophylaxis for central vein catheter thrombosis. Intern Med J 2002; **32**:84–8.

24. Kuriakose P, Colon-Otero G, Paz-Fumagalli R. Risk of deep venous thrombosis associated with chest versus arm central venous subcutaneous port catheters: a 5-year single-institution retrospective study. J Vasc Interv Radiol 2002; **13**:179–84.

25. Carr K, Rabinowitz I. Physician compliance with warfarin prophylaxis for central venous catheters in patients with solid tumors. J Clin Oncol 2000; **21**:3665–7.

26. Monreal M, Alastrue A, Rull M et al. Upper extremity deep venous thrombosis in cancer patients with venous access devices. Prophylaxis with a low molecular weight heparin (Fragmin). Thromb Haemost 1994; **75**: 251–3.

27. Green D, Hull RD, Brant R, Pineo GF. Lower mortality in cancer patients treated with low-molecular-weight versus standard heparin [letter]. Lancet 1992; **339**:1476.

28. Bona RD. Thrombotic complications of central venous catheters in cancer patients. Semin Thromb Hemost 1999; **25**:147–55.

29. Haire WD, Lieberman RP. Thrombosed central venous catheters: restoring function with 6-hour urokinase infusion after failure of bolus urokinase. J Parenteral Nutr 1992; **16**:129–32.

30. Savage KJ, Wells PS, Schulz V et al. Outpatient use of low molecular weight heparin (dalteparin) for treatment of deep vein thrombosis of the upper extremity. Thromb Haemost 1999; **82**:1008–110.

31. Frank DA, Meuse J, Hirsh D et al. The treatment and outcome of cancer patients with thromboses on central venous catheters. J Thromb Thrombolysis 2000; **10**: 271–75.

15

Prevention and treatment of thrombosis in cancer patients

Hans Klaus Breddin and Rupert Bauersachs

Introduction

The association of venous thrombosis and cancer was first described by Armand Trousseau in 1865.[1] Many further observations and later clinical trials, including those with different antithrombotic agents, have verified that cancer patients have a higher risk of venous thrombosis than patients without malignancies. On the other hand, venous thromboembolism (VTE) is frequently associated with occult malignancy. Concerning the prevention and treatment of VTE in cancer patients, there remain some major questions:
(1) Do cancer patients undergoing surgery need intensified or prolonged medical prophylaxis?
(2) Do patients with cancer and acute deep venous thrombosis (DVT) or pulmonary embolism (PE) benefit from prolonged or intensified antithrombotic treatment, and which treatment regimen is to be preferred?
(3) Can some antithrombotic agents, such as low-molecular-weight heparins (LMWH), reduce cancer mortality?

Cancer and the risk of venous thrombosis

The presence of active cancer besides other thrombophilic conditions is a persistent risk factor for recurrent VTE. A strong association of VTE with age over 60 years, increasing body weight, and previous thrombosis was described by Kakkar et al.[2] The association with cancer surgery was weaker ($p = 0.04$).[3–7] This has also been shown in recent treatment trials.[8,9] Immobilization, surgery, cytostatic drugs, and indwelling venous catheters, as well as increased procoagulants, probably contribute to the increased risk.[10–12]

The risk may be related to the release of procoagulants from tumor cells, which could cause some degree of resistance to the usual intensities of anticoagulant drugs in patients with cancer.[13] In spite of intensive research, no definite correlation has been established between the plasma levels of different hemostatic markers, such as fibrinogen, platelet count, D-dimer, prothrombin fragments 1 and 2, and others, and the occurrence of thrombosis in cancer patients. Patients with VTE and cancer are at a higher risk of recurrent VTE complications during anticoagulation. It is very likely that the excess risk of VTE after cancer surgery is due not only to the presence of malignancy itself, but also to accumulation of other well-known and common risk factors, including advanced age, debility, extended and complex surgical procedures, and complicated postoperative course. Links between cancer and a high risk of postoperative thrombosis have been reported for gynecological surgery.

VTE as the first sign of cancer

Population-based studies

In a large, population-based Swedish study, Baron et al assessed the cancer incidence amongst 62 000 patients with DVT admitted to hospital between 1965 and 1983. During the first year of follow-up, the standardized incidence ration (SIR) of new malignancies was 4.4%. During the following years also, cancers were diagnosed more frequently than in a noncancer population.[14]

In a similar Danish study, Sørensen et al[15] identified 15 348 patients with DVT and 11 305 patients with PE. The SIR for new cancer was 1.3 for patients with VTE. The risk was higher (SIR 3.0) during the first 6 months of follow-up.

In a veteran population, Saba et al[16] found subsequent cancer in 26.2% of 183 patients with established VTE during the following 5 years, while the incidence was 11.5% in a group of 200 age-matched control patients. The cancer incidence was higher in patients below 60 years of age. The majority of patients were diagnosed with cancer within less than 1 year after their VTE

Prospective trials

A number of prospective trials on the relationship between VTE and subsequent cancer have also been published. Prandoni et al[17] followed 250 patients with symptomtic, venographically proved DVT for 2 years. Of these patients, 145 had idiopathic venous thrombosis, 7.6% developed overt cancer, and 35 patients had confirmed recurrent thromboembolism. The incidence of cancer was less frequent in the patients with secondary venous thrombosis (1.9%).

Hettiarachchi et al[18] studied 400 patients, of whom 70 already had been diagnosed with malignancy. Within the following 6 months, 10 new malignancies were observed in 137 patients with unexplained DVT (7.3%), compared with a relatively low risk (1.6%) in patients with secondary DVT.

Schulman and Lindmarker[19] observed an SIR of 3.4 for new malignancies during the first year after a thromboembolic event, compared with expected numbers based on the Swedish national incidence rates. This ratio remained between 1.3 and 2.2 for the following 5 years. A first cancer was diagnosed in 111 of 854 patients (13%) during follow-up.

Laporte et al[20] observed a cumulative incidence of 10% in 344 patients with proximal DVT with or without PE. Similarly, Taliani et al[21] found newly diagnosed cancer in 32 (7.5%) of 429 patients with VTE during a mean follow-up of 43.7 months.

In conclusion, several population-based and prospective studies have demonstrated that patients with acute idiopathic VTE, particularly those of advanced age, have an increased risk of harboring an occult or inapparent cancer, the diagnosis of which may not be made until several months after the acute VTE episode.

Prognosis of cancer associated with VTE

From a population-based study on 668 patients who had cancer and VTE, Sørensen et al concluded that the combination is associated with an advanced stage of cancer and with a poor prognosis.[22]

Is extensive screening for cancer useful in patients with idiopathic VTE?

Bura et al[23] studied 103 patients with bilateral DVT, of whom 25% had known active cancer and in 19 of whom an unknown malignancy was detected. During the follow-up of a mean of 12.8 months, one further patient developed cancer. The authors concluded that extensive screening for occult malignancy may be useful. However, more data are needed to determine whether and which screening for occult malignancy is warranted in patients with VTE.

Recurrent thromboembolism in cancer patients

Cancer patients with established VTE are more likely to develop recurrent thrombosis than noncancer patients. A large population-based cohort study has confirmed that malignancy is associated with a two- to three-fold risk of recurrent thrombosis.[24] Depending on the presence or absence of antineoplastic therapy, the hazard ratios for recurrent thrombosis were 3.57 and 2.56, respectively. These findings were confirmed in the prospective cohort study by Prandoni et al.[25] In the subgroup of 58 patients with cancer in this study, the overall recurrence rate was 10.3%, compared with 4.7% in patients without cancer. In another prospective cohort study of 738 consecutive patients with a first or second episode of DVT, the 5-year cumulative incidence of recurrent thromboembolism was 21.5%, and the relative risk of recurrence in the presence of cancer versus no cancer was 1.97.[26] Similar rates of recurrent thromboses have been reported in other studies. Bona et al[27] found that the risk of recurrent thrombosis was 0.013 per patient-month of treatment in 104 cancer patients, compared with 0.002 per patient-month in 208 noncancer patients. In a population-based cohort study by Palareti et al,[28] a 6.8% rate of recurrent thrombosis in cancer patients was observed, compared with 2.5% in noncancer patients ($p = 0.06$).

Levitan et al[29] found the probability of readmission within 183 days of initial hospitalization to be significantly higher for patients with VTE and malignancy, as compared to patients with VTE and no malignancy. Patients with VTE and malignancy also had a more than threefold higher risk of thromboembolic disease and death than patients with VTE without malignancy.

Recently, Agnelli et al[30] reported on the @RISTOS project, in which 2373 patients with surgery for cancer were included and followed for 30 days. The overall death rate was 1.75%. VTE was responsible for almost 50% of the deaths.

There are not yet sufficient data available to clarify whether the higher risks for recurrent VTE and possibly also bleeding during the anticoagulation apply to all patients with cancer or to specific groups. It appears that advanced cancer carries an increased risk of recurrence, but also a substantially elevated risk of major bleeding under oral anticoagulation.

Drugs used in the prevention and treatment of DVT

For many years, unfractionated heparin (UFH) was the drug of choice for the prevention and treatment of DVT. LMWH have advantages over UFH. They bind less to plasma proteins, macrophages, platelets, and endothelium,[31] resulting in a longer plasma half-life, better bioavailability, and more predictable pharmacodynamic properties. LMWH therefore can be given once or twice daily in subcutaneous injections. Laboratory monitoring is usually not required. A number of clinical trials have compared UFH administered by continuous intravenous infusion with subcutaneous LMWH.[9,32,33] Dermatan sulfate, which inhibits thrombin via heparin-cofactor II, has been shown to be as effective as UFH. A combination of dermatan sulfate and heparan sulfate (danaparoid, Orgaran) had similar effects.[34] Thrombin inhibitors such as hirudin have not yet been used in trials including cancer patients. After initial treatment with heparin or heparin-related drugs, most patients with acute VTE receive a vitamin K antagonist for the following 3–12 months.

Thrombosis prevention in cancer patients.

In an overview by Clagett and Reisch,[35] 10 trials using low-dose UFH were identified in which the results for cancer patients were reported separately. While low-dose UFH reduced the thrombosis risk in patients both with and without cancer, the DVT risk in malignant disease after prophylaxis was higher. It remained unclear whether changing the heparin dose could improve the thrombosis rate in cancer patients.[36,37]

Many studies with LMWH in patients with abdominal surgery used the ^{125}I-fibrinogen leg scan as endpoint. The European Fraxiparin Study Group[38] prestratified for the presence of cancer, and one other trial[39] was performed in cancer patients only. Patients operated for cancer in the European Fraxiparin Study were older and underwent longer operations than those with benign disease. The results of some relevant trials are listed in Table 15.1.

Each trial showed a trend towards a higher rate of DVT in patients undergoing abdominal surgery for cancer regardless of whether they received LMWH or low-dose UFH. In the clinical endpoint trial by Kakkar et al,[40] treatment with low-dose UFH or LMWH (dalteparin) was followed by very low rates of symptomatic VTE (1.0% and 1.1%, respectively). However, failure of prophylaxis was again more frequent after cancer surgery, compared with patients with benign disease. Danaparoid (750 U twice daily) was compared with UFH in 513 patients with elective surgery for intra-abdominal or intrathoracic surgery. Thromboses were detected by the ^{125}I-fibrinogen uptake. The thrombosis rate was 10.4% in the danaparoid group and 14.9% in the UFH group.[34]

In a multicenter trial, Di Carlo et al[41] compared dermatan sulfate (300 mg intramuscularly) with UFH for 7 days in the prophylaxis of postoperative thrombosis in cancer patients. The thrombosis rate assessed by bilateral phlebography was significantly lower in the dermatan-treated group (15%) than in the UFH group (22%) (Table 15.2). There was no significant difference in bleeding complications between treatment groups. McLeod et al[42] investigated the rate of VTE in 936 patients with colon resections who were randomized to receive either UFH (5000 IU three times daily) or enoxaparin (40 mg once daily) for 5–7 days. Bilateral phlebography was performed after 5–9 days. The rate of VTE (9.4%) was the same in both groups. In cancer patients, the rate of VTE was increased, with a nonsignificant difference between the UFH group (19.9%) and the enoxaparin group (12.5%).

Table 15.1 DVT rates (^{125}I-fibrinogen leg scan) in comparison of LMWH or danaparoid with UFH in general surgery where efficacy was reported separately for patients with malignancy.

Reference	Drug	Cancer surgery (% DVT)		Benign disease (% DVT)	
		LMWH	UFH	LMWH	UFH
European Fraxiparin Study Group, 1988[38]	Nadroparin (Fraxiparin)	15/355 (4.2%)	19/349 (5.4%)	12/605 (2.0%)	23/587 (3.9%)
Gallus et al, 1993[34]	Danaparoid (Orgaran)	25/241 (10.4%)	37/249 (14.9%)		
Nurmohamed et al, 1995[39]	Enoxaparin (Clexane)	36/264 (13.6%)	22/252 (8.7%)	22/454 (4.8%)	23/456 (5.0%)[a]
Bergqvist et al, 1995[49]	Dalteparin (Fragmin) 2500 Xal U/day	14.9%		Approx. 8.2%[a]	
	Dalteparin (Fragmin) 5000 Xal U/day	8.5%		Approx. 3.0%[a]	

[a]Total patient number = 1957.

Table 15.2 Studies on the incidence of deep vein thrombosis in cancer patients using phlebography.

Reference	Drugs used	n	Duration	VTE rate (%)	p
Di Carlo et al, 1999[41]	Dermatan sulfate 300 mg/day UFH	267 254	10 days	15 22	0.033
McLeod et al, 2001[42]	Enoxaparin 40 mg once daily UFH		9 days	12.5 19.9	NS
ENOXACAN study group, 1997[43]	Enoxaparin 40 mg once daily UFH		3 months	14.7 18.2	NS

In the ENOXACAN study,[43] patients with malignancies and elective abdominal or pelvic surgery were randomized to UFH or enoxaparin. Bilateral phlebography was used to detect venous thrombosis. In total, 631 patients were evaluable, and thromboembolic complications occurred in 18.2% of the UFH group and in 14.7% of the enoxaparin group. There was no difference in mortality rate after 30 days (Table 15.2).

Therefore, as stated in the 2001 ACCP Consensus Recommedations,[44] in order to reduce the risk of venous thrombosis, we would suggest that patients with cancer receive low-dose UFH or LMWH when they are confined to bed for any reason and when undergoing low-risk surgical procedures .

Surgery for gynecological cancer

DVT prevention in women undergoing surgery for gynecological malignancy was explored in a number of trials by Clarke-Pearson et al.[45-47] While low-dose UFH twice daily was ineffective in reducing the risk of venous thrombosis, 8-hourly low-dose UFH reduced the DVT rate, and more so if the patients received 2–9 doses of low-dose UFH before surgery.[46] Von Tempelhoff et al[48] studied 60 patients with ovarian cancer, of whom 17 had thromboses. Four of 28 patients on LMWH (certoparin) developed new thrombosis, compared with none of 30 patients receiving UFH during the 9-day postoperative period. Cancer mortality was 21.4% in the LMWH group and 37.5% in patients who had received UFH (Table 15.3).

Duration of prophylaxis in cancer patients

The optimal duration of initial postoperative thromboprophylaxis also in noncancer patients is still under debate. Recent studies have shown that, in patients with elective hip and knee surgery and patients with hip fracture, prolonged prophylaxis up to 30–40 days significantly reduces the risk of late postoperative thrombosis.[49]

Abdominal surgery for cancer also carries a high risk of VTE. Bergqvist et al[50] studied the effect of long-term prophylaxis with either enoxaparin 40 mg day subcutaneously or placebo after an initial treatment with enoxaparin in patients operated for abdominal or pelvic cancer. Bilateral phlebography was performed between days 25 and 31. The rate of VTE at the end of the double-blind period was significantly higher in the placebo group (12%) than in the enoxaparin group (4.8%) ($p = 0.02$). The difference persisted at 3 months. There were no significant differences in the bleeding rates between the two treatment

Table 15.3 Deep-vein thrombosis and mortality in patients with gynaecological malignancies.

Reference	Drugs	Method	DVT rate[a]	Mortality rate (%)	P
Clarke-Pearson et al, 1983[45]	12-hourly UFH, start 2 hr preop Controls	125I-fibrinogen	13/78 (15) 12/87 (12)		NS
Clarke-Pearson et al, 1990[46]	8-hourly UFH starting 2 hr before surgery 8-hourly UFH starting 2–9 doses before surgery Controls	125I-fibrinogen	9/104 (9) 4/97 (4) 19/103 (19)		<0.04 <0.001
Clarke-Pearson et al, 1993[47]	EPC during surgery and for 5 days postsurgery 8-hourly UFH starting with admission	125I-fibrinogen	4/101 (4) 7/107 (6.5)		NS
von Tempelhoff et al, 1997[48,b]	LMWH (Monoembolex) bid UFH	IPG/venography	4/28 0/30	21.4 37.5	NS

aPercentages in parentheses.
bPatients with ovarian cancer.
EPC = external pneumatic compression device.
IPG = impedance plethysmography.

groups. Thus, prolonged postoperative prophylaxis with LMWH seems indicated in cancer patients undergoing major surgery, as in other high risk situations. Further studies may confirm these results in patients with other malignancies.

Oral anticoagulation in cancer patients

Oral anticoagulant therapy can be difficult in patients with cancer. Frequent blood sampling may be necessary because diet, medication, gastrointestinal absorption, and hepatic function alter the anticoagulant dose response. This is particularly inconvenient because these patients often have limited venous access. Due to the delayed onset and reversal of action, oral anticoagulants must be discontinued days before an invasive procedure, and therapeutic levels may not be reached again for days after reversal of the anticoagulant effect. Such interruptions in anticoagulation make dose adjustment more difficult. Due to the narrow therapeutic window of vitamin K antagonists, unpredictable fluctuations in the INR may lead to excessive bleeding or recurrent thrombosis.

Levine et al[51] studied the effect of low-dose warfarin in patients with breast cancer receiving chemotherapy. In total, 152 patients received low-dose warfarin (INR of 1.3–1.9) for 6 weeks, and 159 patients were on placebo. Seven thromboembolic events occurred in the placebo group and one in the warfarin group (p = 0.03); major bleedings occurred in two placebo patients and in one patient on warfarin.

Palareti et al[28] compared the outcome of 95 patients with malignancy on oral anticoagulants with that of 733 patients without malignancy. On the basis of 744 patient-years of treatment, there was a higher rate of thromboembolic complications in cancer patients (6.8%) than in non-cancer patients (2.5%). However, the total bleeding rate was significantly higher in cancer patients (21.6%) than in the noncancer group (4.5%).

A cancer patient who develops recurrent thromboembolism with subtherapeutic INR can be treated acutely with UFH or LMWH and then be given oral anticoagulant therapy to ensure that the INR is maintained between 2.0 and 3.0. Patients who develop documented recurrent VTE while on therapeutic oral anticoagulant therapy represent a difficult therapeutic challenge. The options for 'retreatment' of the acute episode with UFH or LMWH include continued oral anticoagulant therapy at a higher INR target range, or LMWH at doses higher than those for the usual prophylactic regimen. Several regimens have been proposed: half of the therapeutic dose, the full therapeutic dose, or a dose between these two doses. Further studies are necessary to clarify this important point.

The use of an inferior vena caval filter alone should be considered only very rarely—perhaps only in patients with active bleeding or in those at very high risk of bleeding. In a randomized trial conducted in France, the use of a vena caval filter reduced the rate of recurrent PE over the short term nonsignificantly, but at the expense of a significant increase in recurrent DVT during longer follow-up.[52] Therefore, anticoagulation should be administered whenever possible. But the question remains open whether permanent filters are useful, or not.

The effect of LMWH on VTE recurrence in cancer subgroups from larger trials of acute VTE treatment

Cancer patients with established venous thrombosis have a higher risk of developing recurrent VTE than noncancer patients.[53,54] In a number of studies, the effects of different antithrombotic regimens in patients with acute VTE and cancer have been reported. Usually, the rate of VTE is presented for the total study population only. Patients are normally not stratified to different treatment regimens according to different types of cancer.

Short-term treatment with LMWH and cancer mortality rate

In several studies published in the mid-1990s,[55–57] in which LMWH were used for usually 1 week, a reduction was seen in the cancer mortality rate during the 6-month follow-up. These observations, followed by several meta-analyses,[32,33] supported the hypothesis that a brief treatment with LMWH may reduce cancer mortality in comparison to UFH. It has to be mentioned that patients in these trials were not stratified for different types of cancer. This limits the value of the single studies—but even more so that of the meta-analyses—because it is extremely unlikely that all cancer types may benefit from a specific form of anticoagulation. In some subsequent studies, similar results were obtained, but in many other trials no LMWH effects on mortality were found[9,58,59] (Tables 15.4 and 15.5). In the CORTES trial,[9] 375 patients with acute DVT were treated with UFH, while 762 received reviparin (for the majority, 12 600 IU) in either one or two daily subcutaneous injections. The 374 patients with single daily injections received reviparin for 21 days. Between 10.6% and 14.4% of the patients in the different treatment groups had cancer. Cancer mortality within 3 months was 1.6% in the UFH group and 1.84% in the two reviparin groups, respectively. Clinical recurrence of thromboembolic events occurred in significantly more cancer patients (10.2%) than noncancer patients (0.3%).

Two such trials have been reported. Von Tempelhoff et al[48,60] studied the effect of treatment with certoparin or UFH for 7 days in 185 patients with breast cancer and in 102 patients with pelvic cancer. After a follow-

Table 15.4 Effect of LMWH treatment on VTE recurrence rates in the total study population and in cancer subgroups, and on cancer mortality in patients with acute DVT.

Reference	Total population				Cancer patients		
	Drug used		Recurrence[a]	Mortality[a]	n[a]	Thrombosis	Cancer mortality
Hull et al, 1992[55]	Logiparin 175 U/kg once daily	213	6 (2.8)	10 (4.7)	46		15.2%
	UFH	219	15 (6.9)	21 (9.5)	49		28.6%
Prandoni et al, 1992[56]	Nadroparin 13–19 000 U bid	?	?	?	?		6.7%
	UFH						44.4%
Koopmann et al, 1996[57]	Nadroparin 8200–18 400 U bid	202	14 (6.9)	16 (8.1)	36 (18)		8 (4%)
	UFH	198	17 (8.5)	14 (6.9)	34 [17]		8 (4%)
COLUMBUS, 1997[8]	Reviparin weight-adjusted bid	510	27 (5.3)	36 (7.1)	119	Total: 20 (8.6%)	Total: 74 (20.3%)
	UFH	511	25 (4.9)	39 (7.6)	113		
Kirchmaier et al, 1998[58]	Certoparin i.v./s.c.	255	2 (0.8)	16 (6.3)	20 (7.8)		11 (4.3%)
	UFH	130	4 (3.0)	10 (7.7)	9 (6.9)		3 (2.3%)
CORTES, 2001[9]	Reviparin bid	388	7 (1.8)	9 (2.32)	41 (10.6)		5 (1.3%)
	Reviparin once daily	374	13 (3.5)	15 (4.0)	54 (14.4)	10.2%	8 (2.13%)
	UFH	375	24 (6.4)	11 (2.93)	42 (11.2)		5 (1.3%)
Simonneau et al, 1997[59]	Tinzaparin	304		11 (3.6)	34 (11)		4 (1.3%)
	UFH	308		14 (4.5)	26 (9)		2 (0.64%)

[a]Percentages in parenthesis.

Table 15.5 Specific studies on cancer survival.

Reference	Type of cancer	Patients n	Drug	Duration	Survival rate after 1 year		p
Lebeau et al, 1994[61]	Small-cell lung cancer	138 139	UFH s.c. for 5 weeks No treatment	1 year	40% 30%		
FAMOS, 2002[54]	Breast, colorectal, ovarian, pancreas, and others	185 181	Dalteparin Saline	9 months	45% 42%		NS
					Mortality		
Tempelhoff et al, 2000[60]	Breast cancer	94 91	Certoparin UFH	1050 days	9 10	(9.6%) (10.9%)	0.812
	Pelvic cancer	46 56	Certoparin UFH	1050 days	4 15	(8.7%) (28.6%)	0.013
					Thromboses		
FAMOS, 2002[54]	Breast, colorectal, ovarian, pancreas, and others	185 181	Dalteparin Saline	9 months	2.4% 3.5%		NS

up of 650 or 1050 days, there was no difference in mortality between the two treatments in the breast-cancer groups, while the patients with pelvic cancer showed a significant difference in mortality after 650 days. This difference, however, was no longer significant after 1050 days.

In 1994, Lebeau et al[61] reported that patients with small-cell lung cancer treated with UFH for 5 weeks had a higher 1-year survival rate (40%) than nontreated patients (30%). Several hypotheses on possible mechanisms that may reduce cancer mortality in patients treated with anticoagulants, and specifically LMWH, have been published. The only way to verify these hypotheses is to study the effect of anticoagulation in specific cancer types over longer treatment periods.

Effect of extended treatment with LMWH on VTE and mortality

Meyer et al[62] studied the effect of enoxaparin (1.5 mg/kg s.c. once daily) compared with warfarin given for 3 months in 146 cancer patients with VTE. Of the 71 patients on warfarin, 21% experienced a major outcome event within 3 months, compared with 7% of the 67 patients in the enoxaparin group. A combined outcome event was defined as major bleeding or recurrent VTE within 3 months. Of the 71 evaluable patients on warfarin, 21% had a major outcome event, compared with 10.5% of the patients on enoxaparin. The differences, however, were not statistically significant. There were six deaths due to haemorrhage in the warfarin group and none in the enoxaparin group. In another recent study (CLOT),[63] cancer patients with acute VTE were treated with dalteparin (200 IU/kg s.c. once daily) for 5–7 days and a coumarin derivative for 6 months, or with dalteparin alone for 6 months. Of the 336 patients on oral anticaogulation, 53 experienced recurrent VTE, compared with 27 of 336 patients in the dalteparin group. The cumulative rate of recurrent VTE was reduced from 17.4% in the oral anticoagulation group to 8.8% in the dalteparin group. There was no difference in major bleeding between the groups. Although there was no difference in mortality between the treatment groups, in the subgroup of 150 patients with nonmetastatic solid tumors at randomization, 15 of 75 dalteparin patients died, compared with 26 of 75 patients on oral anticoagulation.

In the FAMOS study,[54] patients with advanced solid malignancies without underlying thromboses were randomized to receive either 5000 anti-Xa U of dalteparin subcutaneously daily (382 patients) or saline injections (181 patients). Treatment was scheduled to last 1 year. The thrombosis rates were 3.4% for the placebo group and 2.4% for the dalteparin patients (Table 15.5). There were no significant differences in the survival rates between the treatment groups after a mean observation period of 9 months for the placebo group and 10.3 months for the dalteparin group. However, a post hoc subgroup analysis of those patients who survived longer than 17 months revealed a significantly increased survival in the dalteparin-treated group.[64] Similarly, a post hoc analysis of the CLOT data indicated a survival advantage in the dalteparin-treated cancer patients without metastatic disease at the time of presentation.[65] The results of the MALT study[66] also demonstrated improved survival for cancer patients treated with LMWH. These new results strongly support the need for larger confirmatory trials on the efficacy of long-term LMWH therapy for prolonging survival in patients with lower tumor burden.

It has become very likely that long-term treatment with anticoagulants reduces the frequency of thromboembolic complications in cancer patients. This, however, has to be weighed against the possibly higher incidence of bleeding complications. Long-term treatment with LMWH in patients with nonmetastatic cancer possibly also reduces cancer mortality. New clinical trials are needed in which patients will be stratified according to tumor-cell type and stage as well as other prognostic variables specific to the particular malignancy.

Bleeding risk in cancer patients

Patients at high risk of bleeding

In many institutions, inferior vena caval filters are routinely inserted in patients with a high risk of bleeding. Although there is consensus that tight anticoagulant control is necessary, clinical practice varies. Some clinicians omit the initial bolus of heparin, and some advocate the use of LMWH instead of oral anticoagulant therapy for long-term management. LMWH are attractive because their anticoagulant response is more predictable. They do not require laboratory monitoring, and experimental observations suggest that they cause less bleeding than UFH.[31] The major concern with oral anticoagulant therapy is that poor control would increase the bleeding risk, and most reported cases of intracranial hemorrhage have been associated with over-anticoagulation.

Bleeding risk

An increased bleeding risk of cancer patients on anticoagulant therapy has frequently been described.[67-69] These data were obtained prior to the routine use of INR monitoring and may have been influenced by high-intensity treatment. A large, population-based study also found malignancy associated with major hemorrhage.[70] In this study, most major bleeding occurred when the INR was higher than 4. Palareti et al[28] compared the safety and efficacy of oral anticoagulation in 95 cancer patients with 73 patients without cancer. Total (21.6% vs 4.4%) and major (5.4% vs 0.7%) bleeding were significantly more frequent in the cancer patients. Prandoni et al[71] also demonstrated an increased risk of major hemorrhage in cancer patients: 12.4% major bleedings after 12 months in the cancer group, compared with 4.9% in patients without cancer.

For some special indications, data are still inconclusive, as in patients with metastatic brain tumors. In summary, long-term anticoagulant therapy with vitamin K antagonists is generally associated with a significantly increased risk of major bleeding, compared with patients without cancer.

Patients with cancer have an increased risk of bleeding. Any form of anticoagulation further increases the bleeding risk. Vitamin K antagonists seem to carry a higher risk than LMWH at prophylactic or slightly higher doses. The bleeding risk has to be weighed against the benefit of antithrombotic effects when developing improved antithrombotic regimens in cancer patients.

Conclusions

Cancer patients undergoing surgery need antithrombotic prophylaxis. It is very likely that they benefit from prolonged prophylaxis with LMWH, but further studies have to clarify whether this applies to all types of cancer. The duration of anticoagulation, the choice of the best antithrombotic agent, and the optimal dosage should be identified in future studies.

Studies on the treatment of patients with acute DVT, including cancer patients, have demonstrated that LMWH reduces VTE recurrence. However, with the regimens used thus far, VTE recurrence is still markedly more frequent in the cancer population than in patients with benign diseases. Apparently, there is still room for improvement in the treatment of acute VTE in cancer patients

Long-term treatment of cancer patients with or without previous DVT may result in a reduction of VTE and thereby also have effects on cancer mortality. Further studies in this area are needed.

While some data in nonstratified populations have shown a reduction in cancer mortality in patients with acute VTE treated with LMWH for very short periods, further studies—particularly prospective trials in patients with well-defined tumor types—did not show similar results. However, several recent trials have made it likely that prolonged treatment with LMWH in patients with nonmetastatic tumors may reduce cancer mortality.

References

1. Trousseau A. Phlegmasia alba dolens. In: Clinique medicale de l'Hôtel Dieu de Paris, Vol 3, 2nd edn (Baillière: Paris, 1865) 654–712.

2. Kakkar VV, Howe CT, Nicolaides AN et al. Deep vein thrombosis of the leg. Is there a 'high risk' group? Am J Surg 1970; **120**: 527–30.

3. Kakkar VV, Murray WHJ. Efficacy and safety of low molecular weight heparin (CY 216) in preventing post-operative venous thromboembolism: a co-operative study. Br J Surg 1985; **72**:765–791.

4. Walsh JJ, Bonnar J, Wright FW. A study of pulmonary embolism and deep leg vein thrombosis after major gynaecological surgery using labelled fibrinogen–phlebography and lung scanning. J Obstet Gynaecol Br Commonw 1974; **81**:311–16.

5. Huber O, Bounameaux H, Borst F et al. Postoperative pulmonary emobolism after hospital discharge. An underestimated risk. Arch Surg 1992 **127**:310–13.

6. Mousa SA. Anticoagulation in thrombosis and cancer: the missing link. Semin Thromb Hemost 2002; **28**:45–52.

7. Sutherland DE, Weitz IC, Liebman HA. Thromboembolic complications of cancer: epidemiology, pathogenesis, diagnosis, and treatment. Am J Hematol 2003; **72**: 43–52.

8. The COLUMBUS Investigators. Low-molecular-weight heparin in the treatment of patients with venous thromboembolism. N Engl J Med 1997; **337**:657–62.

9. Breddin HK, Hach-Wunderle V, Nakov R et al. Effects of a low-molecular-weight heparin on thrombus regression and recurrent thromboembolism in patients with deep-vein thrombosis. N Engl J Med 2001; **344**:626–31.

10. Prandoni P, Lensing AWA, Cogo A et al. The long-term clinical course of acute deep venous thrombosis. Ann Intern Med 1996; **125**:1–7.

11. Gouin-Thibault I, Achkar A, Samama MM. The thrombophilic state in cancer patients. Acta Haematol 2001; **106**:33–42.

12. Donati MB, Falanga A. Pathogenetic mechanisms of thrombosis in malignancy, Acta Haematol 2001; **106**:18-24.

13. Rickles FR, Levine MN. Epidemiology of thrombosis in cancer, Acta Haematol 2001; **106**:6–12.

14. Baron JA, Gridley G, Weiderpass E et al. Venous thromboembolism and cancer. Lancet 1998; **351**: 1077–80.

15. Sørensen HAT, Mellemkjær L, Steffensen FH et al. The risk of a diagnosis of cancer after primary deep venous thrombosis or pulmonary embolism. N Eng J Med 1998; **338**:1169–73.

16. Saba H, Khalil F, Morelli GA et al. Relationship of thromboembolism (TE) to subsequent cancer diagnosis: a study in a veteran population. Thromb Haemost 2003; Suppl 1: Abst P0836.

17. Prandoni P, Lensing AW, Buller HR et al. Deep-vein thrombosis and the incidence of subsequent symptomatic cancer. N Engl J Med 1992; **327**:1128–33.

18. Hettiarachchi RJ, Lok J, Prins MH et al. Undiagnosed malignancy in patients with deep vein thrombosis: incidence, risk indicators, and diagnosis. Cancer 1998; **83**:180–5.

19. Schulman S, Lindmarker P. Incidence of cancer after prophylaxis with warfarin against recurrent venous thromboembolism. Duration of anticoagulation trial. N Engl J Med 2000; **342**:1953–8.

20. Laporte S, Mismetti P, Quenet S et al. Predictive factors of cancer discovery after deep-vein thrombosis: an 8-years follow-up study. Thromb Haemost 2003; Suppl 1: Abst P0819.

21. Taliani MR, Agnelli G, Prandoni P et al. Incidence of newly diagnosed cancer after three months or one year of oral anticoagulation for a first episode of idiopathic venous thromboembolism. Thromb Haemost 2003; Suppl 1, Abst P0817.

22. Sørensen HT, Mellemkjær L, Olsen JH et al. Prognosis of cancers associated with venous thrombembolism. N Engl J Med 2003; **343**:1846–50.

23. Bura A, Cailleux N, Bienvenu B et al. Bilateral deep-vein thrombosis and cancer: propspective study of 103 patients. Thromb Haemost 2003; Suppl 1: Abst P0830.

24. Heit JA, Mohr DN, Silverstein et al. Predictors of recurrence after deep vein thrombosis and pulmonary embolism. A population-based cohort study. Arch Intern Med 2000; **160**:761–8.

25. Prandoni P, Villalta S, Bagatella P et al. The clinical course of deep-vein thrombosis. Prospective long-term follow-up of 528 symptomatic patients. Haematologica 1997; **82**: 423–8.

26. Hansson PO, Sorbo J, Eriksson H. Recurrent venous thromboembolism after deep vein thrombosis: incidence and risk factors. Arch Intern Med 2000; **160**:769–74.

27. Bona RD, Hickey AD, Wallace DM. Efficacy and safety of oral anticoagulation in patients with cancer. Thromb Haemost 1997; **78**: 137–40.

28. Palareti G, Legnani C. Lee A et al. A comparison of the safety and efficacy of oral anticoagulation for the treatment of venous thromboembolic disease in patients with or without malignancy. Thromb Haemost 2000; **84**:805–10.

29. Levitan N, Dwlati A, Remick SC et al. Rates of initial and recurrent thromboembolic disease among patients with malignancy versus those without malignancy. Risk analysis using Medicare claims data. Med Baltimore 1999; **78**:285–91.

30. Agnelli G, Bolis G, Capussotti L et al. A clinical outcome-based prospective study on venous thromboembolism in cancer surgery: the @RISTOS project. Thromb Haemost 2003; Suppl 1: Abst OC191.

31. Weitz JI. Low molecular weight heparins. N Engl J Med 1997; **337**:688–98.

32. Siragusa S, Cosmi B, Piovella F et al. Low-molecular-weight heparins and unfractionated heparin in the treatment of patients with acute venous thromboembolism: results of a meta-analysis. Am J Med 1996; **100**:269–77.

33. Gould MK, Dembitzer AD, Doyle RL et al. Low molecular weight heparins compared with unfractionated heparin for treatment of acute deep vein thrombosis. A meta-analysis of randomized controlled trials. Ann Intern Med 1999; **130**:800–9.

34. Gallus A, Cade J, Ockelford P et al. Orgaran (Org 10172) or heparin for preventing venous thrombosis after elective surgery for malignant disease? A double-blind, randomised multicentre comparison. Thromb Haemost 1993; **70**:562–7.

35. Clagett GP, Reisch JS. Prevention of venous thromboembolism in general surgical patients. Results of a meta-analysis. Ann Surg 1988; **208**:227–40.

36. Törngren S. Optimal regimes of low-dose heparin prophylaxis in gastrointestinal surgery. Acta Chir Scand 1979; **145**:87–93.

37. Cade JF, Clegg EA, Westlake GW. Prophylaxis of venous thrombosis after major thoracic surgery. Aust NZ J Surg 1983; **53**:301–4.

38. Encke A, Breddin HK. Comparison of a low molecular weight heparin and unfractionated heparin for the prevention of deep vein thrombosis in patients undergoing abdominal surgery. European Fraxiparin Study (EFA) Group. Br J Surg 1988; 75: 1058–63.

39. Nurmohamed MT, Herhaege R, Haas S et al. A comparative trial of a low molecular weight heparin (enoxaparin) versus standard heparin for the prophylaxis of post-operative deep vein thrombosis in general surgery. Am J Surg 1995; 169:567–71.

40. Kakkar VV, Cohen AT, Edmondson RA et al. Low molecular weight versus standard heparin for prevention of venous thromboembolism after major abdominal surgery. Lancet 1993; 341:259–65.

41. Di Carlo V, Agnelli G, Prandoni P et al for the DOS (Dermatan sulphate in Oncologic Surgery) Study Group. Dermatan sulphate for the prevention of postoperative venous thromboembolism in patients with cancer. Thromb Haemost 1999; 82:30–4.

42. McLeod RS, Geerts WH, Sniderman K et al. Subcutaneous heparin versus low-molecular-weight heparin as thrombo-prophylaxis in patients undergoing colorectal surgery: results of the Canadian colorectal DVT prophy-laxis trial: a randomized, double-blind trial. Ann Surg 2001; 233: 438–444.

43. ENOXACAN Study Group. Efficacy and safety of enoxaparin versus unfractionated heparin for preven-tion of deep vein thrombosis in elective cancer surgery: a double-blind randomized multicentre trial with venographic assessment. Br J Surg 1997; 84:1099–03.

44. Geerts WH, Heit JA, Glagett GP et al. Prevention of venous throm-boembolism. Chest 2001; 119: 132S–75S.

45. Clarke-Pearson DL, Coleman RE, Synan IS et al. Venous thromboem-bolism prophylaxis in gynecologic oncology: a prospective controlled trial of low-dose heparin. Am J Obstet Gynecol 1983; 145:606–13.

46. Clarke-Pearson DL, DeLong E, Synan IS et al. A controlled trial of two low-dose heparin regimens for the prevention of postoperative deep vein thrombosis. Obstet Gynecol 1990; 75:684–9.

47. Clarke-Pearson DL, Synan IS, Dodge R et al. A randomized trial of low-dose heparin and intermit-tent pneumatic calf compression for the prevention of deep venous thrombosis after gynecologic oncology surgery. Am J Obstet Gynecol 1993; 168:1146–54.

48. Von Tempelhoff GF, Dietrich M, Niemann F et al. Blood coagulation and thrombosis in patients with ovarian malignancy. Thromb Haemo-st 1997; 77:456–61.

49. Bergqvist D, Brumark US, Flordal PA et al. Low molecular weight heparin started before surgery as prophylaxis against deep vein thrombosis: 2500 versus 5000 XaI units in 2070 patients. Br J Surg 1995; 82:496–501.

50. Bergqvist D, Agnelli G, Cohen AT et al (the ENOXACAN II Investigators). Duration of prophylaxis against venous thromboembolism with enoxaparin after surgery for cancer. N Engl J Med 2002; 346:975–80.

51. Levine MN, Hirsh J, Gent M et al. Optimal duration of oral anticoagu-lant therapy: a randomized trial comparing four weeks with three months of warfarin in patients with proximal deep vein thrombosis. Thromb Haemost 1995; 74:606–11.

52. Decousus H, Leizorovicz A, Parent F et al. A clinical trial of vena caval filters in the prevention of pul-monary embolism in patients with proximal deep-vein thrombosis. Prévention du Risque d'Embolie Pulmonaire par Interruption Cave

Study Group. N Engl J Med 1998; **338**:409–15.

53. Hutten BA, Prins MH, Gent M et al. Incidence of recurrent thromboembolic and bleeding complications among patients with venous thromboembolism in relation to both malignancy and achieved international normalized ratio. J Clin Oncol 2000; **18**:3078–83.

54. Kakkar AK, Kadziola Z, Williamson RCN et al, on behalf of the Fragmin Advanced Malignancy Outcome Study (FAMOS). Low molecular weight heparin (LMWH) therapy and survival in advanced cancer. Blood 2002; **100**: Abst 557.

55. Hull RD, Raskob GE, Pineo GF et al. Subcutaenous low-molecular-weight heparin compared with continuous intravenous heparin in the treatment of proximal-vein thrombosis. N Engl J Med 1992; **326**:975–82.

56. Prandoni P, Lensing AWA, Büller HR et al. Comparison of subcutaneous low-molecular-weight heparin with intravenous standard heparin in proximal-vein thrombosis. Lancet 1992; **339**:441–5.

57. Koopman MMW, Prandoni P, Piovella F et al. Treatment of venous thrombosis with intravenous unfractionated heparin administered in the hospital as compared with subcutaneous low molecular weight heparin administered at home. N Engl J Med 1996; **334**:682–7.

58. Kirchmaier CM, Wolf H, Schäfer H et al. Efficacy of a low molecular weight heparin administered intravenously or subcutaneously in comparison with intravenous unfractionated heparin in the treatment of deep venous thrombosis. Int Angiol 1998; **17**:135–45.

59. Simonneau G, Sors H, Charbonnier B et al, for the THÉSÉE Study Group. A comparison of low-molecular-weight heparin with unfractionated heparin for acute pulmonary embolism. N Engl J Med 1997; **337**:663–9.

60. Von Tempelhoff GF, Harenberg J, Niemann F et al. Effect of low molecular weight heparin (certoparin) versus unfractionated heparin on cancer survival following breast and pelvic cancer surgery: a prospective randomized double-blind trial. Int J Oncol 2000; **16**: 815–24.

61. Lebeau B, Chastang C, Brechot JM et al. Subcutaneous heparin treatment increases survival in small cell lung cancer. 'Petites Cellules' Group. Cancer 1994; **74**: 38–45.

62. Meyer G, Majanovic Z, Valcke J et al. Comparison of low-molecular-weight heparin and warfarin for the secondary prevention of venous thromboembolism in patients with cancer: a randomized controlled study. Arch Intern Med 2002; **162**:1729–35.

63. Ley AY, Levine MN, Baker RI et al. Randomized comparison of low-molecular-weight heparin versus oral anticoagulant therapy for the prevention of recurrent venous thromboembolism in patients with cancer (CLOT) Investigators. Low-molecular-weight heparin versus a coumarin for the prevention of recurrent venous thromboembolism in patients with cancer. N Engl J Med 2003; **349**:146–53.

64. Kakkar A, Levine MN, Kadziola Z et al. Low molecular weight heparin therapy and survival in patients with malignant disease. Thromb Haemost 2003; Suppl 1: Abst: P0843.

65. Lee AYY, Julain JA, Levine MN et al. Long-term treatment with dalteparin low-molecular-weight heparin (LMWH) may improve survival in patients with non-metastic malignancy and venous thromboembolism (VTE). Thromb Haemost 2003; Suppl 1: Abst OC004.

66. Klerk CPW, Smorenburg SM, Otten JMMB et al. Malignancy and low-molecular weight-heparin therapy: the MALT trial. Thromb Haemost 2001; Suppl 1: Abst OC195

67. Wester JPJ, de Valk HW, Nieuwenhuis HK et al. Risk factors for bleeding during treatment of acute venous thromboembolism. Thromb Haemost 1996; 76:682–8.

68. Landefeld CS, McGuire E, Rosenblatt MW. A bleeding risk index for estimating the probability of major bleeding in hospitalized patients starting anticoagulant therapy. Am J Med 1990; 89:569–78.

69. Chan A, Woodruff RK. Complications and failure of anticoagulation therapy in the treatment of venous thromboembolism in patients with disseminated malignancy. Aust NZ J Med 1992; 22: 119–22.

70. Gitter MJ, Jaeger TM, Petterson TM et al. Bleeding and thromboembolism during anticoagulation therapy: a population-based study in Rochester, Minnesota. Mayo Clin Proc 1995; 70:725–33.

71. Prandoni P, Lensing AWA, Piccioli A et al. Recurrent venous thromboembolism and bleeding complications during anticoagulant treatment in patients with cancer and venous thrombosis. Blood 2002; 100:3484–8.

16

Antimalignant properties of antithrombotic agents

Clara PW Klerk, Susanne M Smorenburg, and
Harry R Büller

Introduction

Because of the high risk of thrombosis, cancer patients often receive anticoagulants as prophylaxis or treatment. It has been suggested that antithrombotic agents influence cancer progression, but this is still a matter of debate, since it is unclear whether the aberrations in coagulation found in cancer patients are just an epiphenomenon or essential for the progression of cancer.

Fibrin has been found to be an important stromal component in some, but not all, tumors.[1-11] Since most cancer cells do not synthesize fibrin or its precursor fibrinogen, the fibrin around the cells is thought to be derived from extravasation and extravascular clotting of plasma fibrinogen.[1,12] Fibrinogen accumulates extravascularly through increased permeability of vessels around the tumor.[4] Both tumor coagulants and the procoagulant activity of tissue itself make formation of fibrin possible.[13] Fibrin thus formed may influence both primary tumor growth and metastasis, and serve various purposes, such as protection of cancer cells from the host immune system (depending on the density of fibrin deposition), trapping of extravasated plasma proteins in the interstitium, and induction of vessel formation (angiogenesis).[13] Moreover, it has been hypothesized that by forming a clump around the cancer cells in the bloodstream, fibrin may enhance entrapment of the cells in the vessels or aid in their adhesion to the vessel wall.[14] However, the fibrinolytic system has an important role in cancer progression as well: cancer cells produce or stimulate expression of proteolytic enzymes, such as urokinase-type plasminogen activator (u-PA) and gelatinases, in order to cross the extracellular matrix (ECM) and to extravasate.[15-17] Moreover, in the process of angiogenesis, proteolysis of the provisionary matrix is needed.[18] Thus, it appears that the balance between fibrin formation and fibrinolysis is important in cancer progression, and that this balance 'shifts' at the various steps of progression.

If coagulation is important for the malignant process, it is to be expected that drugs altering the coagulation status of the host would be able to influence cancer progression. Since the 1930s, studies have investigated the effects of heparins, vitamin K antagonists (VKA), fibrinolytic agents, and platelet aggregation inhibitors, both in animal models and in patients with malignancy. Some of these have shown promising results. However, it is known that many antithrombotic agents have other properties apart from their effects on coagulation. Because of these various effects, the cancer may be affected by different mechanisms at the same time, making it difficult to extrapolate the results of in vitro studies and animal studies to the situation in man.

Recent clinical results have renewed the discussion of whether agents affecting coagulation can influence cancer progression. In 1999, a meta-analysis was published that calculated and compared the mortality rates of cancer patients with venous thromboembolism (VTE) who were initially treated with low-molecular-weight heparin (LMWH) versus those who were treated with unfractionated heparin (UFH).[19] In this analysis, the survival of cancer patients was significantly better when they were treated with LMWH compared with UFH. These findings gave rise to a revived interest in the application of antithrombotic agents to influence cancer progression.

In this chapter, after briefly discussing the findings of experimental studies, we will evaluate the clinical data on the antimalignant effects of antithrombotic agents, including anticoagulants (heparin and VKA), thrombolytics, and various agents with antiplatelet aggregation effects.

Anticoagulants

Heparins

After intravenous administration, the anticoagulant effect of heparin is instantaneous; therefore, UFH and, more recently, LMWH are often used when this immediate effect is required, such as in the prophylaxis or initial treatment of VTE.[20] Heparins are members of the glycosaminoglycan family, which comprises chains of alternating residues of D-glucosamine and auronic acid.[21] Through either chemical or enzymatic depolymerization of UFH, smaller fragments of UFH called LMWH are derived.[20,22] LMWH has anticoagulant activity similar to UFH, but exhibits an anti-factor F-Xa to anti-IIa ratio of 4:1 to 2:1, versus 1:1 for UFH.

Experimental studies

Effects on cancer progression have been studied for UFH, but not so much for LMWH, in various animal models, and it appears that these agents do not affect the cancer by their anticoagulant properties alone. UFH and, to a lesser extent, LMWH bind to a wide variety of proteins and other molecules via electrostatic interactions; therefore, these heparins exert many other biological activities besides their anticoagulant effect.[20] In a recent review, the numerous findings of animal studies have been analyzed and the actions of heparin on the various stages of cancer progression have been described.[23]

Several steps in cancer progression were found on which heparin could have an effect, such as cancer-cell proliferation, activity of the host immune system, angiogenesis, migration of cancer and endothelial cells, invasion of cancer and endothelial cells, and adhesion of cancer cells to vascular endothelium. In fact, experimental studies have found that UFH exerts a variety of positive and negative effects on cancer progression. Because of the complex interaction between cancer and UFH and the existence of both enhancing and inhibiting effects, the overall effect in man is difficult to predict. Possibly, the balance of effects is different in various types of cancer. The effects of UFH and LMWH are often similar, but sometimes they are contradictory. For instance, UFH and high-molecular-weight heparin appear to enhance the binding of angiogenic growth factors to their receptors, whereas LMWH inhibits this binding.[23] Moreover, studies have shown that UFH and LMWH can also influence the structure of the fibrin matrices, resulting in stimulatory and inhibitory effects, respectively, on in vitro angiogenesis.[24]

Clinical trials

As mentioned above, important information on the effects of anticoagulants in cancer has been derived from studies on the treatment of VTE in the general population with different types of anticoagulants. The standard treatment is a course of heparin followed by a VKA, such as warfarin or acenocoumarol, for secondary prophylaxis. Considering the subgroup of cancer patients with VTE, a meta-analysis found an improved survival in cancer patients treated initially with subcutaneous LMWH when compared with those treated with intravenous UFH.[19] In the 629 cancer patients treated (306 LMWH-treated versus 323 UFH-treated), the pooled odds ratio (OR) for 3-month mortality was 0.61 (95% confidence interval [CI] 0.40–0.93) in favor of LMWH. In these studies, a wide variety of cancer subtypes were present.

Of course, these results in cancer patients with VTE may not be applicable to cancer patients without VTE. However, a study performed in patients with breast or pelvic cancer surgery, in which patients were randomized to prophylactic UFH or LMWH perioperatively, also found an improved long-term survival with LMWH on day 650—relative risk (RR) 0.37 (95% CI 0.17–0.79)—but not thereafter.[25] A subanalysis revealed that it was specifically the survival rate of patients with endometrial and ovarian carcinoma that was improved by LMWH treatment, while breast-cancer survival did not seem to be affected by the kind of heparin used in the perioperative period.[25]

Although the meta-analysis was retrospective and the prospective study found improvement only during a limited time interval, the results of these studies suggest either a negative influence of UFH or a positive influence of LMWH (or both) on survival in (some types of) cancer. Therefore, we analyzed the results of clinical studies that compared UFH versus placebo or no treatment in patients with cancer without VTE. These trials reported contradictory results, and a systematic review of all methodologically sound studies found no convincing evidence of either positive or negative effects of UFH on survival of patients with malignancy.[26] One multicenter, randomized trial that compared survival in patients with small-cell lung carcinoma (SCLC) who received chemotherapy alone or in combination with UFH found better survival in the latter, with a 3-year survival rate of 11% versus 6% in controls.[27] Two other randomized trials, however, which studied the effect on survival of prophylactic UFH after resection for colorectal cancer, found no overall effect on survival.[28,29] Other studies were found to have a less robust methodology, making their results less reliable.

These inconclusive data make it difficult to interpret the effect seen in the studies comparing LMWH with UFH. Since there is no evidence that UFH is detrimental to cancer survival, it is probably appropriate to hypothesize that LMWH may be beneficial. This hypothesis is supported by data from the recent study by Meyer et al comparing the standard therapy of short-term LMWH followed by warfarin treatment with long-term therapy with LMWH.[30] In the 3-month follow-up of this study, 22.7% (17 of 75) died in the warfarin-treated group (of which 6 deaths were due to major hemorrhage) and 11.3% (8 of 71) in the LMWH-treated group (no deaths due to major hemorrhage). However, this difference did not reach statistical significance, possibly because of the small number of patients studied. At present, no data from clinical trials specifically addressing the effects of LMWH on survival of cancer patients without VTE are available. However, two studies have been performed recently evaluating these effects. One study investigated the effect on cancer survival of a prophylactic dose of LMWH during 1 year. The other studied the effect of 2 weeks of LMWH in a therapeutic dose followed by 4 weeks of half this dose of LWMH. Results will be available soon for both studies.

Vitamin K antagonists (VKA)

Experimental studies

In most of the approximately 20 animal studies performed on this subject, VKA reduced the number of metastases.[31-34] Colucci and colleagues[32] found that the dietary induction of vitamin K deficiency had the same antimetastatic effect on Lewis lung-carcinoma cells as warfarin. Both also inhibited cancer-cell procoagulant activity (PCA). When vitamin K was administered together with warfarin, both the antimetastatic effect and the effect on PCA of the cancer cells were reversed. But when prothrombin complex concentrate was administered, this did not have an effect on cancer-cell PCA. The effect on metastases was not tested.[32] These results suggest that VKA exert their anticancer effect primarily through the induction of vitamin K deficiency, influencing cancer-cell PCA in addition to the systemic coagulation factors. McCulloch and George did test the effect of restoring factors II, VII, IX, and X in animals inoculated with mammary carcinoma cells and receiving VKA. The antimetastatic effect of VKA was reversed by the restoration of these factors at the time of cancer-cell inoculation. When the factors were administered 12 hours later, this reversal was no longer attained.[33] Therefore, these experiments show that, unlike heparins, VKA appear to exert their anticancer effect primarily through their anticoagulant effect. Moreover, coagulation appears to be only important or sensitive to inhibition in the first 12 hours that the cancer cells circulate in the bloodstream.

Clinical trials

Several clinical trials have investigated the effects of VKA on the survival of cancer patients. However, as with the studies on UFH, not all these studies have a comparable robustness of methodology. When only the properly randomized studies are taken into account, in which the study groups were treated equally besides the VKA intervention and in which dosages and duration were specified,[35-39] a systematic review revealed that there was no statistically significant difference in survival in cancer patients treated with VKA versus controls.[40] When the relative risk (RR) was calculated from the level-one data of the systematic analysis, a pooled RR of 0.95 (95% CI 0.86–1.05) was found. However, an analysis of a subgroup of patients with SCLC revealed an almost statistically significant trend towards improved survival (RR of 0.87 [95% CI 0.74–1.01]).[40] This is especially interesting since UFH and urokinase (which will be discussed below) were also found to be beneficial in this subgroup of patients.[27,41] One hypothesis that has been put forward to explain this phenomenon is that the susceptibility to agents that inhibit thrombin formation (or enhance the dissolution of the fibrin that is formed by thrombin around the tumor) is dependent on the tumor's own ability to form thrombin.[42] This would explain why SCLC, which has been found to generate thrombin,[43] was found to be susceptible to VKA, whereas colon cancer, which has not been found to generate thrombin locally, was not.[42]

Thrombolytic agents

Experimental studies
In animal experiments, positive effects have been reported with thrombolytic agents. Here the emphasis has been on metastasis, and not so much on effects on the primary tumor. Brown and colleagues report that, when streptokinase was administered 30 minutes after inoculating rats with mammary carcinoma cells, the result was a reduction of pulmonary seeding compared with untreated controls.[44] For recombinant tissue-type plasminogen activator (rt-PA), similar results were obtained. This suggests that, at least in metastasis, some influence could be expected from administration of thrombolytic agents. However, when the effects on spontaneous metastasis were studied, only metastases of Lewis lung-carcinoma cells were found to be inhibited by synthetic peptides based on parts of murine and human urokinase-type plasminogen activator (u-PA).[45] Since some cancer types do appear to react to these agents, there is apparently some tumor-specificity in the sensitivity to thrombolytic agents, similar to that seen in anticoagulants.

Interestingly, several studies have also been performed with agents that inhibit fibrinolysis, some of which showed a positive result as well.[46] Therefore, either there is an optimal balance that can be disturbed both by inhibition and by stimulation of fibrinolysis, or cancer types are sensitive to only one type of these interventions.

Clinical trials
Four randomized studies have been published on the effect of thrombolytic agents on cancer progression.[39,47–49] Two studied the effect of adding urokinase to doxorubicin for the intravesical therapy of superficial tumors of the bladder. No difference was found in response (no response at 16 weeks: 4 of 20 in the treatment group versus 2 of 21 in the placebo group [$p > 0.2$]) or recurrence (all patients in both study arms) when patients were treated with urokinase.[47,48] The other two studies reported on the effect on survival in colorectal cancer. The goals of the studies were to reduce the number of metastases induced during surgery through the administration of thrombolytic agents perioperatively, and thus to improve survival. One investigation studied the effect of postoperative infusion of urokinase and found no effect on survival (4-year survival rate of 69% versus 70% in controls [$p = 0.41$]).[39] The other

one was an interim report on a trial that studied the effect of streptokinase during surgery. Although the numbers were still low, a trend towards better survival was reported in the treated group (3 deaths in 22 due to recurrence in an average of 58 months' survival to date versus 4 deaths in 23 due to recurrence in an average of 34 months' survival to date in controls).[49]

Two other studies with similar study questions yet lacking appropriate control groups were also published. One studied the effect of postoperative infusion of urokinase in the portal vein in patients with colorectal cancer.[50] This was not found to influence survival. The second, a phase II trial, tested the addition of urokinase to chemotherapy for SCLC and found a modest improvement compared with the results normally expected (in patients with limited disease, an 85% response rate and a mean survival time of 26.5 months).[41] In summary, methodologically rigorous studies fail to show a statistically significant effect of thrombolytic agents on cancer progression, but there are some indications that certain treatment schedules may be more effective and some cancers more sensitive to this type of treatment than others.

Antiplatelet drugs

There are an increasing number of data showing that platelets are involved in cancer metastasis (see also Chapter 3). In vitro, several types of cancer cells have been found to induce platelet aggregation—so-called tumor-cell-induced platelet aggregation (TCIPA).[51] Moreover, aggregates of platelets have been found around cancer cells in the bloodstream.[52] Similarly, the administration of cancer cells into the bloodstream of animals has been found to induce thrombocytopenia, which may be induced by consumption.[53,54] It has been suggested that the aggregation of platelets can assist cancer progression. This is supported by the fact that the induction of thrombocytopenia by neuraminidase before the injection of cancer cells diminishes the number of lung colonies.[55,56] Honn et al have discussed the following possible roles of platelets in cancer progression: (1) stabilizing cancer-cell arrest in the vasculature; (2) influencing both intravasal and extravasal cancer cell proliferation by the secretion of various growth factors; (3) enabling or facilitating extravasation of the cancer cells into the tissue; (4) enhancing interactions of cancer cells with the ECM.[57] If platelet aggregation does aid these processes, then inhibition of platelet aggregation is expected to hinder cancer progression. However, with many of the antiplatelet drugs tested, it is not clear how much of their anticancer activity is based on their antiplatelet activity and how much can be attributed to other actions of these drugs.

Platelet aggregation is a complex process. The different antiplatelet agents intervene at various points in this process. Although all inhibit platelet aggregation, their mechanisms of action vary. It can be imagined, therefore, that the effects these agents may have on cancer, apart from affecting aggregation, may differ as well. For example, an important group of platelet aggregation inhibiting drugs are the nonsteroidal anti-inflammatory drugs (NSAIDs), of which aspirin is a well-known example. These drugs work through the inhibition of cyclooxygenase (COX). This results in less substrate for the enzyme that produces thromboxane, which is an important platelet agonist. Thromboxane synthetase inhibitors inhibit this production lower downstream. Other platelet antagonists exert their function through the inhibition of other parts of the process of platelet aggregation. Adenosine diphosphate (ADP) inhibitors and direct thrombin inhibitors inhibit two other important agonists of platelet aggregation. $\alpha_{IIb} \beta_3$ inhibitors bind to the $\alpha_{IIb} \beta_3$ receptor, thereby blocking its binding to fibrinogen, which normally enables platelets to adhere to one another. Finally, drugs that elevate intracellular cyclic adenosine monophosphate (cAMP) levels, such as adenylate cyclase stimulators and phosphodiesterase inhibitors, also inhibit platelet aggregation, although the exact mechanism for this is still unknown.

Research on antiplatelet agents and cancer has focused mainly on NSAIDs. Therefore, in the following paragraphs, the results of experimental studies on these agents are presented and the findings of clinical trials are discussed. Then the mechanisms through which other types of antiplatelet drugs may influence cancer, apart from their antiplatelet activity, will be identified, and the clinical trials with various other antiplatelet agents will be considered.

NSAIDs

Experimental studies

In animal studies, NSAIDs have been found to reduce the incidence or multiplicity of various types of cancer.[58–60] The most important anticancer effect of NSAIDs appears to be exerted through the inhibition of cyclooxygenase-2 (COX-2). This is supported by the fact that specific COX-2 inhibitors, which do not exert an effect on platelet aggregation, are able to reduce cancer incidence in animals.[58,61] Moreover, cross-breeding of a mouse model for familial adenomatous polyposis (FAP) with a COX-2-deficient mouse also resulted in a decrease in intestinal polyposis in these mice.[62] Finally, NSAIDs have also been shown to restore apoptosis in cells where this was suppressed (as happens during tumorigenesis).[63]

Clinical trials

In clinical trials, much attention has been paid to the effects of NSAIDs on cancer, especially colon cancer. Although NSAIDs appear to be effective in reducing the polyps associated with FAP,[64] so far they have not been found to be effective in other populations with an increased risk of colorectal cancer.[65,66]

Epidemiological studies in the general population have shown an association between regular use of NSAIDs and a lower incidence of colorectal cancer.[64] However, the only available prospective, randomized study in a healthy population did not find a reduction in the incidence of colorectal carcinoma associated with aspirin use in a mean follow-up of 5 years in 22 071 male physicians randomized to aspirin or placebo.[67] For other types of cancer, data on the effects of NSAIDs are scarce. Randomized controlled trials showed that the addition of NSAIDs to standard therapy did not have an effect on survival in SCLC, response rate in metastasized malignant melanoma, or recurrence of mammary carcinoma.[68-70] However, a randomized controlled trial testing the effect of prednisolone, indomethacin, or placebo orally until death in undernourished patients with solid tumors found that indomethacin prolonged mean survival by 260 ± 28 days ($p < 0.05$).[72]

Other antiplatelet agents

Experimental studies

Based on experimental studies, the other antiplatelet agents can be expected to influence cancer progression in more ways than just through inhibition of platelet aggregation. Prostacyclin is a natural antiplatelet agent, but has also been shown to decrease primary tumor growth, inhibit formation of vasculature, and prevent the genetic damage induced in bone-marrow cells of mice.[72,73] Thromboxane synthetase inhibitors have been found to block migration effectively, induce apoptosis in migratory glioma cells, and inhibit angiogenesis.[74,75] SR 25989 is a derivative of ADP-inhibiting thienopyridines but does not exhibit any antiaggregant activity.[76] The fact that this substance has been shown to decrease the number of metastases and inhibit angiogenesis suggests that thienopyridines might also influence cancer progression with mechanisms independent of their antiplatelet activity.[76] Disintegrins inhibit $\alpha_{IIb}\beta_3$ receptors but also bind to various other members of the integrin family, such as $\alpha_\nu\beta_3$, which is important in angiogenesis.[77] This may be the mechanism through which disintegrins diminished the growth of the primary tumor, as was seen in some experiments.[77-80] Moreover, there is increasing evidence that integrins such as $\alpha_{IIb}\beta_3$ may mediate information transfer into cells.[81] It is not inconceivable that these receptors have a similar role in cancer cells, which can be influenced by disintegrins and antibodies. Finally, agents that raise intracellular cAMP levels, leading to decreased platelet aggregation, are expected to influence the cell through other mechanisms as well, since cAMP is an important second-messenger molecule, which may also influence a variety of other intracellular processes. Moreover, the phosphodiesterase inhibitor dipyridamole has been found to enhance the anticancer effects of some forms of chemotherapy by inhibiting efflux of the chemotherapeutic agent from the cancer cell or blocking the nucleoside salvage mechanism of these cells.[82,83] Experimental studies have shown for some tumors that the administration of the phosphodiesterase inhibitor pentoxifylline enhances the oxygen supply to the tumor tissue, making these cells more sensitive to radiation therapy.[84,85] Moreover, pentoxifylline was found to reduce the radiation-induced increase of the proinflammatory cytokine tissue necrosis factor α (TNF-α).[86]

The downside of the fact that many of these agents have several mechanisms through which they may influence cancer is that they may also influence the host in various ways, making it difficult to predict the final outcome in man. Therefore, the results of clinical trials with these agents are needed for further conclusions.

Clinical trials

These other types of antiplatelet agents have hardly been studied in man. Dipyridamole has been studied in combination with chemotherapy. Although successful results were obtained in preclinical studies, the clinical results so far are not very encouraging.[87] One exception to this is a study with mopidamol (RA-233), a derivative of dipyridamole. This phosphodiesterase inhibitor or placebo was administered alongside standard therapy in 719 patients with advanced carcinomas of the lung or colon. In patients with limited non-small-cell lung cancer (NSCLC), survival was increased in the mopidamol group by approximately 50%. However, survival in the other tumor categories was not affected by mopidamol.[88]

Pentoxifylline has been studied in combination with both chemotherapy and radiotherapy. In combination with chemotherapy, it was thought to reduce oral mucositis, but this could not be proven.[89] In combination with radiotherapy, it was studied as a response modulator. In RCT in which patients with NSCLC were randomized to receive pentoxifylline or placebo alongside radiation therapy, pentoxifylline was found to induce a trend towards longer survival.[90]

Conclusions

In this chapter, the various experimental and clinical data on the antimalignant properties of antithrombotic agents have been analyzed. There are indications that LMWH may prolong survival in cancer patients, but the results of trials conducted for this specific outcome are still awaited. There are some indications that other agents directed at the coagulation process (VKA and thrombolytic agents) may be beneficial in a subgroup of cancers, but more methodologically strong studies are needed for conclusive answers. Finally, antiplatelet therapy has shown some promising results, although it is disputable which mechanism causes them. For NSAIDs, there is strong evidence that it is a mechanism apart from the antiplatelet action of the drugs that affects the cancer. This remains to be elucidated for other antiplatelet agents.

References

1. Dvorak HF, Senger DR, Dvorak AM. Fibrin as a component of the tumor stroma: origins and biological significance. Cancer Metastasis Rev 1983; 2:41–73.

2. Dvorak HF, Dickersin GR, Dvorak AM et al. Human breast carcinoma: fibrin deposits and desmoplasia. Inflammatory cell type and distribution. Microvasculature and infarction. J Natl Cancer Inst 1981; 67: 335–45.

3. Harris NL, Dvorak AM, Smith J et al. Fibrin deposits in Hodgkin's disease. Am J Pathol 1982; 108: 119–29.

4. Senger DR, Galli SJ, Dvorak AM et al. Tumor cells secrete a vascular permeability factor that promotes accumulation of ascites fluid. Science 1983; 219:983–5.

5. Zacharski LR, Memoli VA, Rousseau SM. Coagulation-cancer interaction in situ in renal cell carcinoma. Blood 1986; 68:394–9.

6. Rickles FR, Hancock WW, Edwards RL et al. Antimetastatic agents. I. Role of cellular procoagulants in the pathogenesis of fibrin deposition in cancer and the use of anticoagulants and/or antiplatelet drugs in cancer treatment. Semin Thromb Hemost 1988; 14:88–94.

7. Costantini V, Zacharski LR, Memoli VA et al. Fibrinogen deposition and macrophage-associated fibrin formation in malignant and non-malignant lymphoid tissue. J Lab Clin Med 1992; 119:124–31.

8. Wojtukiewicz MZ, Zacharski LR, Memoli VA et al. Fibrin formation on vessel walls in hyperplastic and malignant prostate tissue. Cancer 1991 67:1377–83.

9. Wojtukiewicz MZ, Zacharski LR, Memoli VA et al. Fibrinogen-fibrin transformation in situ in renal cell carcinoma. Anticancer Res 1990; 10:579–82.

10. Wojtukiewicz MZ, Zacharski LR, Memoli VA et al. Malignant melanoma. Interaction with coagulation and fibrinolysis pathways in situ. Am J Clin Pathol 1990; 93:516–21.

11. Wojtukiewicz MZ, Zacharski LR, Memoli VA et al. Abnormal regulation of coagulation/fibrinolysis in small cell carcinoma of the lung. Cancer 1990; 65:481–5.

12. Dvorak HF, Dvorak AM, Manseau EJ et al. Fibrin gel investment associated with line 1 and line 10 solid tumor growth, angiogenesis, and fibroplasia in guinea pigs. Role of cellular immunity, myofibroblasts, microvascular damage, and infarction in line 1 tumor regression. J Natl Cancer Inst 1979; 62: 1459–72.

13. Dvorak HF. Tumors: wounds that do not heal. Similarities between tumor stroma generation and wound healing. N Engl J Med 1986; 315:1650–9.

14. Wood S Jr, Holyoke ED, Yokoyama K. Mechanisms of metastasis production by blood-borne cancer cells. Can Cancer Conf 1961; 4: 167–223.

15. Zacharski LR, Wojtukiewicz MZ, Costantini V et al. Pathways of coagulation/fibrinolysis activation in malignancy. Semin Thromb Hemost 1992; **18**:104–16.

16. Schmalfeldt B, Prechtel D, Harting K et al. Increased expression of matrix metalloproteinases (MMP)-2, MMP-9, and the urokinase-type plasminogen activator is associated with progression from benign to advanced ovarian cancer. Clin Cancer Res 2001; **7**:2396–404.

17. Andreasen PA, Kjoller L, Christensen L et al. The urokinase-type plasminogen activator system in cancer metastasis: a review. Int J Cancer 1997; **72**:1–22.

18. Reijerkerk A, Voest EE, Gebbink MF. No grip, no growth: the conceptual basis of excessive proteolysis in the treatment of cancer. Eur J Cancer 2000; **36**: 1695–1705.

19. Hettiarachchi RJ, Smorenburg SM, Ginsberg J et al. Do heparins do more than just treat thrombosis? The influence of heparins on cancer spread. Thromb Haemost 1999; **82**:947–52.

20. Hirsh J, Warkentin TE, Raschke R et al. Heparin and low-molecular-weight heparin: mechanisms of action, pharmacokinetics, dosing considerations, monitoring, efficacy, and safety. Chest 1998; **114**:489S–510S.

21. Choay J, Petitou M. The chemistry of heparin: a way to understand its mode of action. Med J Aust 1986; **114**:7–10.

22. Ofosu FA, Barrowcliffe TW. Mechanisms of action of low molecular weight heparins and heparinoids. Baillieres Clin Haematol 1990; **3**:505–29.

23. Smorenburg SM, Van Noorden CJ. The complex effects of heparins on cancer progression and metastasis in experimental studies. Pharmacol Rev 2001; **53**:93–105.

24. Collen A, Smorenburg SM, Peters E et al. Unfractionated and low molecular weight heparin affects fibrin structure and angiogenesis in vitro. Cancer Res 2000; **60**: 6196–200.

25. von Tempelhoff GF, Harenberg J, Niemann F et al. Effect of low molecular weight heparin (certoparin) versus unfractionated heparin on cancer survival following breast and pelvic cancer surgery: a prospective randomized double-blind trial. Int J Oncol 2000; **16**: 815–24.

26. Smorenburg SM, Hettiarachchi RJ, Vink R et al. The effects of unfractionated heparin on survival in patients with malignancy—a systematic review. Thromb Haemost 1999; **82**:1600–4.

27. Lebeau B, Chastang C, Brechot JM et al. Subcutaneous heparin treatment increases survival in small cell lung cancer. 'Petites Cellules' Group. Cancer 1994; **74**: 38–45.

28. Nitti D, Wils J, Sahmoud T et al. Final results of a phase III clinical trial on adjuvant intraportal infusion with heparin and 5-fluorouracil (5-FU) in resectable colon cancer (EORTC GITCCG 1983–1987). European Organization for Research and Treatment of Cancer. Gastrointestinal Tract Cancer Cooperative Group. Eur J Cancer 1997; **33**:1209–15.

29. Fielding LP, Hittinger R, Grace RH et al. Randomised controlled trial of adjuvant chemotherapy by portal-vein perfusion after curative resection for colorectal adenocarcinoma. Lancet 1992; **340**:502–6.

30. Meyer G, Marjanovic Z, Valcke J et al. Comparison of low-molecular-weight heparin and warfarin for the secondary prevention of venous thromboembolism in patients with cancer: a randomized controlled study. Arch Intern Med 2002; **162**:1729–35.

31. Maat B, Hilgard P. Anticoagulants and experimental metastases-evaluation of antimetastatic effects in different model systems. J Cancer Res Clin Oncol 1981; **101**:275–83.

32. Colucci M, Delaini F, de Bellis Vitti G et al. Warfarin inhibits both pro-coagulant activity and metastatic capacity of Lewis lung carcinoma cells. Role of vitamin K deficiency. Biochem Pharmacol 1983; **32**:1689–91.

33. McCulloch P, George WD. Warfarin inhibition of metastasis: the role of anticoagulation. Br J Surg 1987; **74**:879–83.

34. Neubauer BL, Bemis KG, Best KL et al. Inhibitory effect of warfarin on the metastasis of the PAIII prostatic adenocarcinoma in the rat. J Urol 1986; **135**:163–6.

35. Maurer LH, Herndon JE, Hollis DR et al. Randomized trial of chemotherapy and radiation therapy with or without warfarin for limited-stage small-cell lung cancer: a Cancer and Leukemia Group B study. J Clin Oncol 1997; **15**:3378–87.

36. Zacharski LR, Henderson WG, Rickles FR et al. Effect of warfarin anticoagulation on survival in carcinoma of the lung, colon, head and neck, and prostate. Final report of VA Cooperative Study No. 75. Cancer 1984; **53**:2046–52.

37. Chahinian AP, Propert KJ, Ware JH et al. A randomized trial of anticoagulation with warfarin and of alternating chemotherapy in extensive small-cell lung cancer by the Cancer and Leukemia Group B. J Clin Oncol 1989; **7**:993–1002.

38. Levine M, Hirsh J, Gent M et al. Double-blind randomised trial of a very-low-dose warfarin for prevention of thromboembolism in stage IV breast cancer. Lancet 1994; **343**:886–9.

39. Daly L. The first international urokinase/warfarin trial in colorectal cancer. Clin Exp Metastasis 1991; **9**:3–11.

40. Smorenburg SM, Vink R, Otten HM et al. The effects of vitamin K-antagonists on survival of patients with malignancy: a systematic analysis. Thromb Haemost 2001; **86**:1586–7.

41. Calvo FA, Hidalgo OF, Gonzalez F et al. Urokinase combination chemotherapy in small cell lung cancer. A phase II study. Cancer 1992; **70**:2624–30.

42. Zacharski LR, Memoli VA, Costantini V et al. Clotting factors in tumour tissue: implications for cancer therapy. Blood Coagul Fibrinolysis 1990; **1**:71–8.

43. Zacharski LR, Memoli VA, Rousseau SM. Thrombin-specific sites of fibrinogen in small cell carcinoma of the lung. Cancer 1988; **62**:299–302.

44. Brown DC, Purushotham AD, George WD. Inhibition of pulmonary tumor seeding by antiplatelet and fibrinolytic therapy in an animal experimental model. J Surg Oncol 1994; **55**:154–9.

45. Kobayashi H, Gotoh J, Fujie M et al. Inhibition of metastasis of Lewis lung carcinoma by a synthetic peptide within growth factor-like domain of urokinase in the experimental and spontaneous metastasis model. Int J Cancer 1994; **57**:727–33.

46. Dunbar SD, Ornstein DL, Zacharski LR. Cancer treatment with inhibitors of urokinase-type plasminogen activator and plasmin. Expert Opin Investig Drugs 2000; **9**:2085–92.

47. Lundbeck F, Mogensen P, Jeppesen N. Intravesical therapy of noninvasive bladder tumors (stage Ta) with doxorubicin and urokinase. J Urol 1983; **130**:1087–9.

48. Khan O, Aherne GW, Williams G. Combined intravesical therapy with doxorubicin (Adriamycin) and urokinase in the management of super-

ficial bladder tumours. Br J Urol 1982; **54**:280–2.

49. Thornes RD. Adjuvant therapy of cancer via the cellular immune mechanism or fibrin by induced fibrinolysis and oral anticoagulants. Cancer 1975; **35**:91–7.

50. Wereldsma JC, Bruggink ED, Meijer WS et al. Adjuvant portal liver infusion in colorectal cancer with 5-fluorouracil/heparin versus urokinase versus control. Results of a prospective randomized clinical trial (Colorectal Adenocarcinoma Trial I). Cancer 1990; **65**:425–32.

51. Karpatkin S, Pearlstein E. Heterogenous mechanisms of tumor cell-induced platelet aggregation with possible pharmacological strategy toward prevention of metastases. In: Honn KV, Sloane B, eds. Hemostatic Mechanisms and Metastasis. (Martinus Nijhoff: Boston, 1984) 139–69.

52. Wood S Jr. Pathogenesis of metastasis formation observed in vivo in the rabbit ear chamber. AMA Arch Pathol 1958; **66**:550–68.

53. Hilgard P, Hohage R, Schmitt W et al. Microangiopathic haemolytic anaemia associated with hypercalcaemia in an experimental rat tumour. Br J Haematol 1973; **24**: 245–54.

54. Hilgard P, Gordon-Smith EC. Microangiopathic haemolytic anaemia and experimental tumour-cell emboli. Br J Haematol 1974; **26**: 651–9.

55. Gasic GJ, Gasic TB, Stewart CC. Antimetastatic effects associated with platelet reduction. Proc Natl Acad Sci USA 1968; **61**:46–52.

56. Sindelar WF, Tralka TS, Ketcham AS. Electron microscopic observations on formation of pulmonary metastases. J Surg Res 1975; **18**: 137–161.

57. Honn KV, Tang DG, Crissman JD. Platelets and cancer metastasis: a causal relationship? Cancer Metastasis Rev 1992; **11**:325–51.

58. Harris RE, Alshafie GA, Abou-Issa H et al. Chemoprevention of breast cancer in rats by celecoxib, a cyclooxygenase 2 inhibitor. Cancer Res 2000; **60**:2101–3.

59. Cahlin C, Gelin J, Delbro D et al. Effect of cyclooxygenase and nitric oxide synthase inhibitors of tumor growth in mouse tumor models with and without cancer cachexia related to prostanoids. Cancer Res 2000; **60**:1742–9.

60. Tzanakakis GN, Agarwal KC, Veronikis DK et al. Effects of antiplatelet agents alone or in combination on platelet aggregation and on liver metastases from a human pancreatic adenocarcinoma in the nude mouse. J Surg Oncol 1991; **48**:45–50.

61. Reddy BS, Hirose Y, Lubet R et al. Chemoprevention of colon cancer by specific cyclooxygenase-2 inhibitor, celecoxib, administered during different stages of carcinogenesis. Cancer Res 2000; **60**:293–7.

62. Oshima M, Dinchuk JE, Kargman SL et al. Suppression of intestinal polyposis in Apc delta716 knockout mice by inhibition of cyclooxygenase 2 (COX-2). Cell 1996; **87**:803–9.

63. Chan TA, Morin PJ, Vogelstein B et al. Mechanisms underlying nonsteroidal antiinflammatory drug-mediated apoptosis. Proc Natl Acad Sci USA 1998; **95**:681–6.

64. Thun MJ, Henley SJ, Patrono C. Nonsteroidal anti-inflammatory drugs as anticancer agents: mechanistic, pharmacologic, and clinical issues. J Natl Cancer Inst 2002; **94**:252–66.

65. Lipton A, Scialla S, Harvey H et al. Adjuvant antiplatelet therapy with aspirin in colorectal cancer. J Med 1982; **13**:419–29.

66. Ladenheim J, Garcia G, Titzer D et al. Effect of sulindac on sporadic colonic polyps. Gastroenterology 1995; **108**:1083–7.

67. Gann PH, Manson JE, Glynn RJ et al. Low-dose aspirin and incidence of colorectal tumors in a randomized trial. J Natl Cancer Inst 1993; 85:1220–4.

68. Lebeau B, Chastang C, Muir JF et al. No effect of an antiaggregant treatment with aspirin in small cell lung cancer treated with CCAVP16 chemotherapy. Results from a randomized clinical trial of 303 patients. The 'Petites Cellules' Group. Cancer 1993; 71:1741–5.

69. Miller RL, Steis RG, Clark JW et al. Randomized trial of recombinant alpha 2b-interferon with or without indomethacin in patients with metastatic malignant melanoma. Cancer Res 1989; 49:1871–6.

70. Olivotto IA, Kim-Sing C, Bajdik CD et al. Effect of acetylsalicylic acid on radiation and cosmetic results after conservative surgery for early breast cancer: a randomized trial. Radiother Oncol 1996; 41:1–6.

71. Lundholm K, Gelin J, Hyltander A et al. Anti-inflammatory treatment may prolong survival in undernourished patients with metastatic solid tumors. Cancer Res 1994; 54: 5602–6.

72. Pradono P, Tazawa R, Maemondo M et al. Gene transfer of thromboxane A_2 synthase and prostaglandin I_2 synthase antithetically altered tumor angiogenesis and tumor growth. Cancer Res 2002; 62: 63–66.

73. Koratkar R, Das UN, Sagar PS et al. Prostacyclin is a potent antimutagen. Prostaglandins Leukot Essent Fatty Acids 1993; 48: 175–84.

74. Kürzel F, Hagel C, Zapf S et al. Cyclo-oxygenase inhibitors and thromboxane synthase inhibitors differentially regulate migration arrest, growth inhibition and apoptosis in human glioma cells. Acta Neurochir (Wien) 2002; 144:71–87.

75. Nie D, Lamberti M, Zacharek A et al. Thromboxane A_2 regulation of endothelial cell migration, angiogenesis, and tumor metastasis. Biochem Biophys Res Commun 2000; 267:245–51.

76. Mah-Becherel MC, Ceraline J, Deplanque G et al. Anti-angiogenic effects of the thienopyridine SR 25989 in vitro and in vivo in a murine pulmonary metastasis model. Br J Cancer 2002; 86: 803–10.

77. Yeh CH, Peng HC, Yang RS et al. Rhodostomin, a snake venom disintegrin, inhibits angiogenesis elicited by basic fibroblast growth factor and suppresses tumor growth by a selective alpha(v) beta(3) blockade of endothelial cells. Mol Pharmacol 2001; 59: 1333–42.

78. Zhou Q, Sherwin RP, Parrish C et al. Contortrostatin, a dimeric disintegrin from Agkistrodon contortrix contortrix, inhibits breast cancer progression. Breast Cancer Res Treat 2000; 61:249–60.

79. Carron CP, Meyer DM, Pegg JA et al. A peptidomimetic antagonist of the integrin alpha(v)beta3 inhibits Leydig cell tumor growth and the development of hypercalcemia of malignancy. Cancer Res 1998; 58:1930–5.

80. Kang IC, Lee YD, Kim DS. A novel disintegrin salmosin inhibits tumor angiogenesis. Cancer Res 1999; 59:3754–60.

81. Hynes RO. Integrins: versatility, modulation, and signaling in cell adhesion. Cell 1992; 69:11–25.

82. Krishan A, Sridhar KS, Mou C et al. Synergistic effect of prochlorperazine and dipyridamole on the cellular retention and cytotoxicity of doxorubicin. Clin Cancer Res 2000; 6:1508–17.

83. Cole PD, Smith AK, Kamen BA. Osteosarcoma cells, resistant to methotrexate due to nucleoside and nucleobase salvage, are sensitive to nucleoside analogs. Cancer

Chemother Pharmacol 2002; **50**: 111–16.

84. Bennewith KL, Durand RE. Drug-induced alterations in tumour perfusion yield increases in tumour cell radiosensitivity. Br J Cancer 2001; **85**:1577–84.

85. Kinuya S, Yokoyama K, Konishi S et al. Improved response of colon cancer xenografts to radioimmunotherapy with pentoxifylline treatment. Eur J Nucl Med 2001; **28**:750–5.

86. Rübe C, Wilfert F, Uthe D et al. Modulation of radiation-induced tumour necrosis factor alpha (TNF-alpha) expression in the lung tissue by pentoxifylline. Radiother Oncol 2002; **64**:177–87.

87. Kohne CH, Hiddemann W, Schuller J et al. Failure of orally administered dipyridamole to enhance the antineoplastic activity of fluorouracil in combination with leucovorin in patients with advanced colorectal cancer: a prospective randomized trial. J Clin Oncol 1995; **13**:1201–8.

88. Zacharski LR, Moritz TE, Baczek LA et al. Effect of mopidamol on survival in carcinoma of the lung and colon: final report of Veterans Administration Cooperative Study No. 188. J Natl Cancer Inst 1988; **80**:90–7.

89. Verdi CJ, Garewal HS, Koenig LM et al. A double-blind, randomized, placebo-controlled, crossover trial of pentoxifylline for the prevention of chemotherapy-induced oral mucositis. Oral Surg Oral Med Oral Pathol Oral Radiol Endod 1995; **80**:36–42.

90. Kwon HC, Kim SK, Chung WK et al. Effect of pentoxifylline on radiation response of non-small cell lung cancer: a phase III randomized multicenter trial. Radiother Oncol 2000; **56**:175–9.

Index

Page numbers in *italics* indicate figures or tables.

Printed and bound by CPI Group (UK) Ltd, Croydon, CR0 4YY

23/10/2024

01777674-0007